BEYOND DOG MASSAGE

A Breakthrough Method for Relieving Soreness and Achieving Connection

JIM MASTERSON

WITH ROBIN ROBINETT, DVM

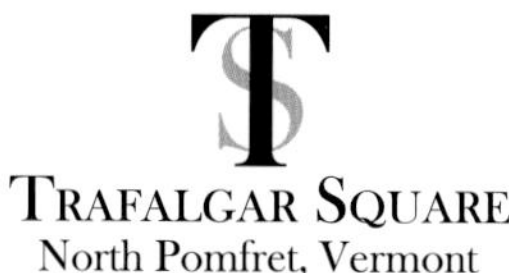

Trafalgar Square
North Pomfret, Vermont

First published in 2023 by
Trafalgar Square Books
North Pomfret, Vermont 05053

Library of Congress Cataloging-in-Publication Data

Names: Masterson, Jim, author. | Robinett, Robin, author.
Title: Beyond dog massage : a breakthrough method for relieving soreness and achieving connection / Jim Masterson with Robin Robinett, DVM.
Description: North Pomfret, Vermont : Trafalgar Square Books, 2023. | Includes index. | Summary: "A lifelong horse person, Jim Masterson developed his method for the purpose of releasing tension and improving movement in the performance horse. An interesting benefit was that it led to improved communication and trust, and a better overall relationship with the horse. Since dogs go with horses "like peanut butter and jelly," Jim says, it was only natural that he began to use his bodywork on canines, too. The techniques used in the Masterson Method rely on reading and following the subtle changes in the dog's body language as you work with him. Once you learn to read his body language, you will be "on the same page" and communication is established. Your dog recognizes that you understand what his body language is saying, that there is no threat to his well-being, and that he feels better when you work with him. In these pages you will learn the steps to incorporating the Masterson Method in your dog's life, bringing happiness to both of you"-- Provided by publisher.
Identifiers: LCCN 2022055997 (print) | LCCN 2022055998 (ebook) | ISBN 9781646011377 (hardback) | ISBN 9781646011384 (epub)
Subjects: LCSH: Dogs--Diseases--Alternative treatment. | Massage for animals. | Veterinary physical therapy. | Dogs--Health. | Dogs--Effect of stress on.
Classification: LCC SF991 .M243 2023 (print) | LCC SF991 (ebook) | DDC 636.7089/5822--dc23/eng/20230215
LC record available at https://lccn.loc.gov/2022055997 LC ebook record available at https://lccn.loc.gov/2022055998

Illustrations by Deanna R C Montero Sculpture Equine Anatomy

All photographs by Stephanie Goddard White Horse Photography except: p. xi and appendices (courtesy of Robin Robinett); figs. 1.4, 1.11 A & B, 4.9 B, 4.18 & B, 4.19, 4.20, 5.36 A & B, 6.38 A-C, 6.39, 6.40 A-C, 7.9, 7.19 B, 7.18, 7.20 A-D (Amanda Barnett-Guidry Photography); figs. 1.18 A-D, 4.5 B, 4.11, 4.12, 5.24, 5.25, 5.26, 5.27, 6.19, 6.20, 6.25, 7.13 A-D, 7.14, 7.15 A & B (Geoff Northridge)

Book design by Lauryl Eddlemon
Cover design by RM Didier
Index by Andrea Jones (JonesLiteraryServices.com)

Printed in China

10 9 8 7 6 5 4 3 2 1

Contents

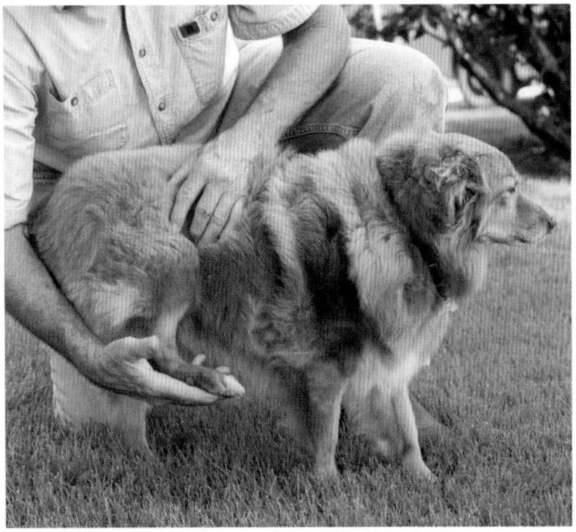

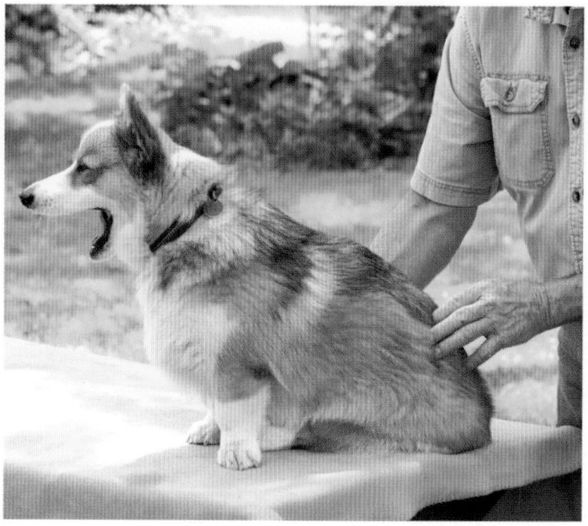

Foreword
by Meg Sleeper, VMD, DACVIM

As an international endurance rider (an equestrian sport based on controlled long-distance races), I have been fortunate to meet many amazing and talented people and I am grateful for the enrichment they have brought to my life. Some of them have also bettered me and my horses and improved our athleticism, but a few have gone beyond helping me and my horse as individuals to actually foster a deeper relationship between us. Jim Masterson is one of these extraordinary people.

It was a gift to have met him (now over a decade ago!!) and to have the opportunity to learn from him. Through his Masterson Method® training and books such as *Beyond Horse Massage*, he opened the door and enabled each of us to help all the horses in our lives, fostering a stronger relationship and a deeper bond.

How amazing that *Beyond Dog Massage* is now available so that we can do the same for the dogs we love! You will find the techniques helpful if your dog is a competitor in agility, flyball, scent work, or obedience—or if he is mostly a contender for the best spot on your sofa after dinner. Jim's methods will improve your dog's range of motion and comfort to allow him to be his best. For older dogs, it is a fabulous adjunct to maintain comfort, while minimizing the need for medications. And add to these benefits the enhanced bond that will develop in your relationship as you use the techniques.

This book is an amazing gift for all dogs, and especially the people who love them.

Meg Sleeper, VMD, DACVIM (Cardiology)
Member United States Endurance Squad
2004, 2006, 2008, 2010, 2012, 2014, 2016

Preface
by Jim Masterson

Like most horse people, I can't remember a time when I didn't have a dog. Dogs and horses seem to go together like peanut butter and jelly. And sometimes, like peanut butter and jelly, you can't get enough.

As the Masterson Method has grown over the years and as more people learn to use these techniques with their horses, I hear from more and more people, both horse and dog, about their experience using the Masterson Method with their dogs—both about their dogs' responses to these techniques and about the changes they're seeing in their dogs. These range from dogs recovering from injuries or physical issues to dogs with behavioral or emotional issues that have learned to relax and trust human touch.

Also, I've heard about positive impacts on the owners themselves. Once you learn to observe and recognize the responses of your dog—or horse—to your touch, you'll find yourself interacting with all animals on that more sensitive and observant level. It just happens automatically. I found this out early on while working with performance horses. I was soon unable to touch, pet, or interact with a horse without observing and gauging his response to not just my touch, but to how I approached him. This was happening soon with dogs. I couldn't touch them without looking for similar responses.

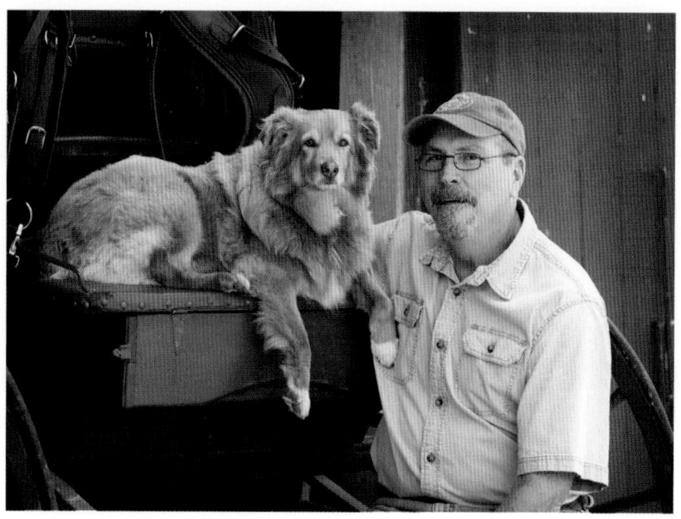

Although I noticed that it relaxed the dogs, the physical benefits that are demonstrated in the horse weren't as apparent to me with dogs at first—possibly because the dogs weren't competing so there was nothing to compare it with. But when working with dogs with specific physical issues, the owners often reported improvements in their movement and comfort.

I may also have had the mental block at first that dogs are predators and horses are prey animals, both with completely different nervous systems, so therefore my techniques wouldn't work well with dogs. But as it turns out, I was wrong. (Score another case of Animal: 1—Human: 0.)

Both horses and dogs are instinctual survival animals. They both ignore and block out physical tension and pain in order to make it through life. It's just that one accumulates tension in the body when running *away* from something in order to survive, and the other accumulates tension when running *toward* something in order to survive.

I decided then that it was time to look at the idea of sharing what I'd learned with dog owners by writing another book. No small undertaking. Fortunately, I was able to pair with Dr. Robin Robinett, a veterinarian and veterinary chiropractor who has been using Masterson Method Techniques with both her large and small animal clients for years. You're holding the practical result of this collaboration in your hands. It's our hope that this book brings you practical results with your canine partner as it has with ours.

Learning how to pay attention and respond to dogs' and horses' responses to touch has changed how I approach and relate to virtually all mammals that I come into contact with, both quadruped and biped (the latter would be us). It's my wish that you experience this valuable side benefit, too.

Jim Masterson
Fairfield, Iowa

Preface
by Robin Robinett, DVM

I always find it interesting to learn how people became who they are. How many people are doing what they dreamed of doing as kids? I do believe that the people we meet help steer us on our pathways through life and are put there for a purpose. I believe that things happen for a reason.

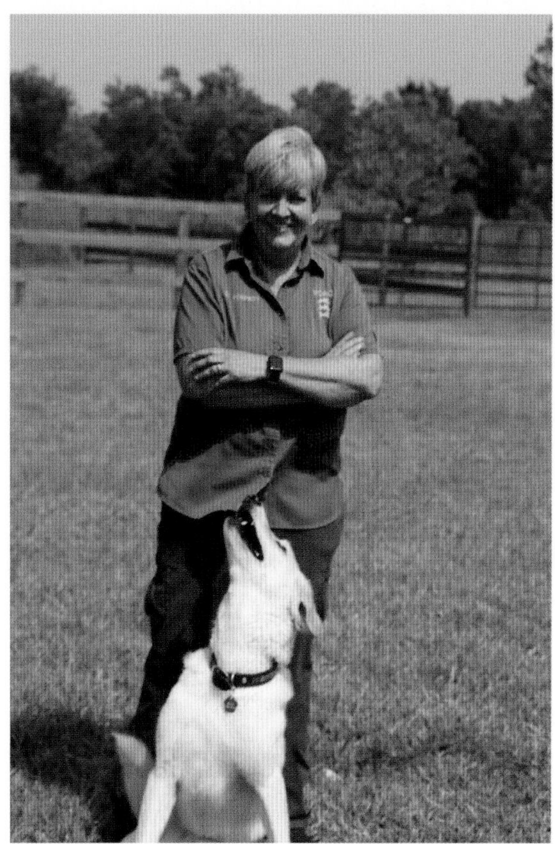

Some of my earliest memories are of begging my parents to get us a family dog. I would go over to my neighbor's house and play with their dog. I didn't think their kids played with or cared about Max, the Dachshund. Since I was shy, I enjoyed playing with him much more than playing with the other kids. (I have always felt more comfortable around animals than people.) Finally, when I was four, my parents gave in and brought home a Dachshund puppy of our own. It was love at first sight! The puppy was given the name of Snookelmyer Von Sweibocken of Robinschoven by my dad or, as we called him, "Snooky."

My parents told me that I had to help take care of Snooky and I had to do my chores before playing with him. My brother, who is two years older than I, thought it was funny that I would wash dishes and do other chores just so that I could feed the dog. He thought that feeding the dog was a chore, but to me it was an important part of taking care of Snooky and was a privilege.

Then came the day I got to go with my mother to take Snooky to the veterinarian for his puppy shots. At dinner that night I made the announcement that I was going to be a veterinarian when I grew up.

After college, when I was accepted to the College of Veterinary Medicine at Texas A&M, my plan was to become an equine-only or a mixed-animal, primarily equine veterinarian upon graduation. I had grown up riding and my main interest was lameness and sport horse medicine, but there were no jobs available at equine-only clinics and only a few positions at mixed animal clinics at that time. I took a position as an associate at a mixed animal clinic near Lubbock, Texas, that did small animal and equine medicine. After working 45 days straight and being on call almost every night and weekend, I gave my boss notice.

I left feeling like a failure for quitting after my probation period, but my favorite clinician at Texas A&M convinced me I was not a failure but smart for not staying and becoming burned out. Unfortunately, many young veterinarians get burned out working like this their first year or two and leave the profession.

I accepted a job as a shelter veterinarian for the Houston SPCA, doing spay and neuter surgeries, examining and treating sick animals, and examining and assisting with abuse cases. Working at the SPCA was never something that was in my plans, but ended up being a great experience, increasing my confidence in myself and improving my surgical skills. I left the SPCA when I opened a clinic with another veterinarian, who had been a high school friend. The clinic was mostly small animals, but I also provided equine mobile services. During this time one of my horse-trainer clients (who had been one of my trainers when I was riding in high school) had an equine chiropractor working on her horses. This individual had no training and sometimes hurt the horse more than helped him. I was called to examine a horse that had become injured during his "chiropractic treatment." After telling my trainer she should find someone who was properly trained to do chiropractic, she challenged me to do it.

In 1994, I went to San Antonio for the American Association of Equine Practitioners Annual Conference, and attended a lecture on equine chiropractic by Sharon Willoughby, who was a veterinarian and chiropractor. She had a school called Options for Animals, that trained chiropractors and veterinarians how to adjust animals. I attended Options for Animals and became certified in animal chiropractic in 1996.

In 1997, I started a mobile veterinary chiropractic service and did small animal veterinary relief until 2006. I stopped doing relief work in 2006 because I was so busy with the chiropractic services. In 2006, I took the Veterinary Basic Acupuncture course at the Chi Institute in Florida (now the Chi University) and became certified in acupuncture in 2008. In October 2008, I opened my "dream": Veterinary Chiropractic and Rehabilitation Clinic. Services included chiropractic, acupuncture, and rehabilitation for dogs, cats, and horses.

In 2013, at the Animal Rehabilitation Institute in Florida, taking an equine rehabilitation certification course, I met Becky Tenges, an instructor for the Masterson Method. I actually had a copy of the book *Beyond Horse Massage* by Jim Masterson but had not had time to really look into it much before the class. I learned that Becky was going to be teaching a course near Austin, Texas, so I invited her to Houston after she finished teaching. She came and spent three days with me at my clinic, and we worked on horses together. We discussed and shared techniques for examining and working on horses.

Before Becky left, I scheduled her to come back and teach a Masterson Method weekend course a few months later. And this was how I started my journey of incorporating the amazing, light touch techniques of the Masterson Method into my chiropractic techniques in order to adjust animals and help correct their muscular imbalances and compensations.

My education continued with taking the Advanced Five-Day Masterson Method course. Then in May 2021, I got to meet and work with Jim Masterson to become the first Masterson Method Certified Veterinary Practitioner. The Masterson Method was developed on horses, but I had started incorporating some of the work into my other chiropractic techniques for dogs and cats. Talking and working with Jim, we began to discuss and work on the Masterson Method Techniques for dogs.

It has been a privilege to assist on this project and work with Jim. He has such a calm, soothing presence with horses and dogs; they respond so well to his techniques. With a wonderful sense of humor, Jim is an amazing person and a pleasure to work with. I hope everyone enjoys this book and that all dogs benefit from the Masterson Method.

Robin Robinett, DVM
Houston, Texas

PART ONE

The Masterson Method

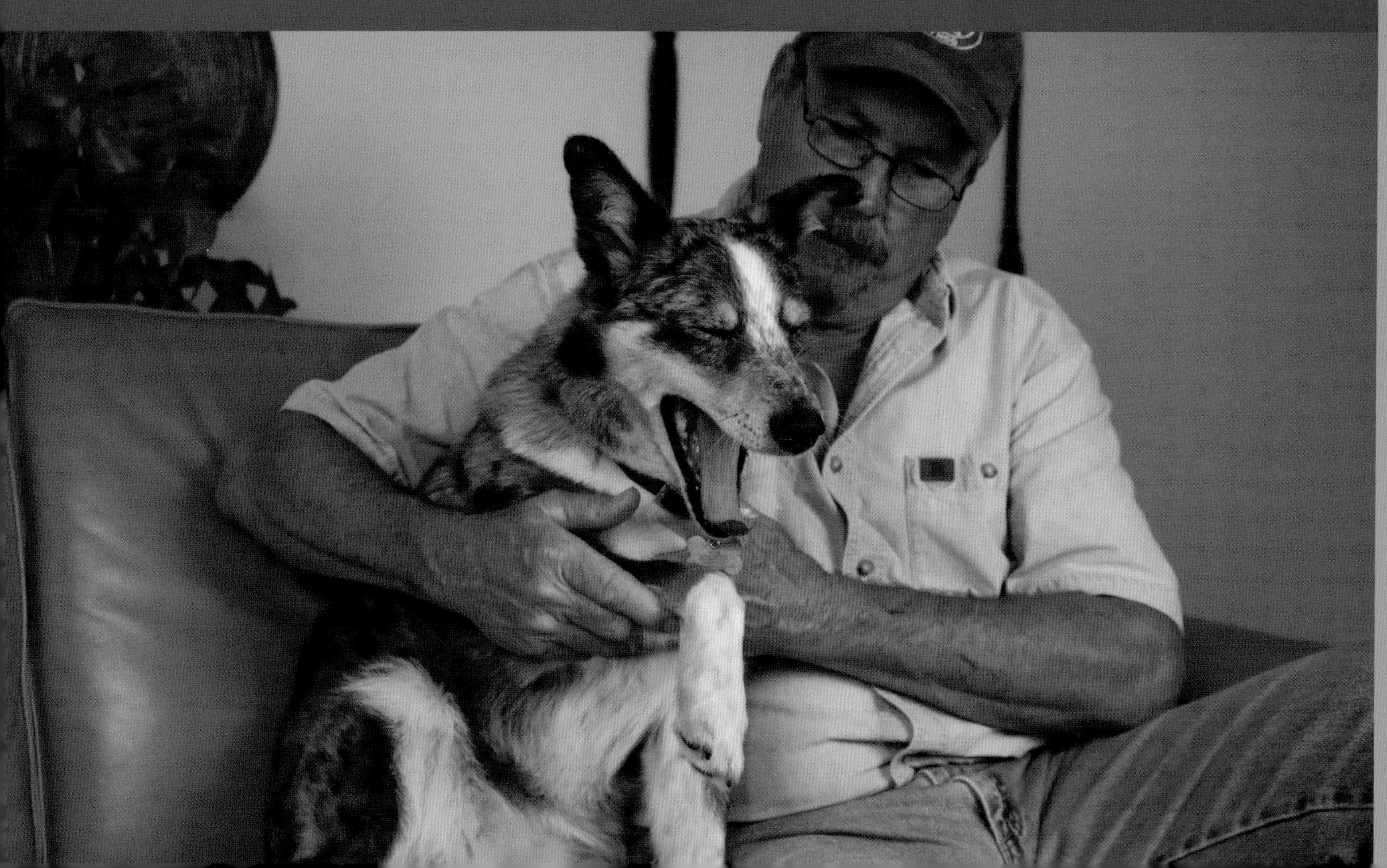

1

CHAPTER 1

What Is the Masterson Method®?

The Masterson Method is an interactive method of animal bodywork that follows and uses the animal's responses to your touch to find and release tension in areas of his body that affect movement, comfort, and longevity.

It was developed for the purpose of releasing tension and improving movement in the performance horse. The Masterson Method proved to be effective because with it, the horse participates in the process. It's a method in which you work *with* the horse, not *on* the horse. An interesting benefit that comes with using this method is that it leads to improved communication and trust, and a better relationship with the horse. Another interesting feature is that it works with other animals. And it's teachable.

As with horse owners, horse trainers, and horse therapists, dog owners, dog trainers, and dog therapists can learn techniques that will improve movement, comfort, and longevity and open new levels of communication and enhance their relationship with their animals.

The Techniques used in the Masterson Method all rely on reading and following the subtle changes in the dog's body language as you work with him. Once you learn to read his body language, you and he are on the same page. Communication is established. When you use this body language to help the dog release his tension, trust is developed and a relationship is formed. The dog recognizes that you understand what his body language is saying and there is no threat to his well-being.

The Masterson Method is very practical, easy to use, and results-oriented. You see the results in the dog's responses during the bodywork, and in behavior, comfort, and movement afterward.

What Causes Tension in the Dog's Body?

Dogs develop tension in the body from many sources:

- Work, and overwork or overexertion.
- Play, and overplay or overexertion (fig. 1.1).
- Compensation for other issues such as joint, ligament, systemic, or intestinal issues.
- Past accidents, incidents, or injuries.
- Fear or trust issues.
- Age.

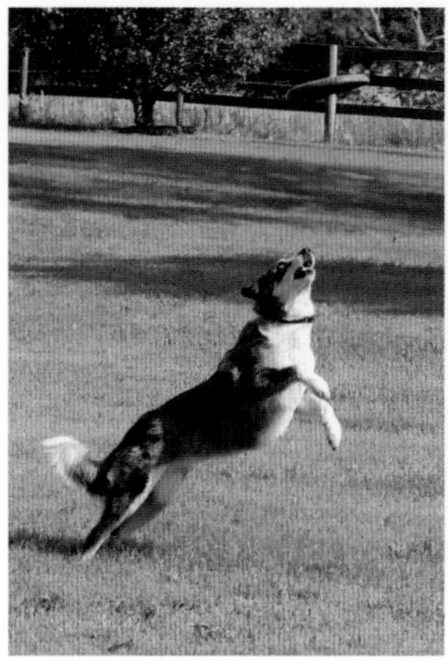
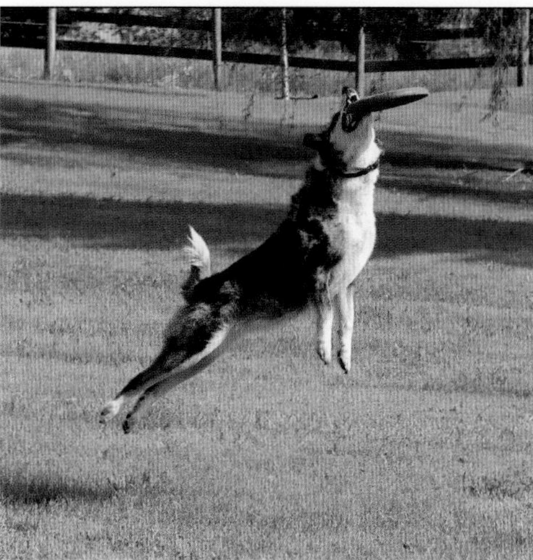
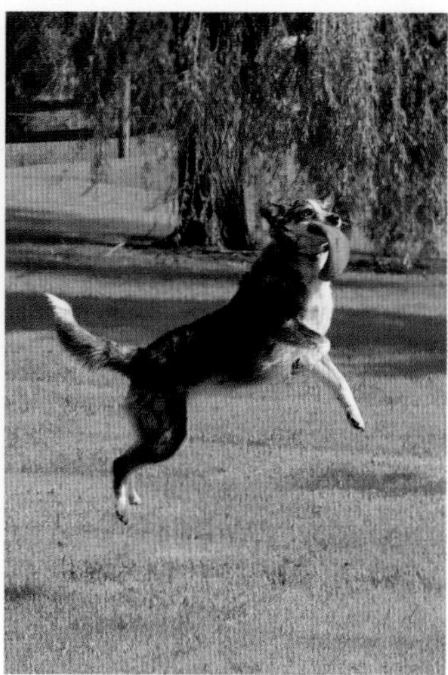

1.1 Play, and overplay or overexertion, can cause tension in the dog's body.

How Do Dogs Deal with Physical Tension or Discomfort in the Body?

Whether prey or predator on the survival scale, the physically stronger and less vulnerable animal has a better chance of survival than the physically weaker or more compromised. As with most animals, dogs are naturally programmed to ignore, block out, and cover up any physical signs of weakness or discomfort in order not to be placed at the *lower* end of the "fitness" scale—that is, at the *top* of the menu! Their nervous system is programmed, to whatever degree they're able, to "cover it up and get on with it"—the *sympathetic nervous system* for people who like bigger words. (See next page for the *parasympathetic nervous system*.)

How Does the Masterson Method Help the Dog Release This Tension?

By working with the dog's natural instincts and the dog's body language, you can help the dog's body to release tension.

The dog communicates through subtle and not-so-subtle changes in behavior and body language. When you learn to recognize changes in behavior and body language that correlate to where the dog is holding pain or tension, you can help him to release it.

When you use levels of pressure that don't trigger the dog's natural tendency to cover up physical signs of weakness or discomfort, and follow subtle changes in the dog's behavior and body language as you do this, you allow the dog to communicate where he is holding tension, and you allow that part of the dog's nervous system that relaxes and releases tension to let go of it—the *parasympathetic nervous system*.

In a sense, you are bringing and keeping the dog's awareness to that area until the part of the dog's nervous system that blocks out pain and tension (the *sympathetic* nervous system) starts to subside, and the part that relaxes and regenerates (the *parasympathetic* nervous system) begins to release the tension.

Creating Trust Through Communication

One of the major benefits to using the Masterson Method with your dog is the bond of trust that develops once your dog understands you're listening to him on his own level, which dogs don't often experience with humans. Most of us miss what our dogs are experiencing in their interactions with us because we're missing the subtle physical level of body language that they use to communicate.

It's one thing to "get" what your dog is telling you, but when you soften or change what you're doing in direct response to what he's telling you, the dog "gets that *you* get what he's saying," and the level of trust that develops becomes exponential.

What Types of Dogs Benefit from the Masterson Method?

- All dogs with physical tension and discomfort.
- Working dogs that need to increase range of motion, and improve speed and mobility.
- Dogs that are resistant to any type of pressure.
- Dogs with behavioral issues that stem from physical discomfort, pain, abuse, or poor training.
- Any dog that needs help to connect and build trust with humans.

The Masterson Method can be learned by anyone with a hand or finger, an eye or two, a willingness to slow down and observe the dog—and the ability to be patient!

Three Different Categories of Techniques

There are three different categories of techniques used in this book. I outline them briefly here, then describe each category in detail, beginning on page 7.

1 Search, Response, Stay, Release

The first category is called *Search, Response, Stay, Release* (*SRSR*). These are techniques that use little or no pressure to find and release tension at specific points on the dog's body (fig. 1.2).

- ***Search*** very lightly (using no pressure) with your fingertips over specific areas of the dog's body.

- Watch for a ***Response***—a subtle change in the dog's behavior—as you search (see p. 8).

- ***Stay***—keep the dog's attention on that spot by resting your fingers there lightly (again, no pressure) until the dog shows you a sign that he has let go of tension.

- ***Release***—this is that sign, a larger *Response* or change in behavior, that you are looking for (see p. 11).

Although *Search, Response, Stay, Release* can be used to find and release tension anywhere in the body, in each chapter you'll be directed to use *SRSR* on specific points or areas that commonly hold tension in the part of the body being discussed.

2 Movement Techniques

In the second category are techniques we call *Movement Techniques*—relaxed range-of-motion techniques (see p. 13). These Techniques ask for gentle movement in different areas of the dog's body while these areas are in a state of total relaxation (fig. 1.3). When you move a muscle, joint, or junction of the body through a range of motion in a state of relaxation—meaning the muscles are totally relaxed during the movement—the muscles and connective tissue involved in the movement release tension. The key to using the *Movement Techniques* is to feel the moment when the dog's muscles begin to brace or tense, then to relax your

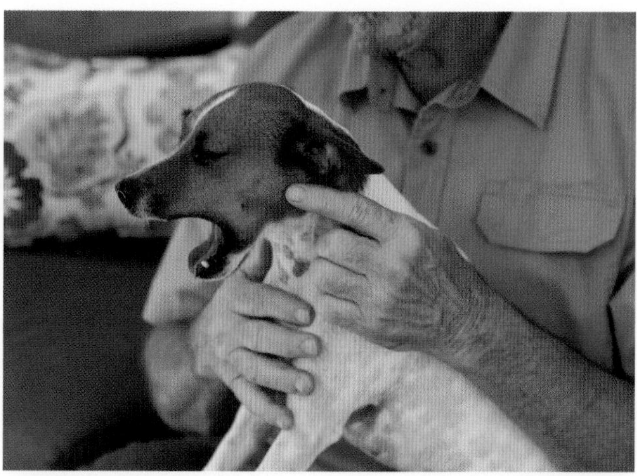

1.2 Terrier showing a release of tension in the TMJ using a *Search, Response, Stay, Release* Technique.

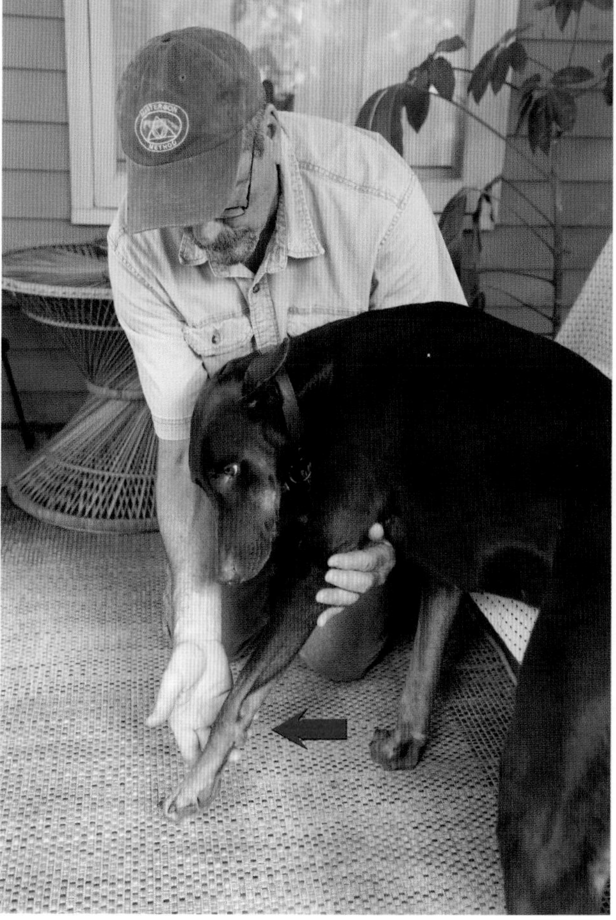

1.3 Moving the forelimb through a range of motion while in a relaxed state using a Movement Technique.

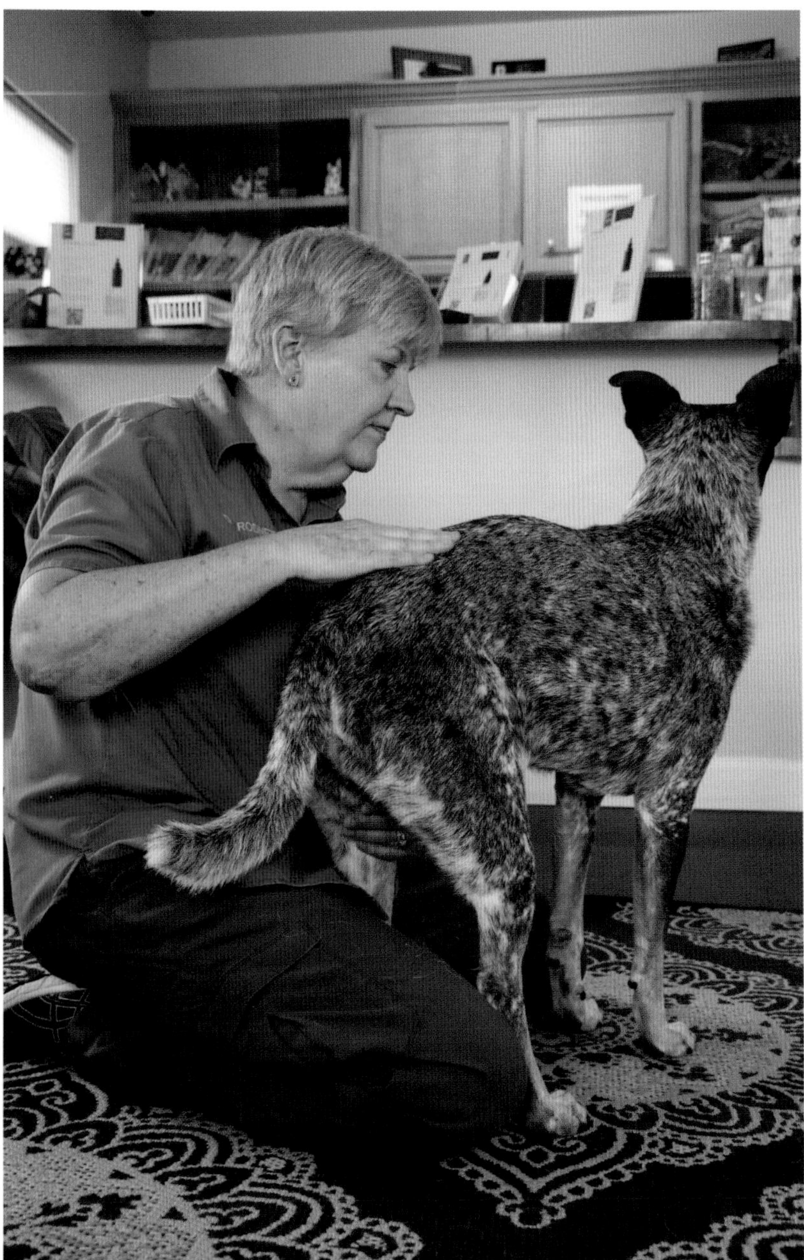

1.4 Releasing tension in the pelvis using a *Hold, Wait, and Melt Technique.*

hands and "yield" to the bracing when it happens, thus allowing the muscles to release the tension (see p. 15).

By feeling your way through the movement, you find *where* the dog is holding tension, and by softening and yielding, you help the body *release* the tension. By watching for *Responses* as you do this, you get added, visual confirmation of *where* and *when* tension has been released.

3 Hold, Wait, and Melt (HWM)

In the third category are what we call *Hold, Wait, and Melt* (*HWM*) *Techniques* (fig. 1.4). These are used to release tension in the connective tissues of larger structures or junctions, such as the pelvic junction and scapula-trunk junction. They are similar to *SRSR* in that they bring the body's awareness to tension, except they are focused on larger structures and junctions.

Communication Through Touch and Response

- All Masterson Method Techniques rely on the use of very gentle and soft hands.
- All Masterson Method Techniques use levels of pressure or touch that stay under the dog's bracing response.
- All Masterson Method Techniques rely on reading and following the dog's *Responses* to your Touch. This allows the body to communicate *where* it's holding tension, and *when* it's released it.

Now I'll talk about the *Levels of Touch* we use, and the *Responses* we look for.

Levels of Touch

As mentioned earlier, the levels of touch or pressure used in all these Techniques are soft and gentle. The reason for this is that the dog's body can block out or brace against even the slightest amount of pressure, especially when there is discomfort or tension underneath it. Here are the different levels:

Scan to view Levels of Touch video

- **Air Gap**—The first level of touch we call *Air Gap*, which is absolutely no pressure and little or no contact (fig. 1.5). This level can range from *barely* touching the skin, to *barely* touching the hair, to holding the hand or fingertips a few inches *away* from the skin or hair. In most cases, your hand or fingers won't even be touching the skin. *Air Gap* is

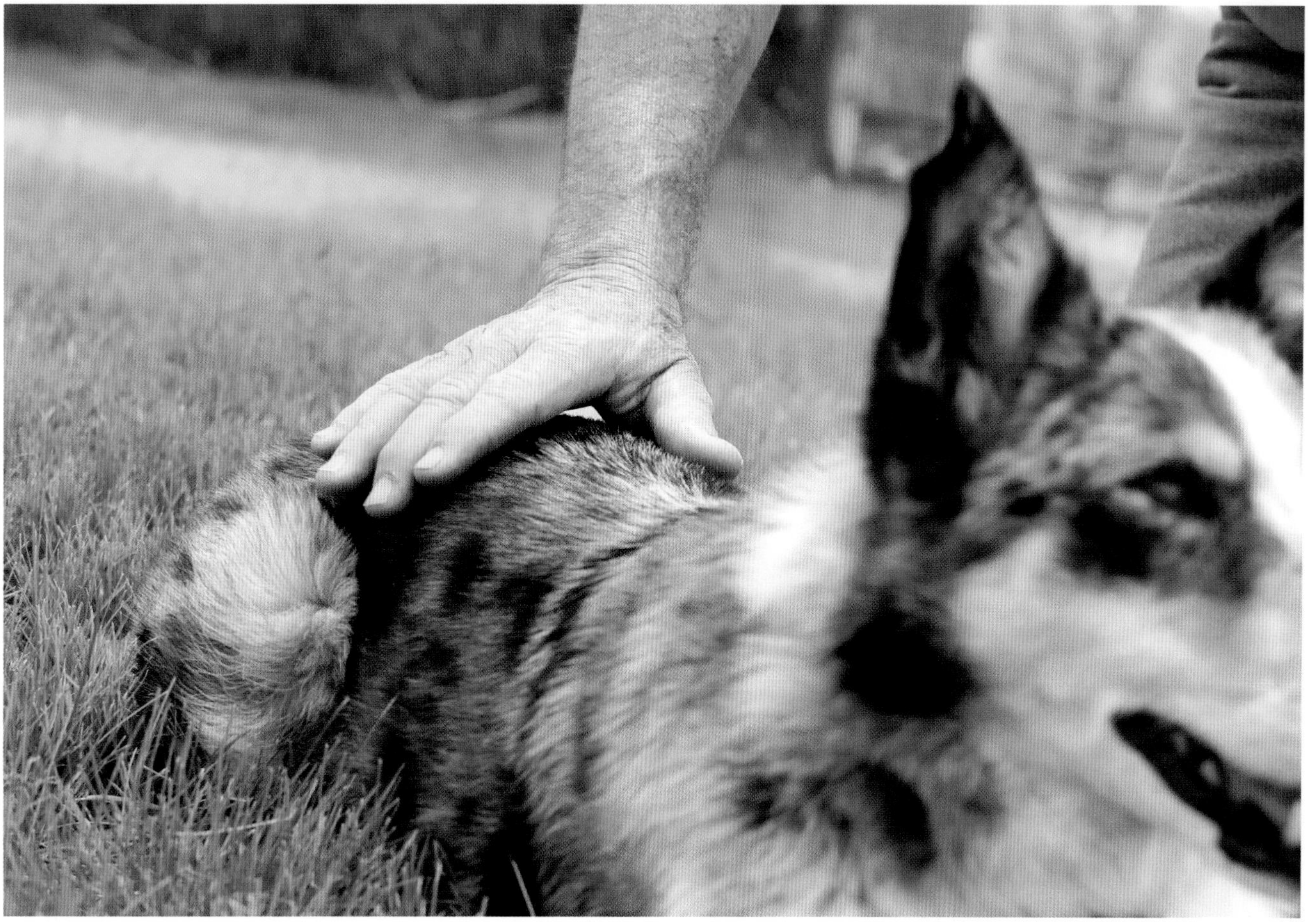

1.5 ***Air Gap*** **pressure (no pressure).**

Scan to view Types of Responses video

the level of pressure used in *Search, Response, Stay, Release* Techniques.

- **Egg Yolk**—The second level is called *Egg Yolk* (fig. 1.6). This is about the amount of pressure needed to barely indent or move the yolk of a raw egg on a plate. It can also equate to the amount of pressure it would take to indent a fresh marshmallow sitting on a plate (*not* one of those hard, stale ones that has been sitting in the cupboard for months!).

We use these Levels of Touch, or *non-pressure* as I like to refer to them, to:

1 Search the dog's body to find where it is holding tension.

2 Help the dog's body release the tension.

Responses

Search Responses

A *Response* is a shift in behavior. It is any subtle shift in behavior (and this is the key) *that correlates with what you are doing with your hands.*

Search Responses are what you will look for during the SRSR process as we *Search* (see p. 11).

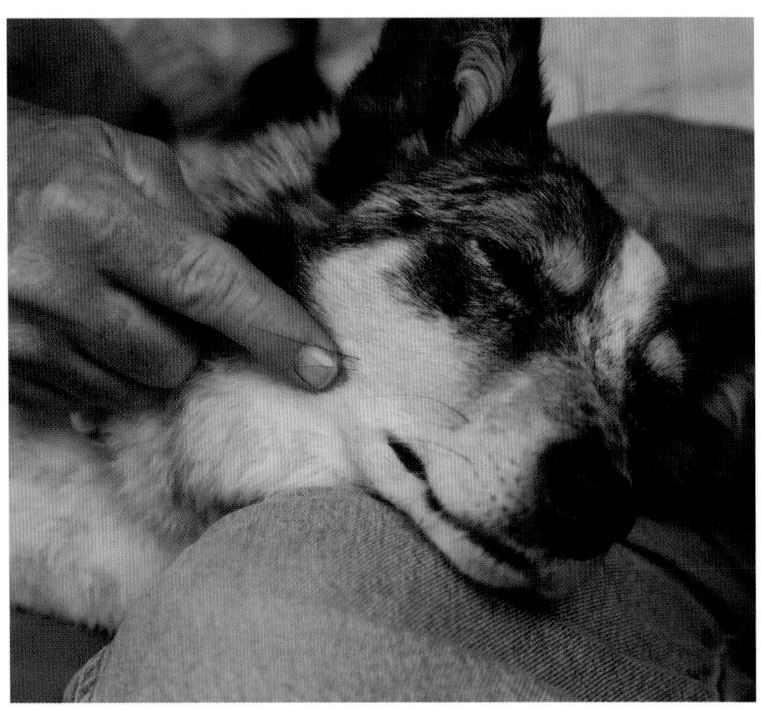

1.6 *Egg Yolk* pressure.

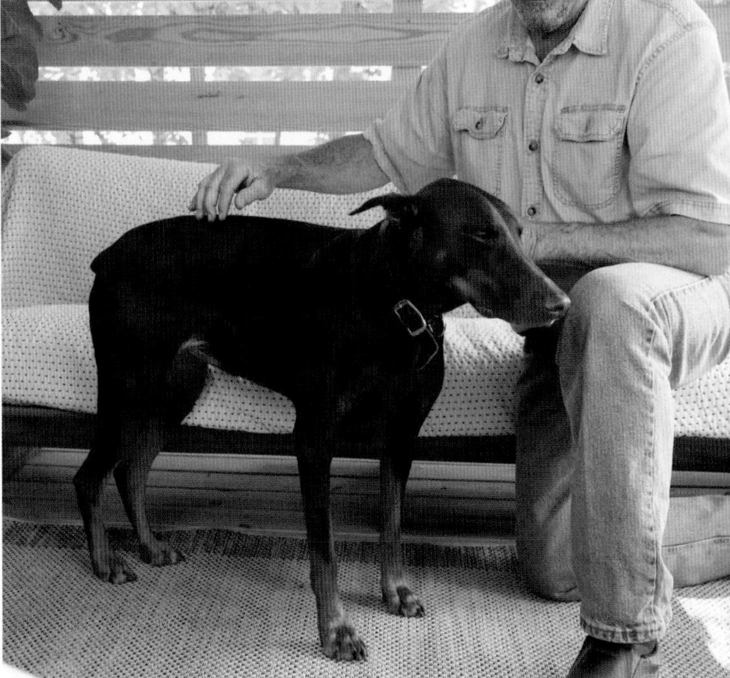

1.7 In this case, as my fingers go over an area where this dog is holding tension, she blinks.

They are an indication from the dog of underlying tension in that area.

The most common and easiest-to-read *Response* is the *eyelid blink;* however, there are a number of different subtle shifts in behavior that can be *Responses*. The following *Responses* are indications that the dog is holding tension in the part of the body that you are working on:

- Eyelid blink or gentle "squint" (fig. 1.7).
- Ear twitch or movement.
- Movement of the dog's head—both looking away from you or at you (figs. 1.8 A & B).
- Change in breathing.
- Small fidgeting or looking uncomfortable.

Release Responses

Release Responses are the sign of a *Release* of tension. They are generally larger *Responses*, and include:

- Licking and chewing (fig. 1.9).
- Sighing or letting out breath.
- Yawning (fig. 1.10).
- Sneezing.
- Lying down or "flopping" over (figs. 1.11 A & B).
- A large fidget (fig. 1.12).

Once you've learned to use the correct level of touch, how to recognize the dog's responses, and the correlation between your touch and the dog's response, following the steps outlined below will get you started on this interactive journey. So, let's go!

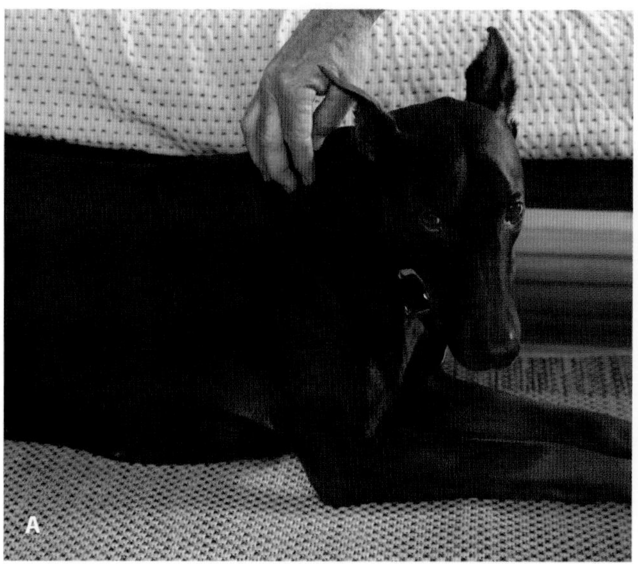

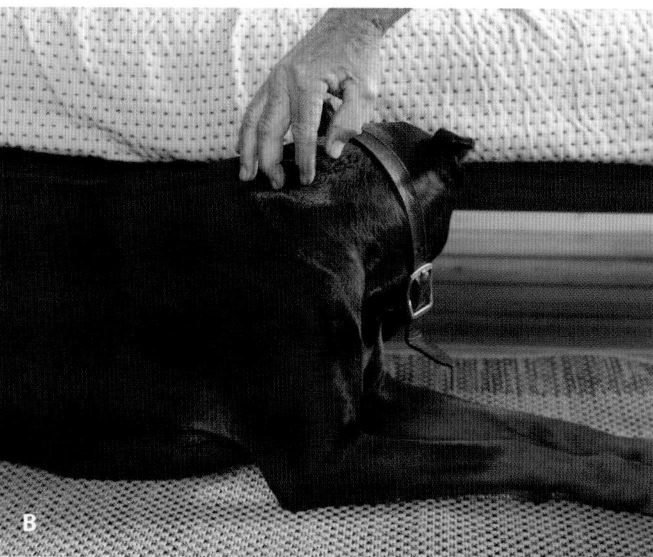

1.8 A & B Here, as my fingers go over an area where the dog is holding tension (A), she turns her head away (B).

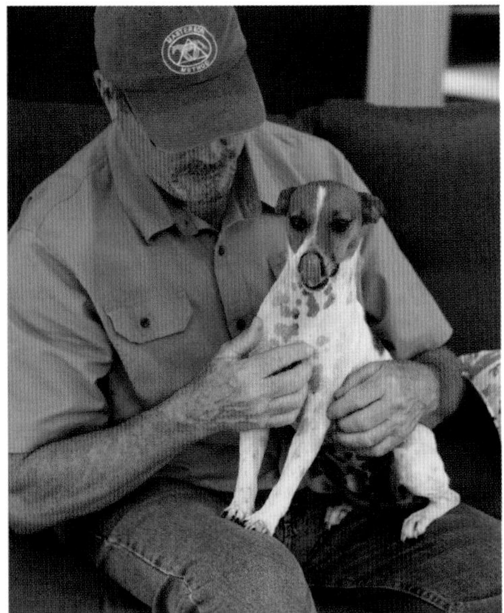

1.9 **Licking and chewing is a sign of releasing tension.**

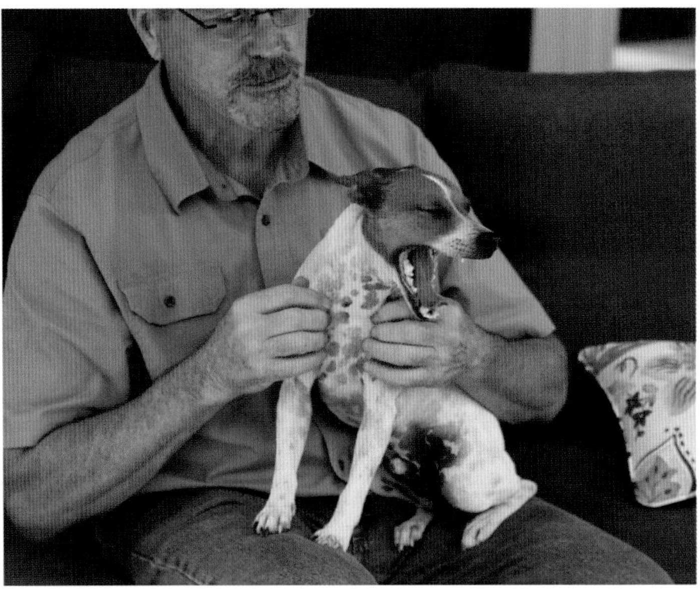

1.10 **Yawning as a sign of releasing tension.**

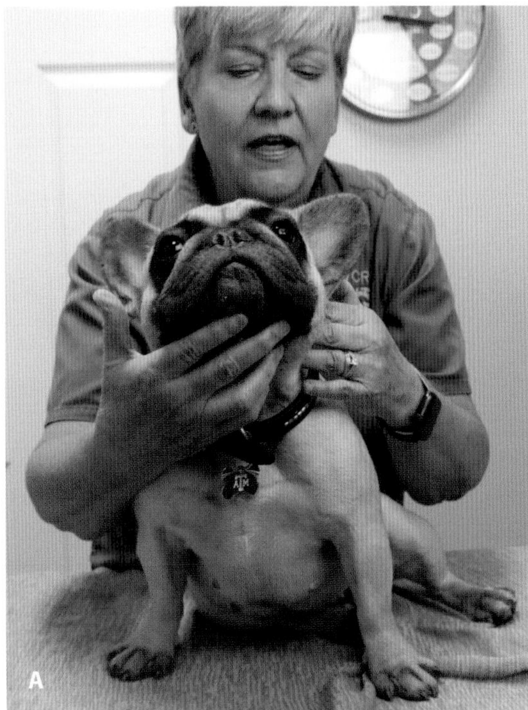

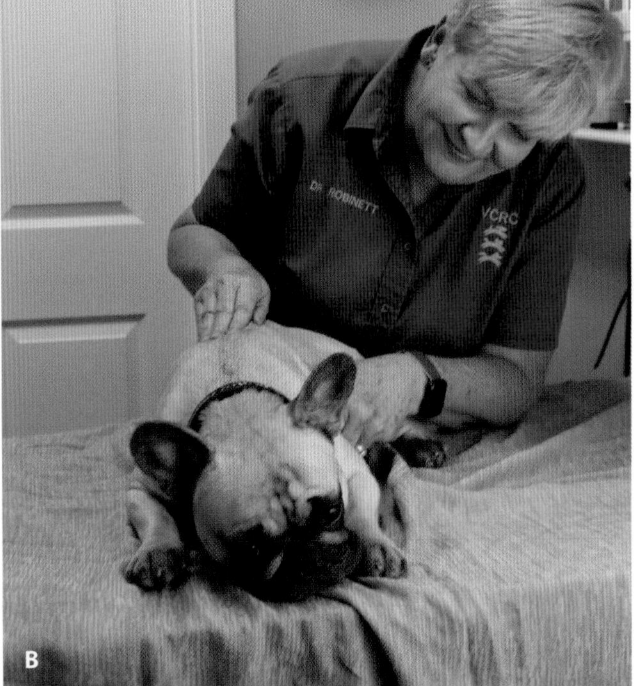

1.11 A & B One minute, she's up (A); next minute, she's down (B).

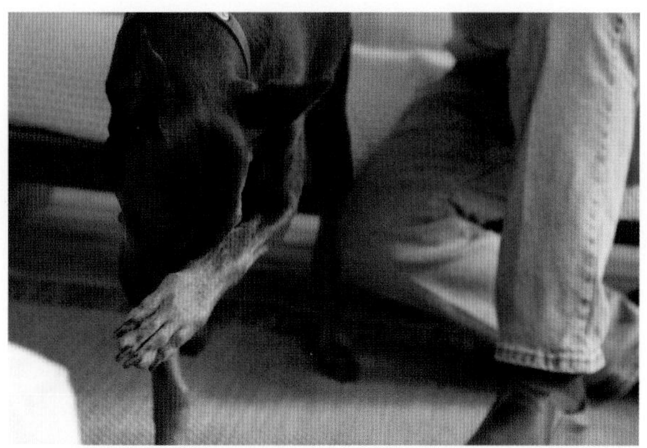

1.12 A large fidget or change of behavior can indicate a release of tension.

What Is Meant by "Fidget"?

A fidget can be defined as any subtle shift or change in behavior that the dog shows during the process. Some common fidgets:

- Looking away or at you ("dirty looks").
- Fussing in any way.
- Wanting to move or walk away.
- Reaching around and scratching, stretching, or flexing the body.

Sometimes a fidget will occur during the *Search* part of the process. This is a sign that you've brought the dog's attention to something that he has been blocking out and may be a little uncomfortable. It is physical tension or discomfort that the dog has been naturally dealing with by "covering it up and getting on with it."

If the fidget comes during the *Stay* (see p. 11) part of the process, it may be part of what's to come—the *Release*. This will make more sense to you once you've started doing this with your dog.

How Search, Response, Stay, Release (SRSR) Works

Scan to view Search, Response, Stay, Release video

Search—To *Search,* slowly run two or three fingertips softly over the dog's body using *Air Gap* (non-pressure). *Air Gap* means touching the hair but not the skin (fig. 1.13).

Response—As you *Search*, you watch for a subtle *Response.* A *Response* is any subtle or not-so-subtle change in behavior that correlates to what you are doing with your hands—your touch (fig. 1.14).

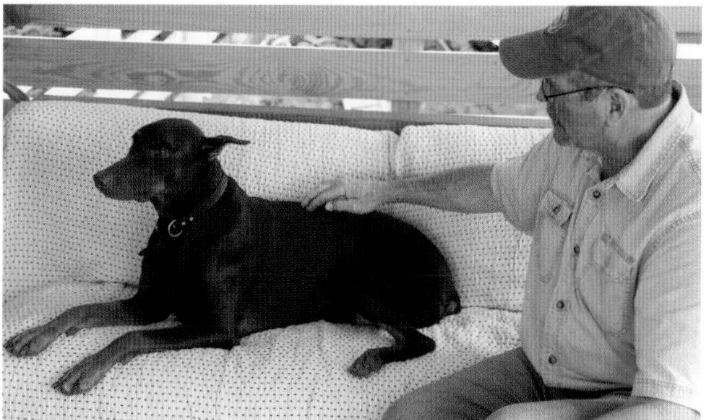

1.13 Search.

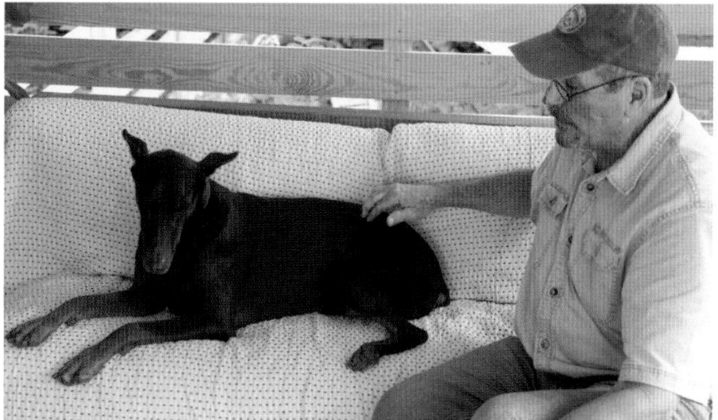

1.14 Response.

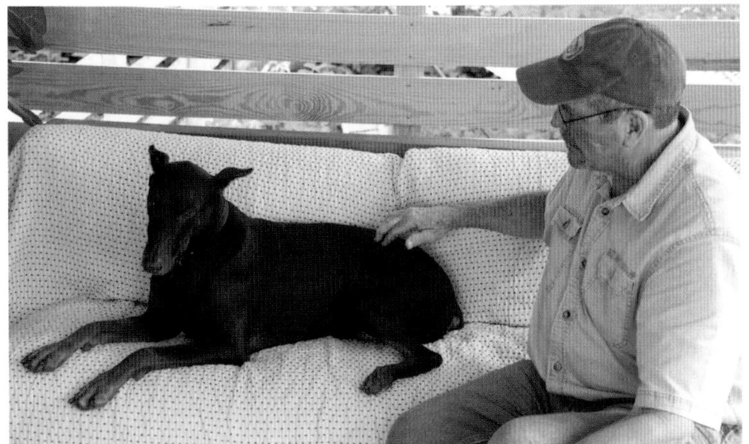

1.15 Stay.

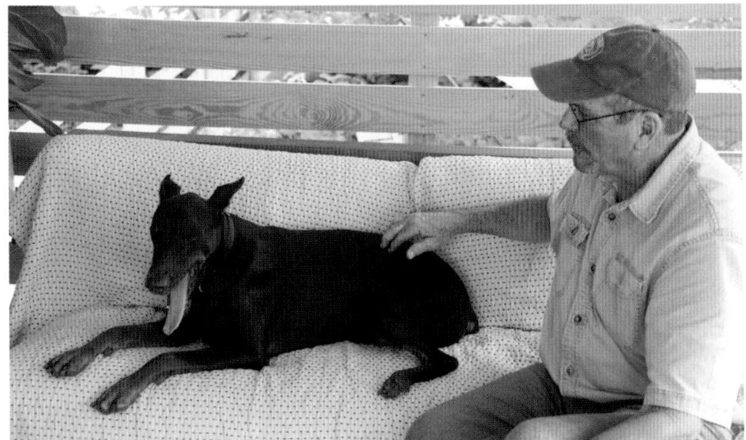

1.16 Release.

I gave you a list of common *Responses* on page 9.

Stay—When you get a *Response* (blink, or ear or head movement), stop and hold your fingertips lightly on that spot doing *nothing* (see p. 5). Nothing means no pushing, poking, petting, rubbing, massaging. This is the hard part for us humans.

You *Stay* there, and *Stay...Stay...Stay...* (remember to breathe) until the dog gives a larger *Response* (fig. 1.15), which indicates what comes next.

Release—Remember that a *Release* is a larger *Response* such as a large sigh, licking and chewing, a yawn or yawns, lying down or flopping over if the dog is standing or sitting up (see list of *Release Responses* on p. 9). These signs mean that his body has released some of the tension he was holding in this area (fig. 1.16).

What's Happening During the SRSR Process

- *Searching* lightly brings the dog's awareness to an area of tension that he has been blocking out for survival purposes (via his *sympathetic nervous system*).
- The subtle *Response* tells you that he is feeling tension in the area underneath your fingers.

Dogs Are Like People: Not All Are the Same

Dogs have different ways of responding. Some respond more readily; others are more guarded and give you hardly anything, then after you have walked away, they will show the *Release*. But there is almost always some kind of *Response*, and soon you will get good at recognizing even the subtlest change that signifies progress.

- *Staying*, or keeping your fingers lightly on that area, keeps the dog's awareness on the tension in a way that his nervous system is unable to brace against or block out. If you keep his attention on it long enough and light enough, his nervous system will begin to let the tension go (via the *parasympathetic nervous system*). However, if you use pressure on the area, his sympathetic survival system will block it out and he will *not* let the tension go.
- The larger *Release Response* means that the nervous system has gone from blocking mode to relax, restore, and regenerate mode, and tension is released.

The Importance of Going Slowly

In order for your dog to participate in this process, you must allow him to do so on his own time. Let go of the element of time (throw away the clock) or the dog won't respond. You are following the *dog's* agenda. Go slowly in the *Search,* watch for a *Response*, and when you get one, *Stay, Stay, Stay,* until you get a *Release*, or until you are satisfied there is nothing happening in that spot.

How Movement Techniques Work

When you move a dog's muscle, joint, or junction through a range of motion while the muscles and connective tissue are in a relaxed state, tension releases in the muscles and the connective tissue associated with that joint or junction.

The key to this isn't the amount of movement,

How Do I Know if a Change in Behavior Is a Response?

So, you might say, "Dogs always blink, yawn, lick their lips, move their nose, ears, and head. How do I know if it's a *Response,* or they are just blinking, hearing, or smelling something—or responding to some other stimulus?"

The answer is you are not just looking for these behaviors. You are looking for the correlation between what you are doing at that moment with your hand, and the behavior the dog is giving you *then*. That's the key.

One way to know for sure is when you get a change in behavior that you think could be a *Response,* take your hand off, and slowly (and lightly) go back over that spot. If you get a *Response* at the exact same spot, there's a correlation between what you were doing and what the dog is telling you. It's a *Response* to your *Search*.

Pretty soon you'll find that you can easily tell what's a *Response* and what's not.

Another way to tell is when you get what you think could be a *Response*, just *stay* on that spot and see what happens. If you get a *Release,* then it was probably a *Response.*

All it takes is the patience to go slowly and lightly, to watch and wait, and to see what your dog has to say. And remember—*less is more.*

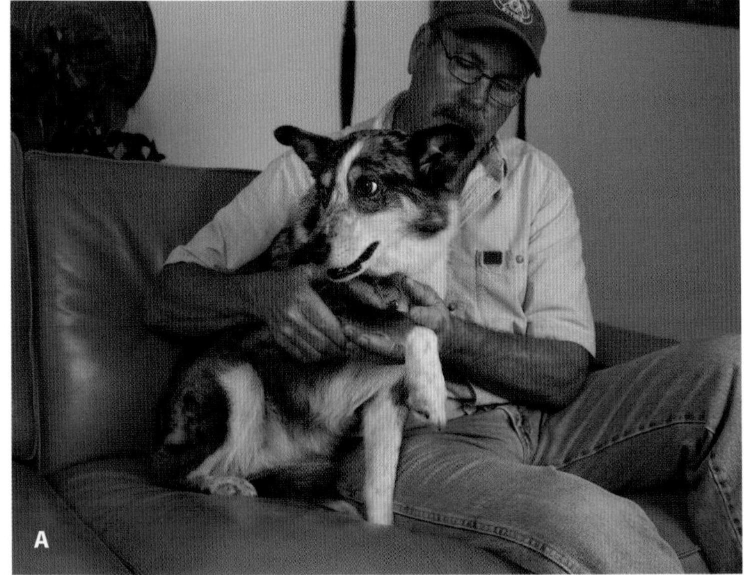

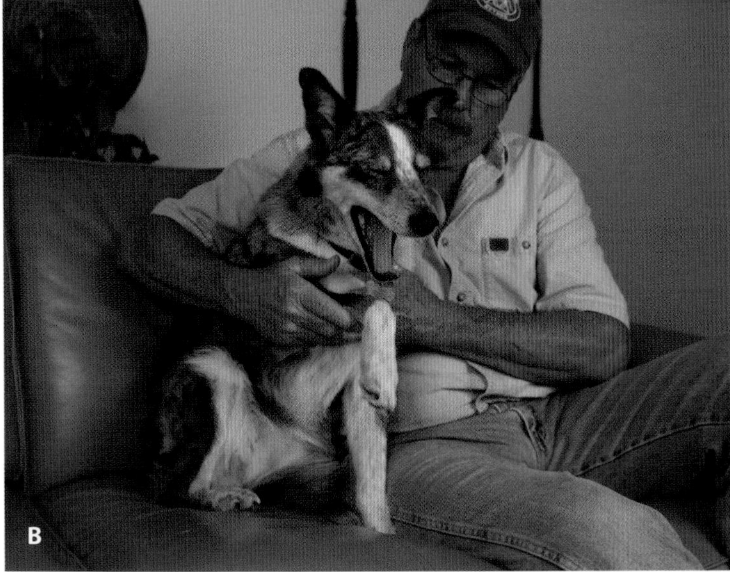

1.17 A & B When I raise the scapula in a relaxed state, there is a moment Nellie gets uncomfortable and starts to tense (A). So I soften my hands and yield to the resistance, allowing her to relax the scapula. She releases the tension and yawns (B).

but the amount of *relaxation* in the movement.

For example, the purpose of this Movement Technique is to wait until the dog's foreleg has relaxed completely into your hand, then to slowly raise the scapula in this relaxed state. If at some point in this range of motion she feels a muscle that is in tension, she will look uncomfortable and tense or start to pull away. When this happens, you will soften your hands and yield to the resistance, allowing her to relax and release the tension (figs. 1.17 A & B).

An interesting part is that relaxed movement helps to find *where* tension is being held. As you ask for—or provide—movement in a relaxed state, the dog will tell you where he is feeling tension: by demonstrating a visual response (blinking or looking away are examples) or by resisting the

A Counterintuitive Way of Working

Our physical reaction to the dog bracing or resisting is often to immediately brace against the resistance.

Once you—and your dog—get used to the Masterson Method's counterintuitive way of responding to resistance and acknowledging to subtle *Responses,* you will experience a new level of communication and interaction with your dog. And the effect of this interaction will spill over into other aspects of your activities together.

movement (tensing, fidgeting, or pulling away). When you come across resistance during a relaxed movement, it can mean the dog is feeling tension or discomfort there, or that he is anticipating or "guarding" against feeling the discomfort.

When this happens, it's important to allow the dog to "un-resist" and relax the tension you're encountering. You do this by softening your hand and *yielding* to the resistance. When you properly yield and soften, the dog will yield and soften, thus releasing tension he's been holding in the muscle or connective tissue associated with that movement.

Asking for relaxed movement and yielding to resistance allows you to both find *and* release tension.

The "No Thumbs" Rule

Any time your thumb is wrapped around a leg, you run the risk of breaking the "No Thumbs" Rule: When your thumb is wrapped around a leg and the dog pulls away, your reaction is to clamp and pull back. The more you are able to handle the legs *without* using your thumbs, the less likely you are to break the rule when the dog pulls away, tenses, or resists. You'll also find that the dog will feel less tense to begin with, the less you rely on using your thumbs when handling the leg.

Touch and Response Applies to Movement

You are also using *touch* and *Response* when asking for movement. In this case the *Responses* from the dog are *palpable* as well as *visual*.

Using your hands to ask for movement is *touch*. When you feel resistance to the movement, this is the dog's *palpable Response* to your touch. At this moment, you soften your hands and *yield* to the resistance. When you soften, the dog also softens or yields to the resistance. When this happens, tension associated with the resistance is released, allowing you to continue with the movement.

How you ask the dog to move is fundamental to the success of this method. If the dog is not in a relaxed state when you ask for movement, then he is, in a sense, *bracing* as he moves. A *relaxed state* means the dog's muscles are completely relaxed, meaning you have the entire weight of the part you are moving—whether it be the limb, the paw, or the head—in your hand. Feel and timing are essential to this. But it can be done!

Try This Exercise

The Principle of Non-Resistance

1 Wrap your hand gently around your dog's paw, then close your eyes (fig. 1.18 A).

2 Ask him to extend his leg toward you. Continue bringing it toward you (fig. 1.18 B).

3 When you feel the dog start to resist or pull, soften your hand slightly. When he feels *you* soften and stop pulling, *he* will soften and stop pulling (fig. 1.18 C).

Scan to view Yielding and Softening video

4 When he relaxes, you can continue the movement toward you. When you give the dog *nothing to resist,* he will stop resisting, and you can then continue with the movement (fig. 1.18 D).

If the dog continues to resist or pulls, it means you are not yielding enough and you're still providing resistance. Simple.

Feel for that moment, when closing your hand around the paw or bringing the paw toward you, when the dog

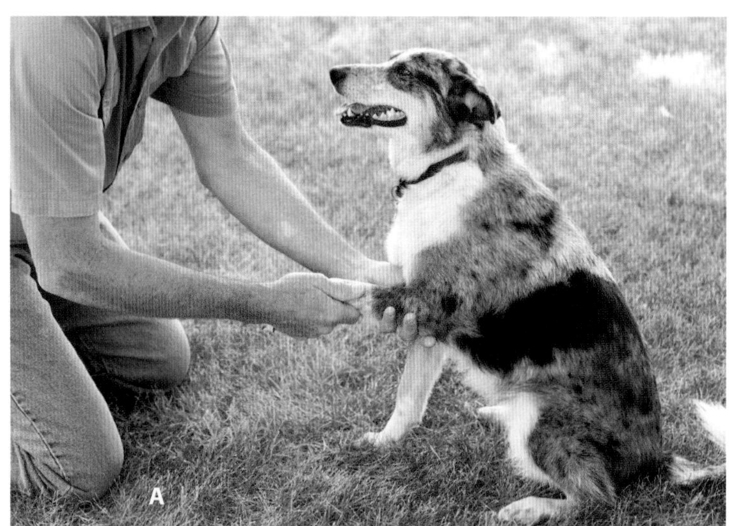

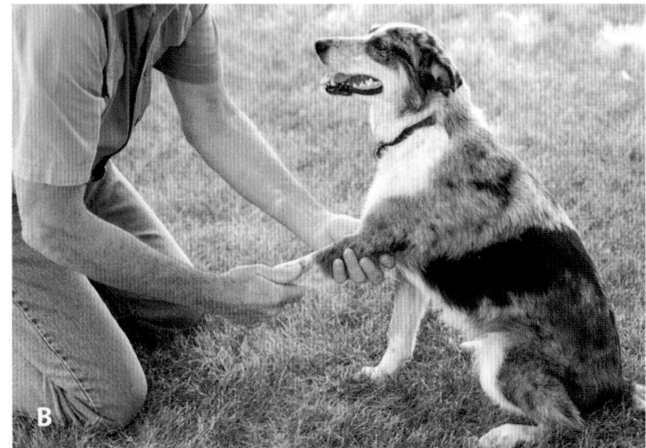

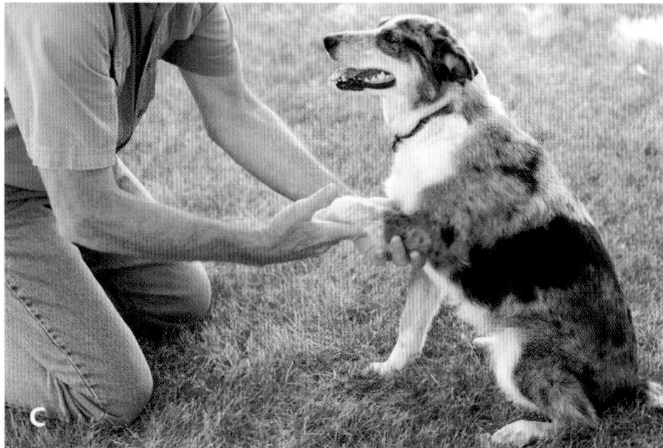

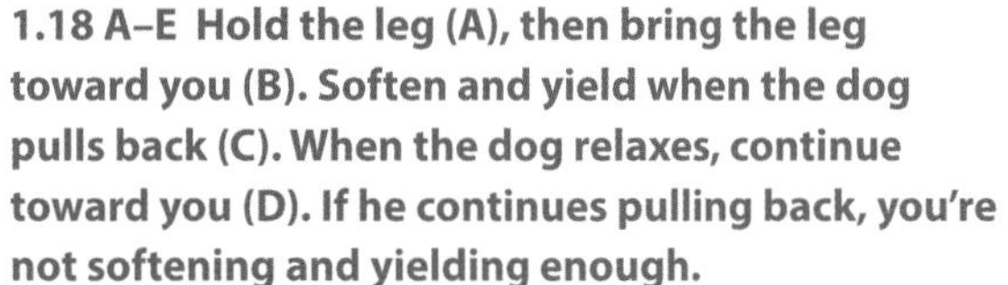

1.18 A–E Hold the leg (A), then bring the leg toward you (B). Soften and yield when the dog pulls back (C). When the dog relaxes, continue toward you (D). If he continues pulling back, you're not softening and yielding enough.

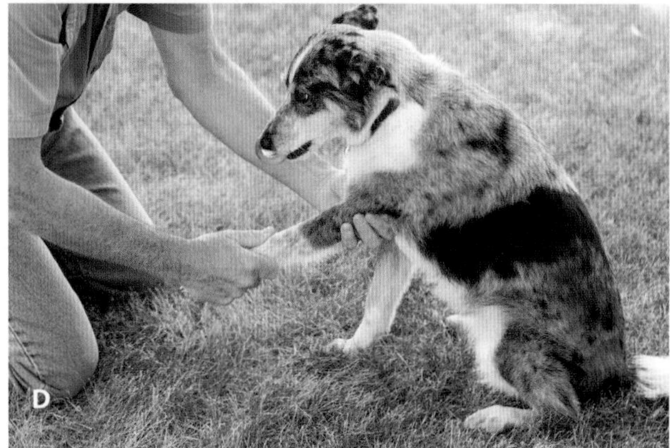

starts to tense or pull away. This is the moment, or even just *before,* at which you need to slightly soften or yield. Any time you ask for movement in a relaxed state on any part of the dog, this is when you need to soften, then continue.

What Does "Resistance to the Movement" Mean?

It means the dog doesn't like it. Wondering why?

The first reason can be that it's strange to him and he doesn't know what you're doing. The second reason can be that the muscles involved in the movement are uncomfortable and he's protecting them. It might also mean that you're doing it too hard, or too fast. In any case, the remedy is for you to *soften* and *yield* enough so you are able to continue the movement without the dog resisting.

When you do this regularly and your dog gets used to it, you'll soon be able to identify where there is actual discomfort or tension in the body, and by softening, help him to release it.

How Hold, Wait, and Melt Techniques Work

Hold, Wait, and Melt is basically applying the use of *SRSR* (p. 4) to release tension in a junction of skeletal structures, or more specifically, the muscles, tendons, and ligaments that are putting tension on the junction. It brings awareness to tension in the connective tissue and provides the stimulus for it to relax and let go, restoring movement and function to the junction.

With *HWM Techniques*, the practitioner places the hand or hands very lightly on specific junctions to bring the dog's awareness to any tension in the junction in a way (meaning using no pressure) that his nervous system is unable to brace against or block out (*Hold*).

The practitioner waits for tension in the connective tissues and muscles of the junction to release (*Wait*).

The release of tension on the junction is indicated by the *Release Responses* described earlier in the book (see p. 9).

Once you get used to this counterintuitive way of working with your dog, you will experience the elation and benefit that comes from being able to read what your dog is telling you through his body language. Once your dog "gets" that you understand what he is telling you, a new level of communication and trust is established that will spill over into other aspects of your relationship.

2

CHAPTER 2

Before You Begin

When and Where

Before you start, it is helpful to know a few things, such as the *ideal* time and place—the working environment—to do the Masterson Method Techniques with your dog.

You will remember, when I was talking about the *Movement Techniques* in the last chapter, I said, "When you move a muscle, joint, or junction of the body through a range of motion in a relaxed state—meaning the muscles are totally relaxed during the movement—the muscles and connective tissue involved will release tension."

The key word here is *relaxed*. The ideal time to do this is any time the dog is *quiet and relaxed*.

This can be while you are:

- Sitting together.
- Petting your dog.
- Talking to a friend.
- Watching TV.
- Reading a (this) book.
- Relaxing in the park, watching nature.
- Waiting (patiently) for your dog to relax.

This can be while your dog is:

- Standing.
- Sitting.
- Lying down.
- Listening quietly and attentively to your every word—or whatever else is going on.

Remember the dog must be *relaxed*, which doesn't necessarily happen:

- At the dog park, while he is running around chasing other dogs.
- In the backyard, with a ball/frisbee/cheeseburger in your hand.
- First thing in the morning, when he's standing over you in bed licking your face, wagging frantically, and waiting for (urging) you to get up.

You get the idea. I take advantage any time either of my dogs is relaxed and resting to search for *Responses*, apply some techniques, and release any tension that may have accumulated during the day from running and playing (my younger dog), or compensating for stiffness and arthritis (my older dog).

Well, that's not entirely accurate. It's not so much that I'm taking advantage of a situation to help my dog as that I'm addicted to doing this and can't help it. As a matter of fact, now that I know what to look for, I'm not physically able to pet or otherwise touch my dog without searching for *Responses* in areas where I know there might be tension, and watching or waiting for a *Release*.

I call these "techniques of opportunity," whenever the dog is in an ideal position for a few minutes of bodywork (figs. 2.1 A–C).

Let this serve as a disclaimer. Doing these Techniques can become addictive and seriously change the nature of your relationship with your dog. You've been warned!

You Can Influence the Environment

It might be that your dog isn't as relaxed as he could be, or is even extremely nervous.

This might be because he's in a *scary* environment with:

- Unfamiliar people.
- Unfamiliar dogs.
- Unexpected or unfamiliar things going on such as loud noises, pouring rain, or thunder..

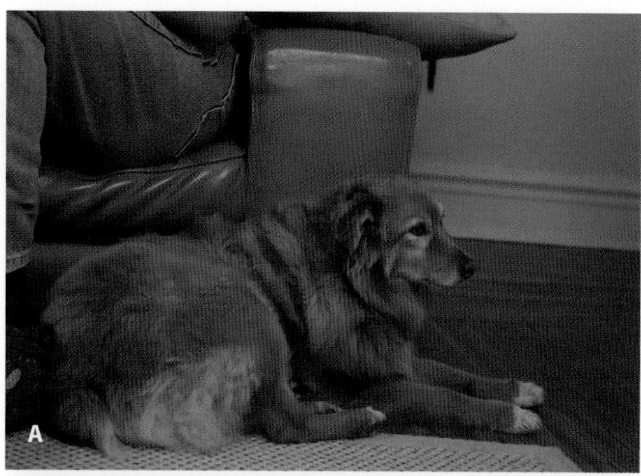

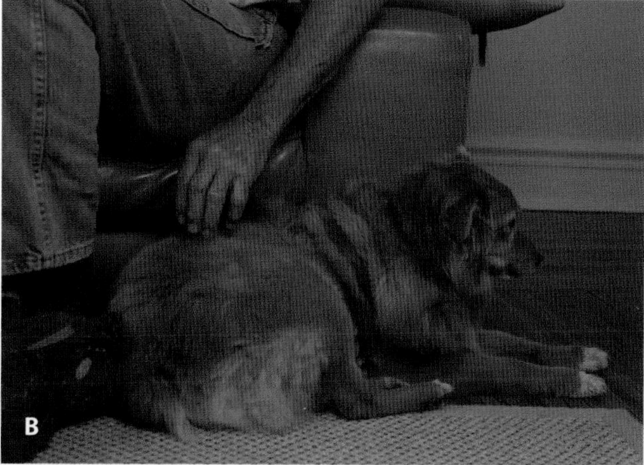

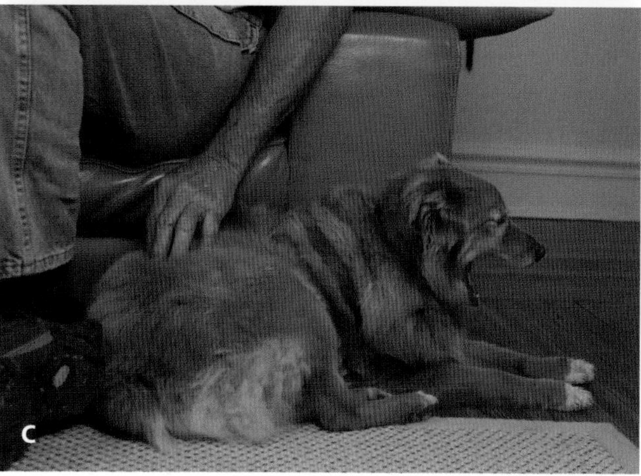

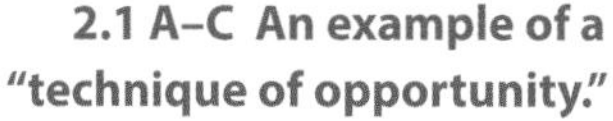

2.1 A–C An example of a "technique of opportunity."

Or it could be because he's in a *fun* environment with:

- Unfamiliar people.
- Unfamiliar dogs.
- Unexpected or unfamiliar things going on such as loud noises, pouring rain, or thunder!

I've noticed that when a dog is in an situation that makes him afraid, it's often not that easy to convince him that it's *not* scary without changing his environment. When a dog is frightened, he's frightened.

You can, however, have an effect on the dog's environment by remembering that relaxation and softness starts with *you*—on the inside as well as the outside. When you are "mentally tense," the dog will be tense. Remaining "mentally soft" creates an environment that allows the dog to relax. Have an intention or "bedside manner" that remains calm, even (or especially) when the dog isn't calm.

Also keep in mind that an animal with physical issues may feel vulnerable and unsafe in a new environment. When you create a calm, relaxed environment for the dog, it helps him to feel safer and more relaxed.

Remain "soft" inside your whole body, not just your hands. Do a conscious check: *hands, arms, shoulders, neck, back*, and *core.* Conscious softness in your body sends the subtle communication to the dog to soften. And remember to breathe!

Let go of expectations and throw away the clock. If you have an agenda or get impatient with the process, your dog will sense it and internally "guard" against it. Anticipating or expecting something to happen before the dog's body decides it's time will get in the way of the dog feeling what is happening.

When there are things going on around you that you can't change, ignore them. If you react to distractions around you, your dog will, too. Be the one to set the tone. You may find this to be as mentally therapeutic for you as for the dog.

Your Intuition

Intuition is a process that gives you the ability to know something directly without analytical reasoning. When your analytical mind is out of the way, you can quiet down and focus on your touch, feel, flow, softness, breathing, yielding, and asking.

While doing *SRSR Techniques*, you might suddenly notice that your mind has stopped thinking or talking to itself and it's just paying attention. In that quiet space a thought might pop into your head like, "I think I'll search here," or "I'm going to ask for a Scapula Movement now."

Listen to the thought. It may have been your intuition. Your mind wasn't analyzing or doubting or debating with itself, the thought just popped into your head.

Move on with whatever you think is the next thing to do. One nice thing about using the Masterson Method is that as long as you're not using pressure or force, and you're paying attention to your dog's *Responses* to the work, you can't really do it wrong. You can only do it better.

And even if you're not into meditating, if you notice at times that your mind isn't busy, you may be doing it.

"Tips" and "What Ifs?" to Get Started

In the next section, Part Two, you'll learn how to use the three categories of Masterson Method Techniques on all different parts of the dog's body. There are step-by-step instructions for the specific bodywork exercises, as well as "Tips" and "What Ifs?" that cover how to deal with individual issues that can arise.

Below are some general "Tips" and "What Ifs?" that are relevant to *all* the bodywork. These will help you get started, and you can look back at them as needed while working with your dog.

Tips on Timing, Order, and Where to Begin

You don't have to address all parts of the dog in one sitting. You can work in one area on one day and a different area on another day.

The Techniques don't have to be done in any specific order, or in the order that they're presented. It is helpful, though, to have the dog release tension in an area using light-touch, *Search, Response, Stay, Release* (SRSR) *Techniques* before doing the *Movement Techniques*, especially when the *Movement Techniques* are initially uncomfortable for your dog.

If you're working on a part of the dog where he is not comfortable, move on to another one, then come back to the uncomfortable area later. Start where it's easiest! If you're not able to do the Techniques on both sides of your dog, don't worry, he won't go around in circles the rest of his life! You also don't have to remain working on one part of the body. When the dog's responses lead you from one area to another, go there.

It's interesting to note that releasing tension in an area on one side of the dog begins the process of releasing tension in the same area on the opposite side, as well as in other areas of the body. In any case, you always follow the dog's *Responses* and his behavior during the process. The dog's body knows how much it needs, and where.

Tips on Softening and Yielding

When doing the *Movement Techniques,* you don't have to let go or take your hand away when you yield—*if* you yield quickly enough and completely. Keep your hand on softly and don't lose contact but "go with" the leg (for example) when you feel it start to tense or pull away. Timing is important here.

It's also important that you learn how to yield *completely*, meaning you have absolutely no pressure on the leg while at the same time continuing to keep your hand very light (almost *Air Gap*, see p. 7) on the dog. When the dog continues to pull after you've yielded, it means you're not yielding completely.

As I've mentioned already, yielding when a dog pulls away is counterintuitive—usually your natural reaction is to tense or pull back when the dog pulls. If you keep this in your mind as you're working, yielding will become your natural reaction, especially when you see that it works. It will also become more natural for the dog once he realizes that there's no resistance when he pulls.

Yield even if you're not sure the dog is tensing. I call it "getting ahead of the dog."

The reason I'm spending time on this is because if you get to the point where you can yield naturally and fluidly, you'll find that the dog will become less guarded and his reactions less intense.

What Ifs?—Search, Response, Stay, Release Techniques

- ***What if my dog becomes uncomfortable when I'm searching in an area?***

As you run your fingers (lightly) over any of the areas of the dog I describe in the pages ahead, you may come across one that is uncomfortable for him. There will probably be different levels of expression of this depending on his level of discomfort there.

- The first thing your dog might do is blink or look around or up at you.
- The second might be to lick your hand or put his mouth to your hand.
- The third, especially if he doesn't know you and he's extremely sore, might be to bite you.

If you're moving your fingers slowly and paying close enough attention, you can often catch the first *Response* and soften or back your hand away slightly before it turns into the second or third. Your dog is telling you that you've found something uncomfortable. If you respond soon enough by softening, it will be easier for your dog to continue. You're also letting your dog know that you're paying attention.

The first thing to do is back your fingers away a few inches, or if needed, entirely away. This will often be enough for the dog to relax again. If this works, then move to a different area. You can come back to this spot later.

This can sometimes happen the first time you work with your dog, before he has experience with what you're doing. Your dog doesn't know what your intentions are, or that he's going to feel better afterward. All he knows is that something is making him uncomfortable. When you soften or back your fingers away, you lessen or take away the sensation. However, three positive things have happened.

1. Now you know where he's sore.
2. You'll be able to come back to this area after he's released tension elsewhere and he may be more comfortable with it.
3. He may already have begun the process of releasing it.

- ***What if my dog wants to walk away?***

There are a few things you can do.

- First is to soften at the first sign of discomfort, or before your dog gets uncomfortable.
- The second is to have one hand resting gently on the dog before you start so that you're able to ask him to remain with you a little longer. There are different ways you can handle this: When working on the front end, you can rest one hand on the dog's chest, or on his shoulder with your thumb

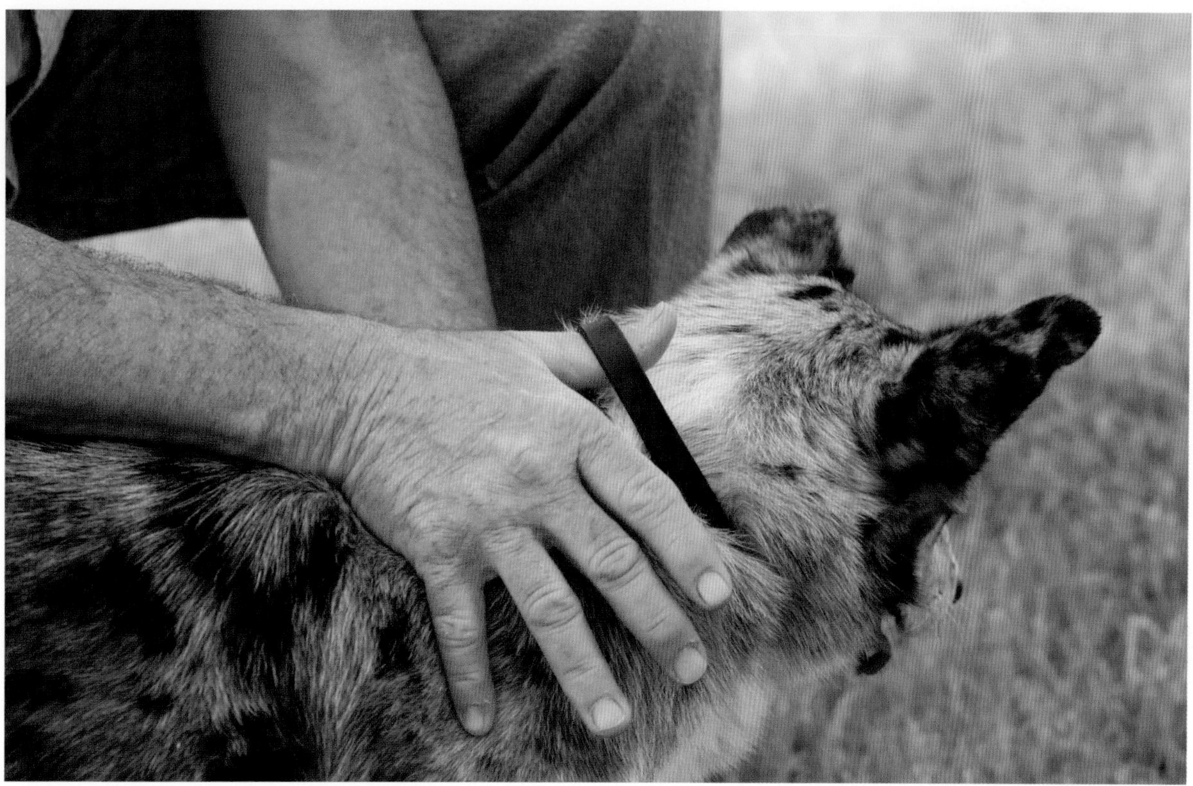

2.2 Holding your thumb under the collar.

under the collar (fig. 2.2). When working on the midsection or hind end, you can have one arm underneath the belly or in front of the hind legs, or you can have someone to help keep your dog "in the neighborhood " (fig. 2.3). If he's comfortable, you can work with the dog on your lap (figs. 2.4 and 2.5).

- Third, you can stop what you're doing, let him settle, then start again in a different area.

If you're paying close enough attention to what your dog is doing, you can often slow down or soften before the dog gets uncomfortable.

Safety Note

Be aware that the dog you are working on may have a serious issue or soreness that you are unaware of, especially if it is a dog new to you (meaning you are new to him), such as a stray or a dog that has come from a rescue situation. We can never be 100 percent sure of a dog's complete history, whether he's been physically or emotionally abused, or if he's experienced an incident or accident or has a health condition that a caring owner is just unaware of. This can impact his level of comfort with the bodywork.

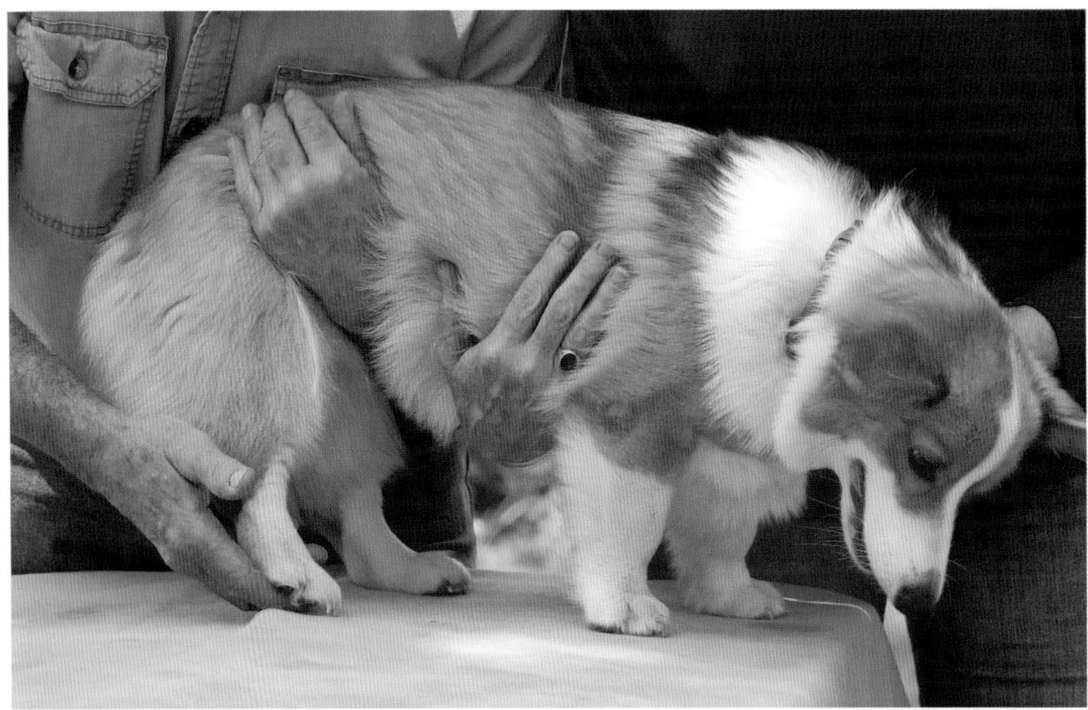

2.3 Having an assistant help.

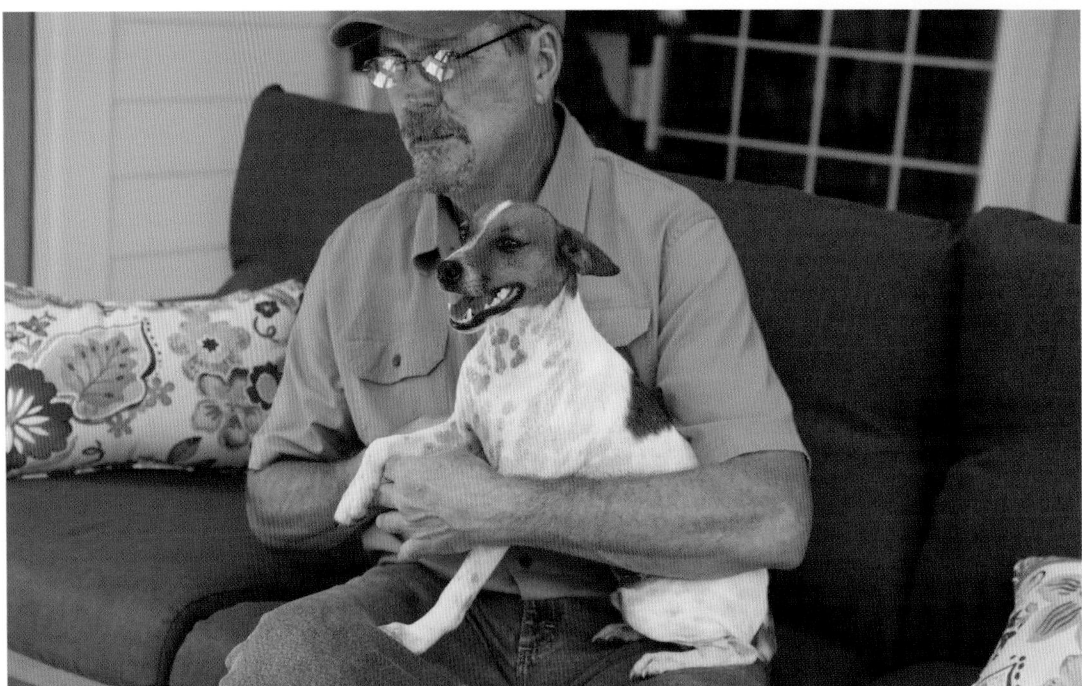

2.4 Working with the dog on your lap.

■ ***What if my dog still wants to walk away?***

Then let him. It's important that you not try to force him to remain if he's uncomfortable, even if you don't think it should be uncomfortable for him. It is counterproductive.

Let him go, and if it's meant to be, he'll come back to you.

Wait…that's a little too much of a cliché. Let's look at this differently: He's your dog. You're his human. He'll come back sooner or later. When he's comfortable, maybe when he's lying down to relax, *that's* your time. Pet him where you normally pet him and start *Searching* there, and don't go immediately where you know he's uncomfortable. Each time you do this he'll get more comfortable with it, especially when he starts feeling the effects of releasing tension he's been holding in. Look at it as a process.

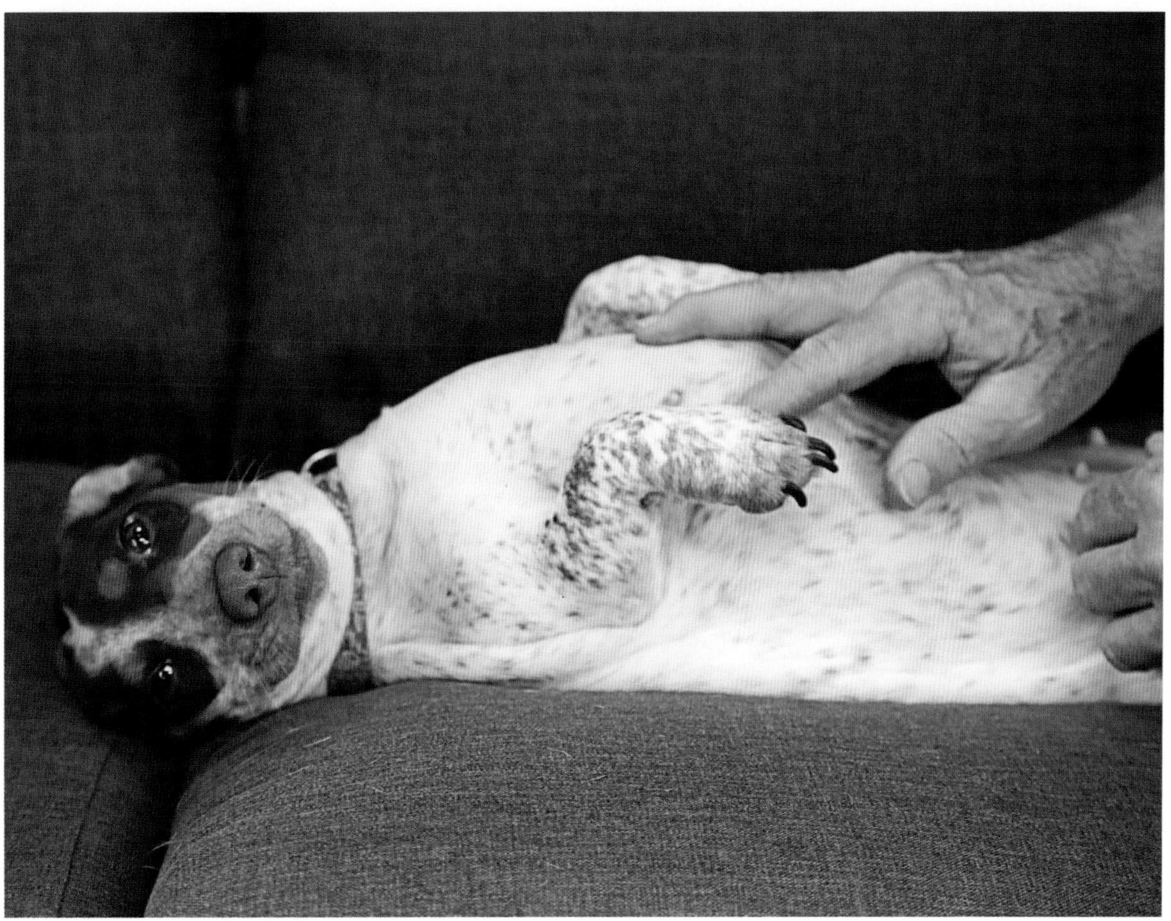

2.5 Work only with soft cuddly dogs who aren't going anywhere!

■ ***What if the opposite happens? What if my dog becomes so relaxed that he flops over or even goes to sleep?***

This can happen, especially when the dog starts releasing deeper tension. When it does, it's still possible to continue *SRSR* on the side that's accessible—as long as your dog doesn't fall asleep. When the dog is "out," he can't respond or show you what's going on. In this case, you'll have to continue later when he's awake. (Besides, he might just need a good nap right about now!)

■ ***What if my dog doesn't give me any responses in general, anywhere?***

Some dogs are very good at blocking out, ignoring, or just not showing any signs of discomfort. Don't take it personally. They're not doing it on purpose. Some dogs are tougher, more independent, or more stoic than others. Others have more hidden physical tension than you might think and are afraid to show it. With these dogs you have to go even slower, lighter, and pay closer attention for even the slightest change in behavior that indicates they're feeling something. These dogs will often become nervous just before or as they *Release*.

There are two more possibilities:

1 You may be too hard, tense, or intense. In this case—*lighten up!*

2 Your dog may not have a lot going on physically. But don't suspect this as a first possibility. Even in day-to-day activity, tension can accumulate in the body.

This is where taking a deep breath and consciously softening yourself internally will help the dog's nervous system to relax. If after 30 seconds or so nothing happens, move on, or let the dog go and see what happens. Often this is where your dog will feel what's released. If so, he might shake his body or start yawning or sneezing. These are signs of a *Release* of tension. If nothing happens, move on to something else.

But remember, if you *Stay* light enough, long enough, the dog's nervous system *has* to let go. It's the law.

Intention

Don't be too strong in your intention that you're going to get a Technique "done." Dogs pick up on your energy and can become confused by your intentions. They can feel threatened if your intention is to "make them sit still so that you can uncover their physical issues." Even if your intention is to help them, if it's too intense it can make them uncomfortable. You have to change your intention from, "I want to find out what's going on so I can help you," to "Let's just sit for a little while," or, "Come sit with me."

What Ifs?—Movement Techniques

■ ***What if my dog doesn't want me to hold his legs?***

It depends on why he's uncomfortable with this.

It may be that it's just not the right time. If he has a lot of energy and wants to move around or play, or if it's close to dinner time, then you have to wait until he's out of energy or finished eating and is more relaxed. Find a time when he's not restless.

If he's still not comfortable, try doing something else that will make him comfortable, then ease into the Technique. If he likes being petted, then pet him—and as you're petting him, slow down and start looking for eye blinks (*SRSR*). And from there, gently slide your hand under his elbow (when doing the forelimb, for example), and search for blinks. And if he remains relaxed, gently move his scapula or foreleg a tiny bit, and soften. Ask again. If you can get him feeling even a little bit of *Release*, then he may stay with you longer. Even if he needs to get up and walk around, he'll come back sooner once he realizes it feels better—or at least that it didn't hurt.

Some dogs may be uncomfortable with this if they've never experienced what you're doing. When you find that this is the case, start with something that's comfortable for them such as being petted, and after the dog has relaxed, sneak in some *SRSR*. You don't have to be in a hurry to get it done at this moment.

■ ***What if at some point while I'm doing a Movement Technique, my dog gets uncomfortable or worried?***

This may be because he's feeling something at that part of the movement. Do the movement slowly enough so you can see or feel signs of discomfort *before* he becomes uncomfortable.

A *visual* response is your dog telling you that you've found something uncomfortable, but he is not yet reacting to it.

A *physical* response is your dog reacting to it by tensing, pulling, or wanting to get away.

How the dog responds will be determined by either the level of discomfort you're finding, or how closely you're paying attention to what the dog is telling you and how quickly you respond to it by softening and yielding.

When you bring the dog's attention to something uncomfortable, the first thing he might do is blink or look around or up at you as he starts to feel something different. Then he might lick your hand or put his mouth to your hand, and finally he might pull his leg away or want to get up and walk away.

When any of these happen, soften and yield. Remove any pressure with your hand while still maintaining very soft contact. If you respond and soften quickly enough, he will relax, release some tension, and it will become comfortable enough for you to continue.

If the dog continues to be uncomfortable, stop, comfort him, and move on to something else. You can come back and do that movement at a later time. If nothing else, you will have just shown your dog that you're paying close attention to what he's telling you and he'll naturally begin to trust you more.

When you come back later, you may find:

- The Technique has released the tension and the dog is comfortable with the movement.
- A Technique you have done elsewhere in the body has helped this to release.
- The Technique has released the tension but the dog is still a little bit distrustful of this movement.
- There is still tension here and the dog is still uncomfortable with it.

When the last is the case, then it could be:

- Something deeper or chronic, and you will have to work on "peeling the layers off."
- Related to something else in the body that needs to be released.
- Something that should be looked at by your veterinarian.

If you find something that is extremely uncomfortable for your dog, don't try to work through it yourself. Ask your veterinarian to check it out. It could need veterinary care.

Bottom line, it's important you don't try to force your dog to stay with you. It's counterproductive. The dog must be relaxed for this to work, and when he's forced to stay, he won't be relaxed. And if he feels trapped, he's not going to want to come back.

Some General Anatomy and Biomechanics

Each chapter in Part Two (p. 33) will have sections on anatomy and biomechanics relevant to the junctions and sections of the dog's body you'll be working with.

Don't be intimidated by the anatomy in this book. You don't have to be an expert in anatomy to get results with this method. The purpose of the anatomy is to give you a vague picture of what you're working on and a general idea of how it all works together, not to give you a headache. More important than memorizing the names of muscles is to have a mental picture of what you're working on and an understanding of some basic biomechanics. Have fun with it.

How Muscles Work

The skeleton is a network of bones connected by *ligaments* and *joints*. Ligaments connect bones to each other to support a joint. They hold structures together and keep them stable. *Tendons* are the sinewy part of the muscles that attach the muscles to the bones. Along with muscles, their function is to move the joint. A *muscle* generally attaches from one bone to another and spans a joint. It does its work by contracting or pulling on the bone. When a muscle contracts, it closes or *flexes* the joint. In order for the joint to open, an opposing muscle must contract to pull it open and *extend* the joint while at the same time, the initial flexing muscle relaxes enough to allow this to happen. The point here is that muscles *flex* and *extend* joints, and they do their work by pulling. A muscle cannot push. It can only contract or pull, and then let go.

While this is a simple description of how the muscles and skeleton work together to create movement, the musculoskeletal system is really a complex network of multi-purpose muscles that work in groups on the skeleton to create coordinated movement in the body.

Muscles accumulate excessive tension through repetitive movement or overexertion. They get tighter and tighter and start to contract more and relax less, which restricts movement and range of motion. The tighter they get, the more resistance the dog encounters and the harder the muscle must work to accomplish a healthy range of motion.

In addition to restricted movement, as muscles get tighter and harder, they lose their flexibility and ability to absorb stress and impact, which leads to muscle, tendon, and ligament injuries and eventually joint injuries and disease.

Releasing tension in muscles keeps them healthy and functioning normally and reduces the risk of damage or injury to them, and consequently, to other parts of the body.

Keeping muscles healthy not only improves movement and flexibility but also helps to maintain the longevity of these structures as well as the comfort and longevity of the dog.

Effects of Unilateral Tension on the Dog's Body

There is an uneven or unilateral effect on the body of repetitive movement and overexertion of muscles. Over time, tension often builds *unilaterally*, meaning more in the muscles on one side than the other.

This unilateral tension can affect straightness in movement but also put uneven pull, or "torque," on key joints or junctions of the body. When joints or junctions become "torqued," it causes other muscles associated with the junction to tighten or spasm. Releasing tension in these key junctions relaxes muscles in other areas of the body.

Balance and Imbalance

When muscles overtighten, they become less effective and less able to do their job. When this happens, other muscles have to work harder in

What Is Fascia?

Fascia used to be a secret. Nowadays everybody who's anybody knows the importance of fascia. "The cat's out of the bag." No, I won't say it. Okay, the *dog's* out of the bag.

Fascia is a thin layer of connective tissue that is woven and wrapped around every muscle fiber, organ, nerve, bone, and other soft tissue in the body. I've heard it described as the "ultimate connective tissue." It's extremely strong yet has an abundance of nerves that make it almost as sensitive as skin.

The importance of fascia, other than that it holds everything together, is that it's a communication system throughout the body. It's through this communication system that the dog can tell you where he's holding tension, and he can release tension when the muscles get the signal back that it's okay to let go. That's how fascia works for us.

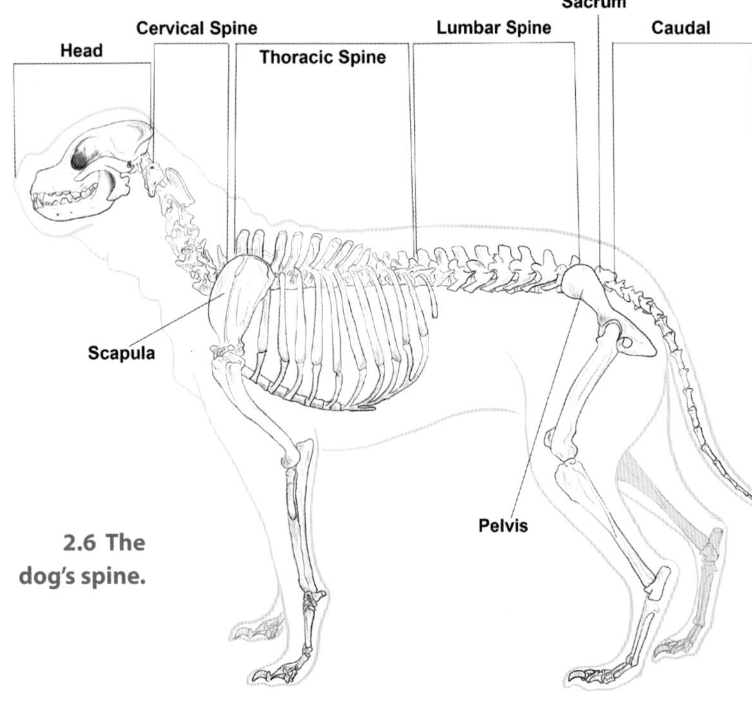

2.6 The dog's spine.

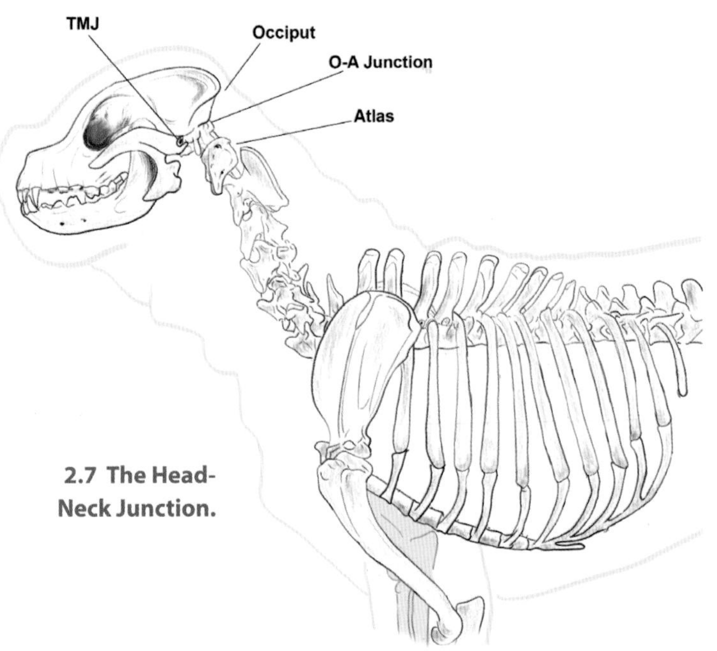

2.7 The Head-Neck Junction.

order for the body to do its job. When muscles are working as they should, the body is working in a balanced way. When they're not—well, it's not.

The Skeleton

Movement Techniques (p. 13) use movement of the skeleton to release tension in the muscles, tendons, and ligaments, which takes tension off the joints. So it's helpful to know a little about the skeleton.

Our focus is on the four sections of the spine, the main parts of the body that attach to the spine, and the junctions where they all come together.

The Spine

The dog's spine is divided into four sections (fig. 2.6):

1 The neck, or *cervical spine,* consists of seven vertebrae (C1 through C7).

2 The trunk, or *thoracic spine,* consists of 13 vertebrae (T1 through T13). The thoracic vertebrae have corresponding ribs attached, which form the rib cage.

3 The lower back, or *lumbar spine,* consists of seven vertebrae (L1 through L7).

4 The *sacrum* consists of three fused vertebrae (S1 though S3).

The tail is also technically part of the spine and varies in length, depending on the dog and the breed.

The Head-Neck Junction

The *Occipital-Atlas* (O–A) Junction is where the back part of the head—*the occiput*—joins with the first vertebra of the neck, C1 (also called the *atlas*). This is an important junction (fig. 2.7).

The C7–T1 Junction and Scapula

The C7–T1 Junction is where the last vertebra of the neck or *cervical spine*—called "C7"—joins with the first vertebra of the trunk or *thoracic spine*—called "T1" (fig. 2.8).

The *scapula*, or shoulder blade, attaches to the neck and trunk at this C7–T1 Junction. More on this to follow.

The *thorax,* or trunk, consists of 13 *thoracic vertebrae* numbered T1 though T13. The thoracic vertebrae have 13 corresponding ribs attached on each side, which are connected on the lower end at the *sternum* (breastbone). This forms the rib cage.

It's interesting to note that there is no joint that attaches the scapula and forelimb to the trunk. The scapula and forelimb are connected to the trunk by a muscular attachment (more on that in Part Two—see p. 72). At the bottom of the scapula is the shoulder joint, into which fits the *humerus* or upper arm on the human.

Lumbosacral-Pelvic Junction

The *lumbar back* (lower back) consists of seven *lumbar vertebrae:* L1 through L7. They do not have ribs, but have wide transverse processes, or wings, to which are attached powerful muscles that drive the hind end, and that support this junction (fig. 2.9).

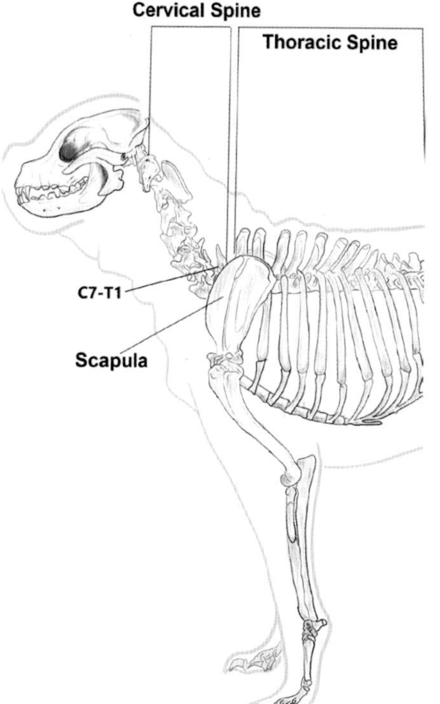

2.8 C7–T1 Junction, scapula, and forelimb.

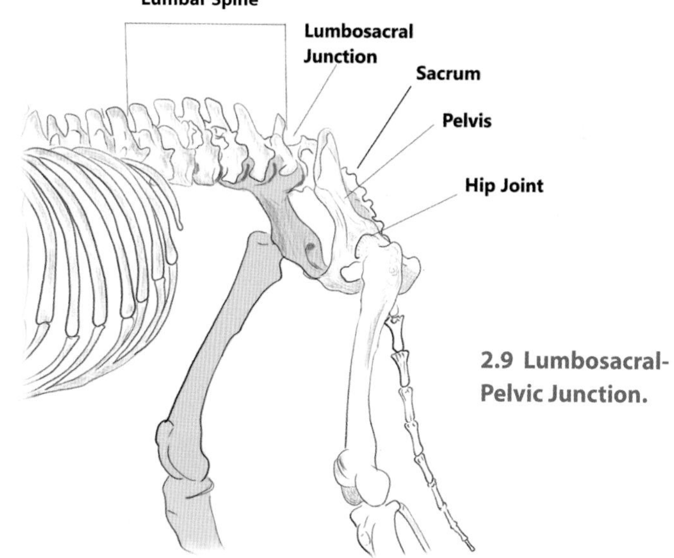

2.9 Lumbosacral-Pelvic Junction.

The *sacrum* consists of three vertebrae that are fused into one bone. It is triangle-shaped, with the point of the triangle pointing to the tail, and the base of the triangle positioned forward, toward the lumbar spine.

The *Lumbosacral Junction* is where the last lumbar vertebra (L7) joins the front of the sacrum.

The *pelvis* is a large structure attached to the hind limbs, as well as many of the muscles that drive the dog forward. The hind limbs attach to the pelvis at the hip joint, which is a ball-and-socket joint. The pelvis is also the structure that connects the hind end of the dog to the spinal column. It does this via the *sacroiliac joint.*

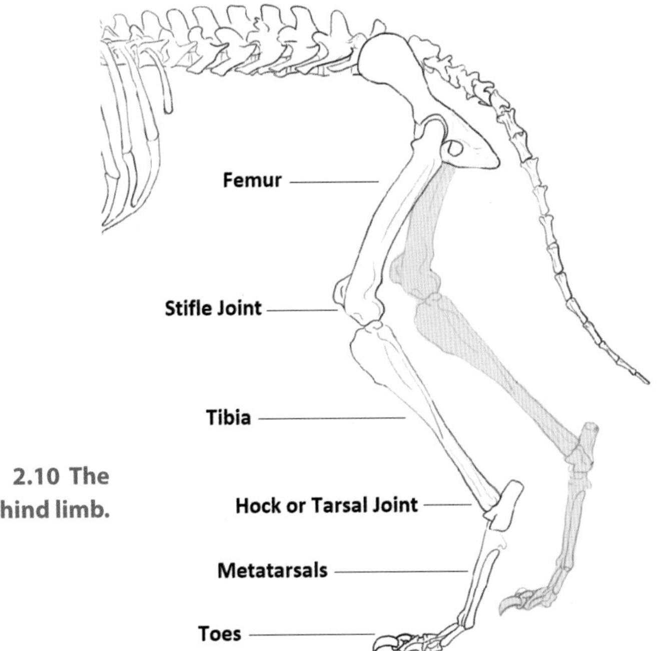

2.10 The hind limb.

It is at this *Lumbosacral-Pelvic Junction* that all the driving forces of the muscles of the hind end transfer into the body.

The Hind Limb

The *hip joint* is a ball-and-socket type of joint that connects the head of the femur or thigh bone to the pelvis. This is known amongst people who know Latin as the *coxofemoral* joint. It is an important junction through which a lot of force is transferred from the hind limbs to the body (fig. 2.10). The next bone of the leg after the *femur* is the *tibia,* which would be our lower leg. The joint between them is called the knee in humans, or the *stifle* in dogs. The stifle is complex in that it has a sliding bone, the *patella,* and *patellar* and *cruciate ligaments* that hold it all together.

At the lower end of the *tibia,* the next joint is called the *hock*, or *tarsal joint.* That "pointy" part of the hock facing backward is called the *calcaneus.* The hock is equivalent to our ankle, except in the dog it's a lot more mobile and more involved in propelling the dog forward.

Below the hock, between the hock and the paw, are the four *metatarsal* bones. *Meta* = "beyond." *Tarsal* = "hock." *Metatarsal* = "beyond the hock." (See, you're "speaking" Latin already!) The metatarsals would be the four bones of our foot leading to our toes, or *phalangeal* bones, which constitute the toes of the dog's paw.

You'll read more about the limbs, how they attach to the body, and the muscles that make them work in Part Two.

PART TWO

Using The Masterson Method Techniques

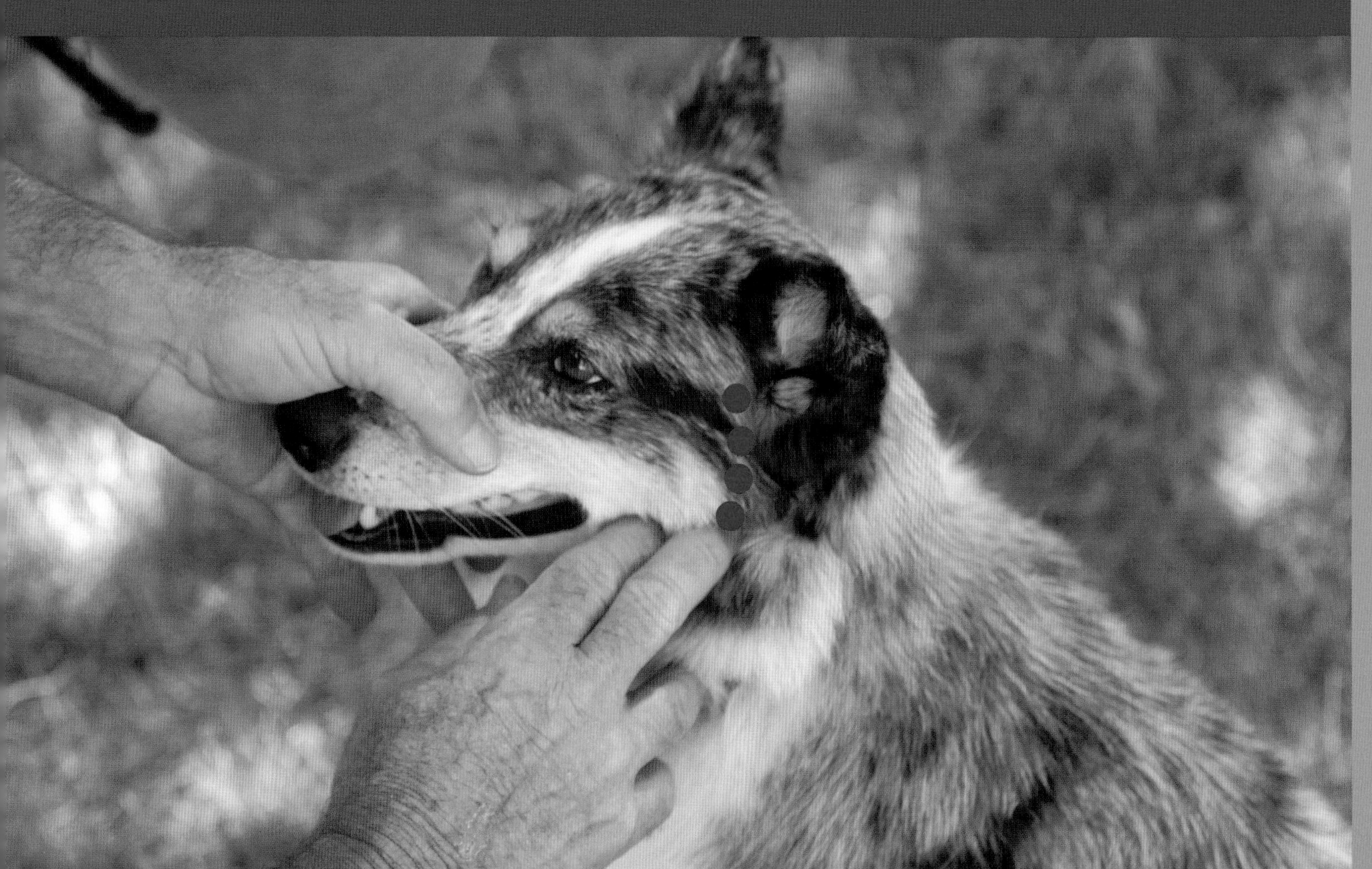

3

CHAPTER 3

The Bladder Meridian Technique

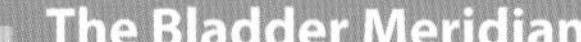

■ The Bladder Meridian

Before You Begin

GOAL: To apply *Search, Response, Stay, Release (SRSR)* to the dog's Bladder Meridian.

RESULT:

- Establishes the connection and basis of communication between you and your dog.
- Relaxes both you and your dog, setting the tone for the interaction.
- Helps you identify areas of the body where your dog may be holding tension.
- Helps the dog's nervous system to start releasing the tension.

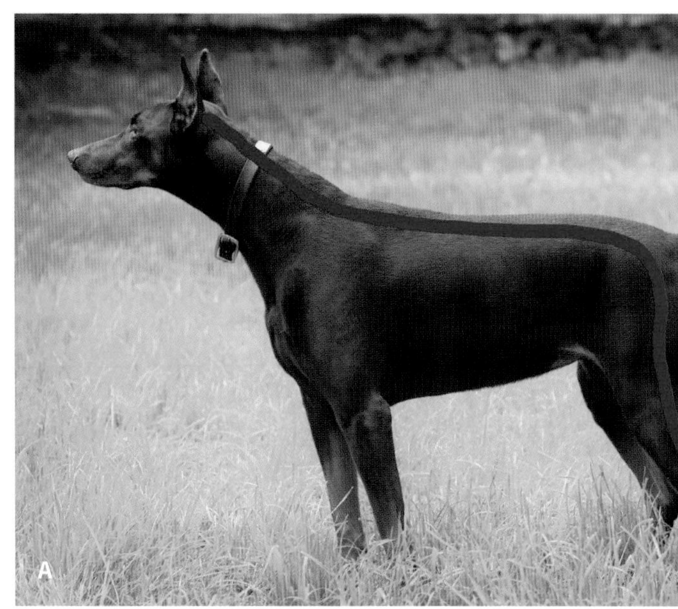

A

More Anatomy and the Effects of Releasing Tension

In Traditional Chinese Medicine, there are 12 primary *meridians*, or energy pathways, on each side of the body. The *Bladder Meridian* is the one we focus on.

There are many reasons to work on the Bladder Meridian with your dog.

- It is one of the major meridians in that it has a unique effect on balancing the entire meridian system.
- It has a calming effect on both you and your dog, preparing him for the bodywork exercise that follows.
- It establishes a basis for communication between you and your dog, giving you a sense of how your

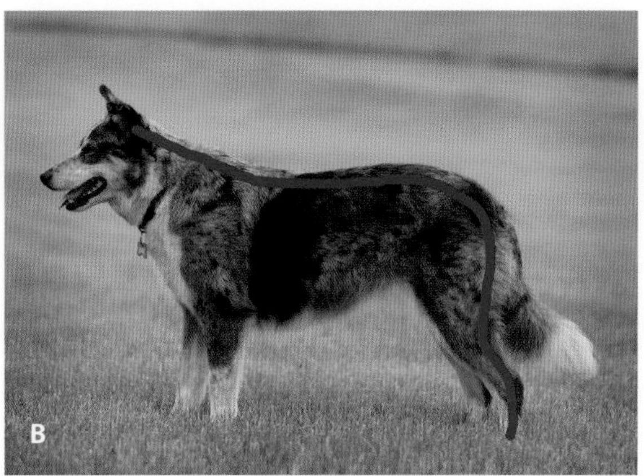

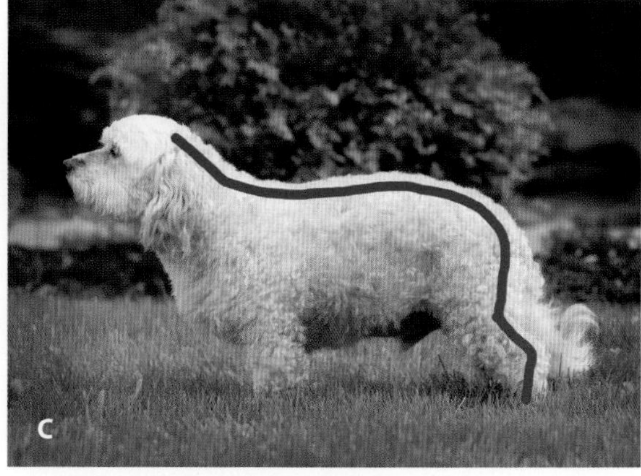

3.1 A–D **The Bladder Meridian.**

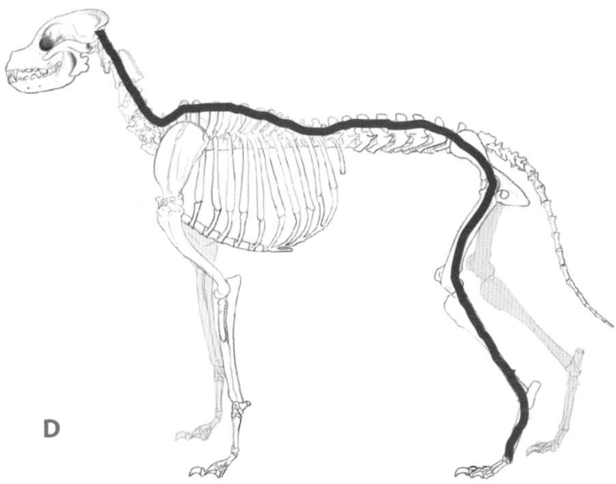

dog is going to respond to your touch, and showing him what he can expect from this interaction with you. His nervous system learns to respond to your touch in a way that bypasses his survival or defense response.

- It lets you know where your dog is blocking out tension or discomfort and allows his nervous system to begin releasing the tension associated with the discomfort.

WHERE YOU WORK

There is a Bladder Meridian on each side of the dog's body (see figs. 3.1 A–D on pp. 34–35).). Each begins just behind the eye and runs between the bump at the top of the head and the ear. From there it continues down the top of the neck on each side of the spine, along the back on each side of the spine until it reaches the tail. Then it follows the outside edge of the hind leg, along the side of the hock, terminating on the outside toe of each hind paw.

Tips

Rule 1: *Go softly*. Use *Air Gap* pressure (non-pressure), keeping your hand soft, and your arm and shoulder relaxed, with the flat of your fingertip or fingertips barely touching the hair or skin. Run them slowly along the meridian, watching the dog's subtle responses to your touch.

Quick Overview: Step-by-Step

SRSR ON THE BLADDER MERIDIAN

Before you start, breathe, and consciously relax and soften your neck, shoulders, arms, and hands. It doesn't matter on which side you start. It's best to begin at the head so you can keep track of where your dog might be holding tension, but it's effective no matter where on the Bladder Meridian you start.

With Nellie (see below), I sit on the dog's left side and start behind the right ear. You'll notice I'm *Searching* with the right hand, using the other hand to gently keep the dog with me.

SEARCH

Step 1. Sit in a comfortable position with your dog (fig. 3.2 A).

Step 2. Place the tips of one or two fingers together (keeping your arm and hand soft) above the ear on one side (fig. 3.2 B). Lighten your fingers to the level of *Air Gap* (p. 7).

Step 3. Keeping your fingers at *Air Gap* and watching the dog's eye, gently and slowly run your fingers down the Bladder Meridian. Go at a pace that's slow enough so you don't miss a *Response* from the dog, but not so slow that the dog is not paying attention.

RESPONSE

Step 4. Watch for a *Response*—a subtle change in behavior such as a *blink* that indicates the dog is feeling something (fig. 3.2 C). When you get a *Response*…

STAY

Step 5. Stop and rest your fingers over that spot, keeping your hand soft and the pressure light, waiting for a *Release* (fig. 3.2 D). This may take one second or one minute. Be patient, breathe, and relax until you get…

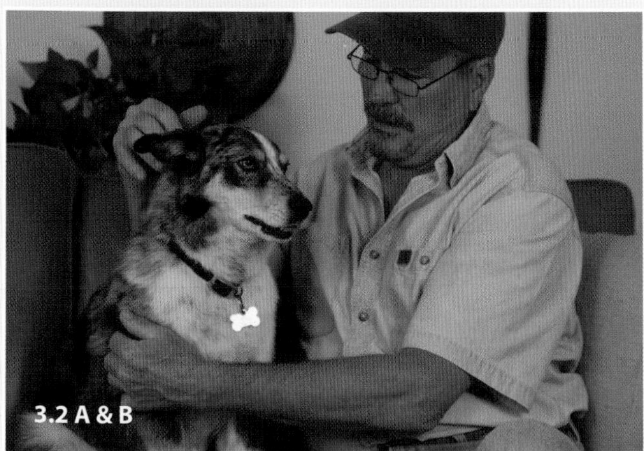

3.2 A & B

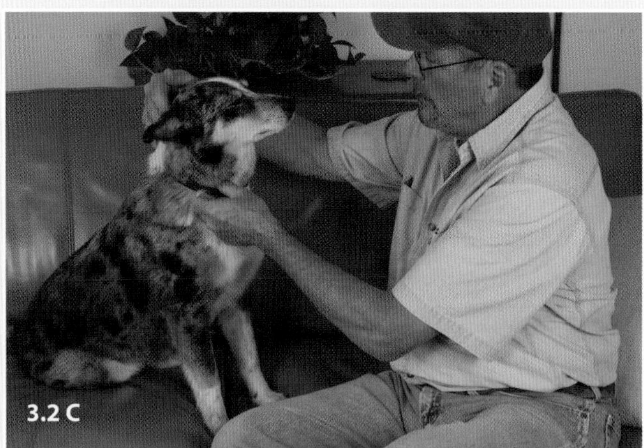

3.2 C

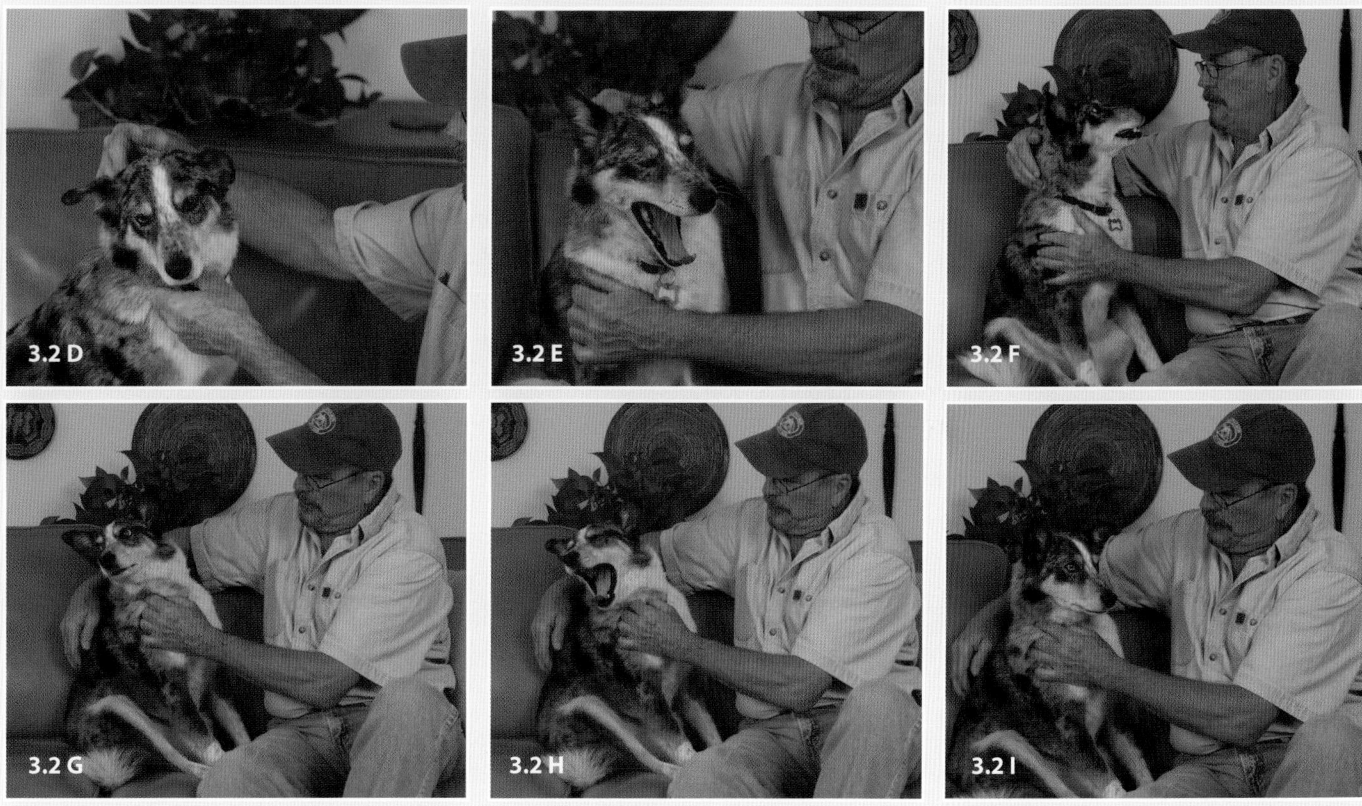
3.2 D 3.2 E 3.2 F 3.2 G 3.2 H 3.2 I

RELEASE

Step 6. A *Release* is a larger *Response*, such as licking and chewing, sneezing, yawning, or fussing, fidgeting, or wanting to step away (fig. 3.2 E).

Step 7. After you get a *Release* (or not) continue slowly (I said, *slowly!)* down the meridian, searching for responses down the side of the neck, over the shoulder and along the back (fig. 3.2 F)…

Step 8. …until you get another *Response* or change in behavior, such as a blink, or the dog looking away (fig. 3.2 G)…

Step 9. *Stay* until you get a *Release* (fig. 3.2 H).

Step 10. Continue over the rump, down the back side of the leg, down the outside of the hock, down the side of the ankle, and to the outside toe (fig. 3.2 I). Each time you get a *Response, Stay* until you get a *Release* (or not), then move on. When you are finished, give your dog a short break to feel any changes. If your dog is still awake, repeat on the other side.

Rule 2: *Go slowly*. Forget about the clock when doing this exercise. If you are anticipatory or anxious, the dog will sense it. Take a deep breath and move your hand very slowly along the meridian, watching for subtle responses in his eyes, movement of the ears, or fidgeting.

Rule 3: *Pay attention to what your dog is telling you.* Watch the eye or body for a *Response*. The main thing to look for is the eye to blink; however, every dog is different. Some are stoic and may only give a tiny blink or movement of the ear or head. Others are more trusting and sensitive. They may give a clear blink or multiple blinks as you go over a spot under which he is feeling something. Some may become nervous and look around at you or away from you when you find something, or even look surprised. A *Response* is any shift in behavior that indicates the dog feels something under your finger.

When you get a *Response*, stop moving your hand and rest it there (remaining at *Air Gap* pressure), and wait for a larger *Release Response* (see p. 11). Note that the dog may look away or become anxious as he feels tension letting go. This is usually followed by some sign of relief or relaxation. Any larger change in behavior indicates a *Release*. Once the dog shows a *Release Response*, move on to the next blink.

Staying can be the easiest (or hardest) part of the process. It can take 10 seconds, or it may take a whole minute. Throw away the clock and any expectations you have. Just wait and give the dog a chance to feel what's going on. *Stay* until you get a *Release*—or not. Stop and hold your hand on a spot at any time if you sense that staying there might bring a *Release*. If it doesn't, move on.

You can start over, or in a different place. You can switch hands, use both hands, stop and begin again, or retrace and go back over an area or spot. If you only get part of the meridian done, or only one

Reminder

A *Response* is any shift in behavior that correlates with what you are doing with your hand. *Responses* indicate that the dog is feeling something under your finger as you *Search* and can include:

- An eyelid blink or gentle "squint."
- An ear twitch or movement.
- A movement of the head.
- A change in breathing.
- A fidget.

Release Responses indicate a release of tension and include:

- Licking and chewing.
- Sighing or letting out a breath.
- Yawning.
- Sneezing.
- Lying down or flopping over. (Don't panic! He's just relaxing!)
- Shaking the head or whole body.
- Any type of fidget, such as looking away or at you (with a curious or worried look), fussing in any way, wanting to move or walk away, or reaching around and scratching or chewing.

side, don't worry. As said earlier, your dog won't go round in circles for the rest of his life if you only get one side done.

You may softly adjust the level of pressure (no more than *Egg Yolk* (p. 8), change fingertips or hands, or slow down as you get *Responses*. Don't worry that you aren't doing it "right." If you're not using pressure and you're being patient, you can't do it wrong. You can only do it *better*. And don't be concerned that you might hurt your dog. If you're not using pressure, you can't hurt your dog. As a matter of fact, if you're worrying about anything, it only causes your dog to worry. So don't worry—be happy!

Note: If you practiced nothing else but the Bladder Meridian Technique on your dog on a regular basis, it would make a noticeable difference in his comfort, behavior, and relationship with you.

What Ifs?

- ***What if I'm not exactly on the Bladder Meridian line or on the right point?***

Don't be too concerned about being on the exact location of a point. Your dog will tell you where it is. Not all points are in exactly the same place on all dogs, and not all dogs have the same thing going on. Just *Search* in the area of the points and your dog will tell you where to *Stay*. (You may have to get used to your dog telling you what to do, but once you get over that, everything will be fine.)

How Slow is "Slow"?

As you watch the dog's eyes, you will start to notice that there is a certain speed at which he stays tuned in or connected to your fingers. Too fast, and you leave the dog behind; too slow, and the dog gets bored and stops "listening."

To give you an idea of how fast or slow you should be running your hand down the meridian, use the back of your hand, and the "One crocodile, two crocodile, three crocodile" technique:

- Hold your left hand in front of you with the palm of your hand facing you.
- Place one fingertip of your right hand lightly on your wrist, barely touching the skin (might as well start practicing *Air Gap* now).
- Move your fingertip slowly from your wrist to the fingertips of your left hand, counting "One crocodile, two crocodile, three crocodile..." It should take six to eight "crocodiles" to get from your wrist to your fingertips. This is about the speed you should move your hand along the dog's bladder meridian. (If you have large or long hands, do eight crocodiles, with smaller hands, do six.)

Note: If the thought of crocodiles bothers you, you may substitute "doggy treat."

It's always an experiment. You're *Searching* areas of your dog's body, paying attention, and waiting to see what will happen. When you find something, your dog may show you *Release Responses* quickly, or not so quickly, or not at all. If not, move on to the next place or point. The dog may not have had anything there to release, or he released and chose not to tell you about it yet. He may show you a little farther on. Don't have an agenda or any set expectations, or your dog may sense it and brace internally.

If your dog gets uncomfortable with what you're finding and wants to walk away, you can soften or stop *Searching* and ask him to stick around a little longer, but if you make him stay and he's uncomfortable, then the part of the dog's nervous system that blocks out tension will take over, and the part that releases tension will not work. There's an "old" saying, "You can lead a dog to *Responses* but you can't make him *Release*…"

- ***What if I get a Response and Stay, then don't get a Release?***

First of all, be patient and allow the dog time to feel what is going on and time to be comfortable releasing. You are following your dog's agenda, not yours.

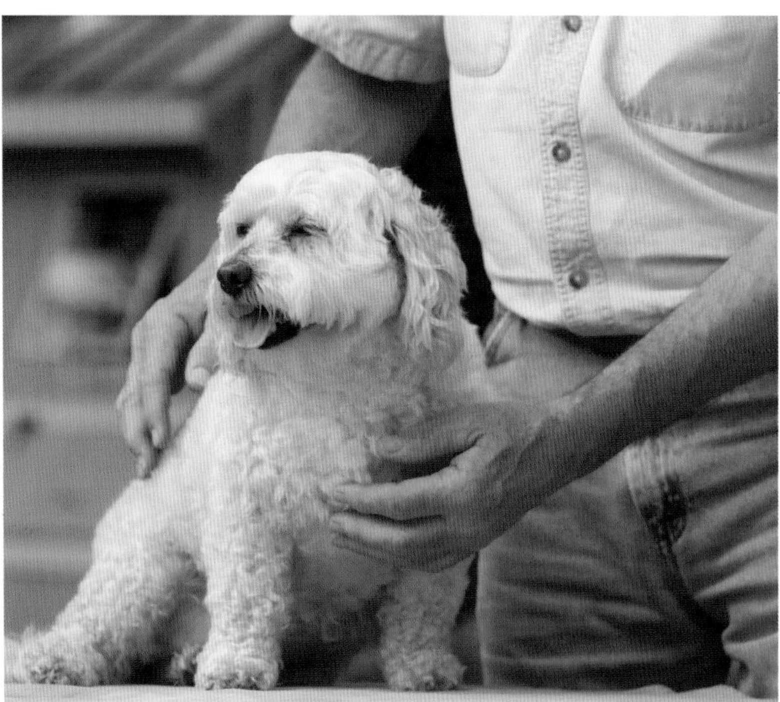

Less Is More

If some of this seems counter-intuitive to you, it is. The less pressure you use, the deeper the dog feels it, and the more you get done. This lightness is what allows the dog to participate in the process. *Less is more.*

3.3 Use as little pressure as possible.

Not all dogs respond alike, especially at first when they're not sure what you're up to. The more you do this, the more the dog will become comfortable with it. Stoic or worried dogs will often hold in the visual signs of *Release*—that is, they *Release* but don't "tell" you. As *Releases* accumulate, the dog will sometimes let them out all at once when your hand gets farther down the body.

Some dogs—especially at first—won't show signs of *Release* at all until after you stop, or step back, or he walks away from you. Some are more expressive and trusting; some are more stoic. With the stoic dogs, you may have to watch for more subtle *Responses* and give them more time.

Second, keep your hand soft. If you feel nothing is happening, try softening your hand more, or even taking your fingertips slightly off the hair. Watch your dog's eyes as you do this. If you see them soften, it means you should go lighter. No matter how light you think your pressure is, lighten it even more.

- ***What if nothing is happening? How long should I wait on a point or spot?***

If after 20 or 30 seconds your dog doesn't respond, move on. It doesn't mean you're doing it wrong, or your dog isn't cooperating. It could be he's not yet ready to release the tension here; or he's released it and isn't telling you yet. Dogs respond differently.

Move on, possibly returning to this spot later.

When in Doubt, Go Softer

If you *Stay* long enough and light enough, the dog's nervous system will have to release tension. It's the law!

- ***What if I can't tell if my dog is blinking at something else, or in response to what I'm doing?***

If you're not sure your dog has blinked at a spot in response to your touch, move your finger a few inches back and slowly go over that spot again. If he blinks on the same spot, there is a correlation between what you're doing and what the dog is doing.

Dogs lick, chew, yawn, blink, and fidget all the time. With this exercise, you are looking for the correlation between your touch and your dog's behavior or response to it. This is where the communication starts.

- ***What if my dog starts to fuss or wants to walk away?***

If the dog has been sitting quietly and you've been *Searching* and found something, and after *Staying* for a few seconds, the dog wants to move or walk away, the first thing to do is soften your hand, even backing your fingers away just a little bit so that you're not even touching the hair.

When he relaxes, you can continue with what you were doing. If you soften a little, it may make him comfortable enough to stay with you. When in doubt, go softer.

If he's still fussy, you can gently reassure him or ask him to stay with you, but don't force the dog to stay if he doesn't want to. When he needs to move away, let him. When he feels trapped at all, this method won't work.

If he shows signs that he's uncomfortable every time you go over a specific area, skip that area, and come back to it later. You might find the next day that there's some improvement and he's better with it.

Often, the dog wants to move away because he's feeling tension releasing and it's a little uncomfortable or unfamiliar. By this time, however, the *Release* has often already happened. If you let him go and give him a minute or two, he'll often be more comfortable and come back for more if you ask him—or even on his own, if you give him the space. This is something you do *with* the dog, not *to* the dog.

Feeling the tension is part of the process of releasing it. Picture Dr. Phil in your mind saying, "You've got to feel it to heal it!" He's right. (Now you can let that picture go!)

Bodywork vs. Training

It's important to get out of "training mode" while doing bodywork with the dog. You're asking the dog to feel things that he may not have been feeling for a while, and you're asking him to let you know through changes in behavior. Things that you might not consider "good" behavior—such as walking away when you want him to stay next to you—are good when you consider that you're asking the dog to "tell" you what he's feeling.

In other words, it's not fair to ask the dog to tell you what he's feeling, then correct him when he tells you.

Points and Meridians

The locations of acupressure points and meridians on the dog's body are not exact and differ with each body. This is only a general guide to the Bladder Meridian. As you aren't giving an actual acupressure treatment, don't worry that you may not be precisely on the line of the Bladder Meridian. Follow the described path and let your intuition and the dog's *Responses* guide you. There are many books available on canine acupressure for those interested in learning more. You'll now have the added benefit of visual responses from your dog on where and how long to stay on different points!

- ***What if I only work with the Bladder Meridian? How often can I do it?***

You can do a little bit every day if your dog continues to respond. You don't need to do the whole meridian every time. If you do it too frequently or for too long and the dog stops responding, give him a few days off and start up again later. It takes the nervous system time to process changes.

Usually, when you do too much, the dog will stop responding or will go to sleep, in which case he's not feeling anything and it's not working. He's got to feel it for his nervous system to release it.

- ***What if I'm not right on the meridian? Will it still work?***

Don't worry about being exactly on the meridian. The Bladder Meridian is an energy pathway and doesn't run in precisely the same place on every dog. The dog will tell you where to work. Part of this is learning to follow his responses.

Search, Response, Stay, Release can be used to find and release tension anywhere on your dog's body. The Bladder Meridian provides a place for you to start and a path for you to follow.

- ***What if I have more than one dog? Will they all respond the same?***

After doing different dogs, you will notice that all respond differently. Depending on the dog, his sensitivity, and your sensitivity, the length of time you are able to spend doing a Technique can vary.

Dogs and Horses

When I first started trying the Masterson Method with my dogs, I realized it was working with them as well as it did with horses. I was also getting feedback from other people who had taken our *Beyond Horse Massage* courses and were using it on their dogs—and getting good results.

To get a little more experience, I went to a local animal rescue and asked to practice on the dogs there. I was led to a fairly large room, empty except for some cabinets and a chair. A very excited dog was brought in from the kennel. He bounced around the room (and me), smelling a million things and completely uninterested in sitting and relaxing.

Eventually, he calmed down a little and was able to stand next to me and be petted for short periods of time before bouncing around again. I started *Searching* and finding "blinks" in areas around his neck and back. He then ran off to sniff around before coming back for a minute, when I *Searched* more and *Stayed* on these spots for a little longer. Pretty soon the dog was with me more and running off less. Eventually he sat, paid attention, and then licked and yawned. Soon he lay down next to me, and I was able to do more.

When I figured he'd had enough, I went to the office to ask about coming back to the shelter later to do more. I looked down to see the dog standing quietly by my leg. The staff commented that he looked "a little different."

Dogs can be a little more animated working with humans than horses are. I realized there can be a little more to the process of getting a dog you don't know to settle down and relax and "be there." You can allow for the time needed to get him through the process of relaxing with you, or you can take the opportunity to work with him when he's already in a relaxed state. The latter might be easier, but to be honest, I found this experience at the rescue to be a little more rewarding.

Case Study

HOW TO HANDLE FIDGETING

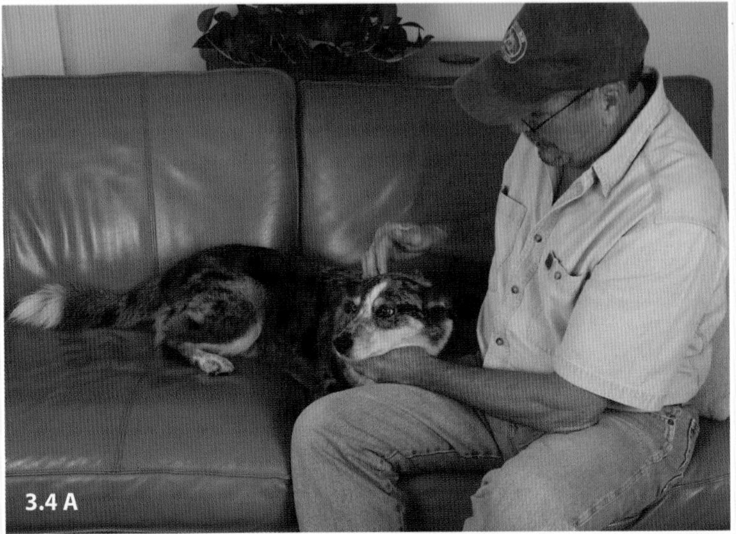
3.4 A

Sometimes work on the Bladder Meridian goes easily, but sometimes the dog can become uncomfortable with the process of feeling and releasing tension and gets a little fussy.

The dog used in the step-by-step instructions in this chapter is my dog Nellie. See how good she was in the photos (see pp. 36–37)? Actually, Nellie is a pretty fidgety girl. To give you an idea of how it can go, I'll show you how our Bladder Meridian session *really* went.

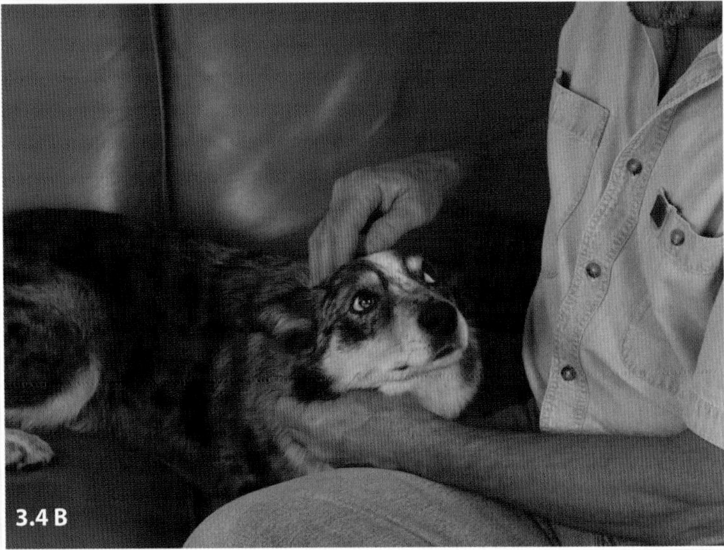
3.4 B

SEARCH AND RESPONSE

I started *Searching* while she was lying down (fig. 3.4 A) and found a *Response* (fig. 3.4 B).

She immediately became fidgety and wanted to sit up. I let her up but asked her to remain with me, gently holding her collar (fig. 3.4 C).

She fidgeted more and wanted to turn away, so I softened my hands even more, and she *Released* (figs. 3.4 D & E).

I continued down the meridian and found another *Response* and *Stayed* (fig. 3.4 F).

After a few seconds, she said, "I'm a little uncomfortable with this, Dad." Well, I made that up, but I softened my hands and was able to gently keep her with me a little longer (fig. 3.4 G)…and she *Released* (fig. 3.4 H).

I stayed soft with her and continued down the Bladder Meridian line. The rest of the session went like this: down…over…twist…stay soft…even softer…and she ends up like this (figs. 3.4 I–N).

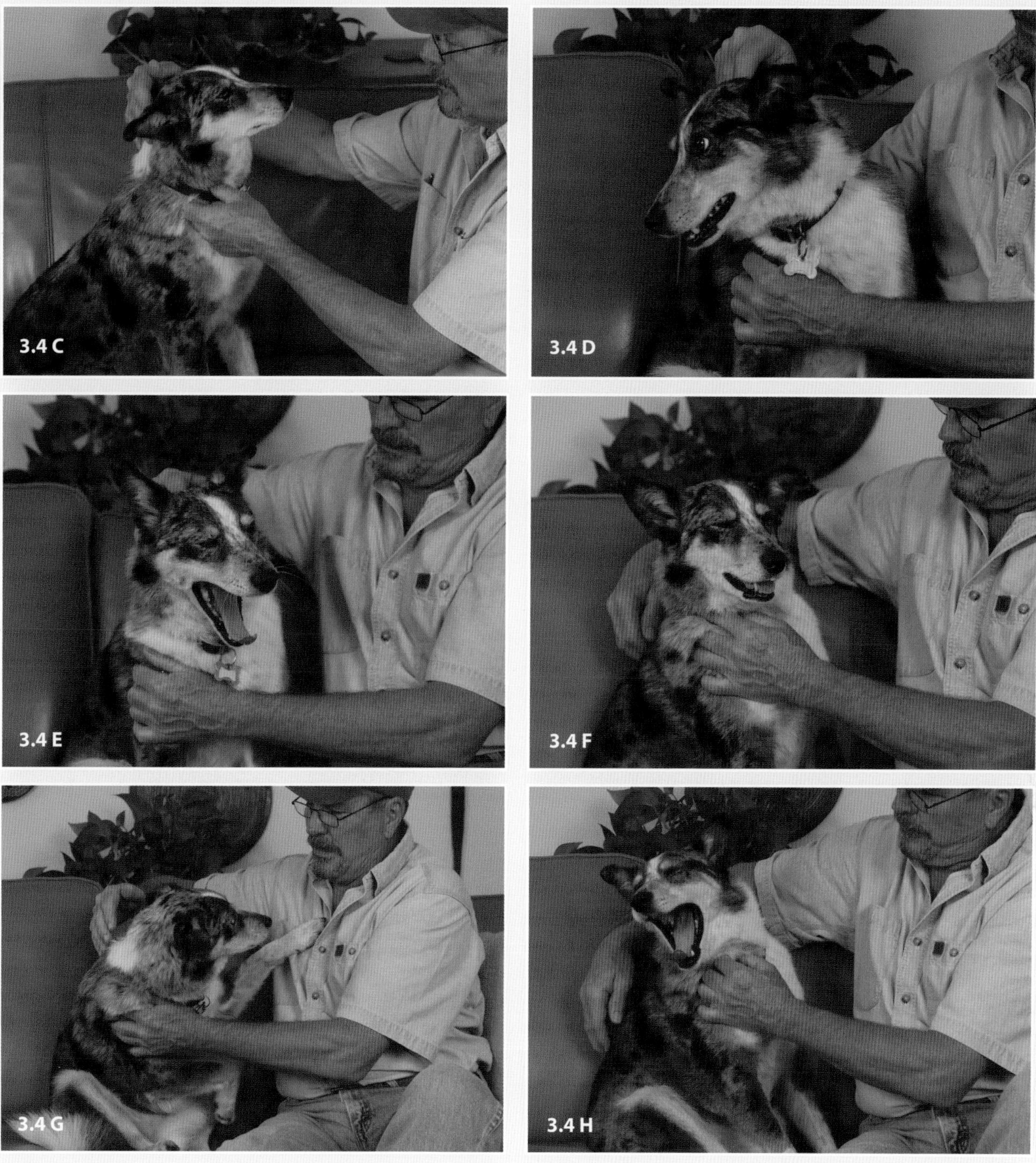

3.4 C

3.4 D

3.4 E

3.4 F

3.4 G

3.4 H

HOW TO HANDLE FIDGETING (continued)

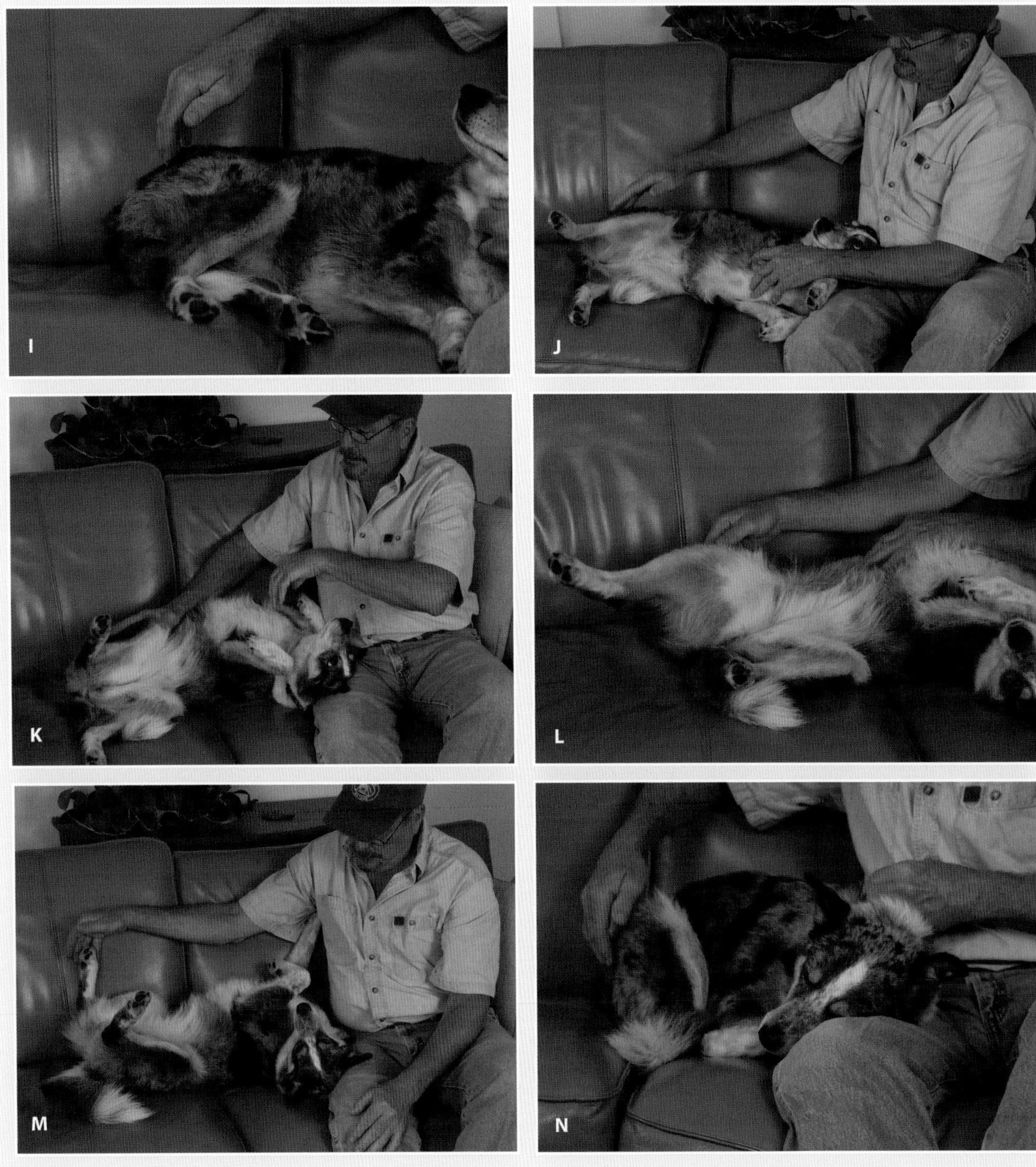

Some are very stoic and take longer to give you a *Response* and *Release*. With these dogs you have to go slower and lighter and pay very close attention to see the subtlest *Responses*. Some are more worried and can show *Responses* in an area but won't *Release* until you move past the area, or until you're done working and step away from them. Some you can only do for short periods of time.

You want to help the dog release tension, but you need to listen to the dog and do it in a way that is the most comfortable for him.

FROM THE VET

Use of the Bladder Meridian in Chinese Medicine

The Bladder Meridian in Traditional Chinese Veterinary Medicine is used very commonly when doing acupuncture in dogs. Many of the acupuncture points along the back section of the Bladder Meridian are Shu points or association points for organs of the body or other parts of the body. The Bladder Meridian points are also used as local points for dogs with Intervertebral Disc Disease (IVDD) or disc problems in the back, and are good to use for any back pain. Most dogs are cooperative about acupuncture along the back.

—*Dr. Robinett*

To Sum Up

It helps to have in mind that any change in your dog's behavior (*Response*) is due to a sensation brought about by bringing his awareness (in a gentle way) to something he has been covering up for survival reasons. Remember, "He's got to feel it to heal it." (There goes Dr. Phil again!)

If you feel there's a chance that a *Response* is connected to what you are doing and the dog is feeling, then *Stay* with it and see what happens. The more you practice, the better you become at this. Be open to trusting that it's working. This creates an opening for it to happen.

Search, Response, Stay, Release is always an experiment. You're *Searching* to see what your dog has to say and waiting to see what his body will do. Don't let expectations, impatience, or doubt get in the way. Doubt the doubt.

4

CHAPTER 4

The Head-Neck (Occiput-Atlas) Junction

This chapter discusses the various areas of the Head-Neck (Occiput-Atlas) Junction that accumulate tension, and offers exercises to release tension in these areas using the three categories of Techniques that I outlined in Part One:

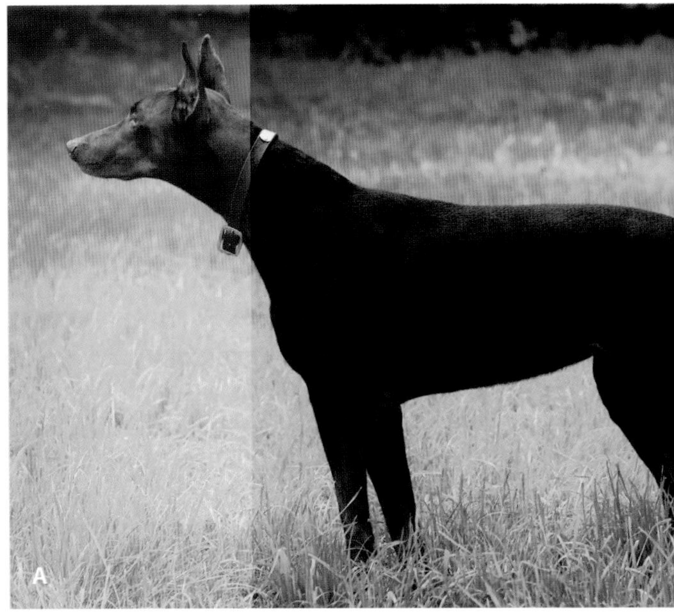

A

Search, Response, Stay, Release (SRSR), page 4; *Movement Techniques*, page 5; *Hold, Wait, and Melt Techniques (HWM)*, page 6.

Search, Response, Stay, Release

TMJ Point, Jawline Groove Points, Occiput-Atlas (O-A) Junction Points

GOAL: To apply the process of *Search, Response, Stay, Release* (SRSR) to the muscles, tendons, and ligaments of the TMJ, the jawline, and the O-A Junction. (To begin these techniques, see p. 54.)

RESULT: Releasing tension in the connective tissue of this junction not only affects this junction

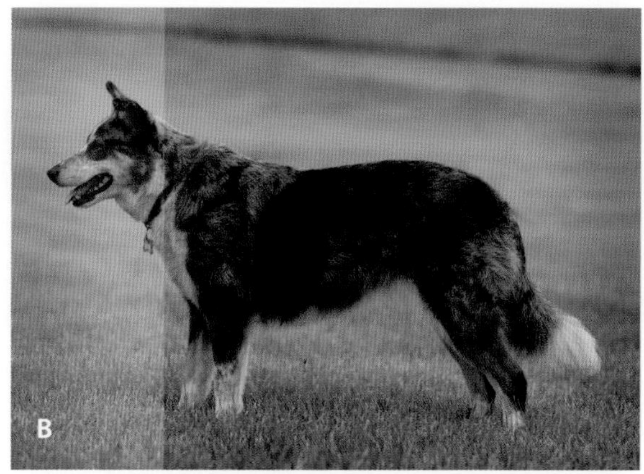

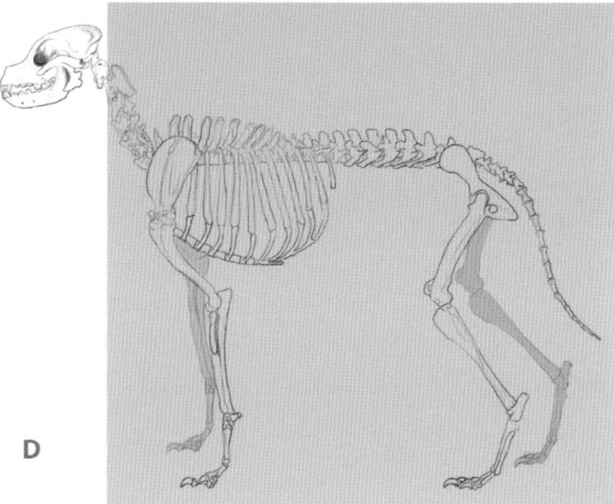

but also is connected to tension in the neck, forelimbs, and hind end.

Movement Techniques

Head Up (Occiput-Atlas) Release

GOAL: To get the dog to relax the weight of his head in your hand and ask for gentle movement of the O-A Junction in a relaxed state. (To begin these techniques, see p. 58.)

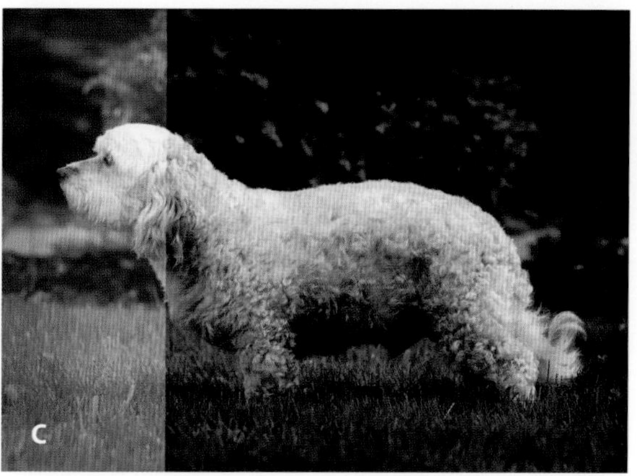

4.1 A–D The Head-Neck (Occiput-Atlas) Junction.

RESULT: Releases tension in the muscles and connective tissues of the O-A Junction, improving movement and suppleness in the junction and neck. Releasing tension in this junction also has a relaxing effect on the entire body.

Jawline Groove and Lateral Cervical Microflexion

GOAL: To apply gentle pressure and ask for movement in the muscles, tendons, and ligaments between the head, neck, and jaw while they are in a relaxed state. Remember, it's not the amount of movement that releases the tension, it's the amount of relaxation.

RESULT: This process releases tension and improves movement in the jaw and TMJ, the occiput and atlas, and the muscles and connective tissue of the cervical vertebrae of the neck.

Hold, Wait, and Melt Techniques

Hyoid Release

GOAL: To apply the process of *Hold, Wait, and Melt* to the muscles and connective tissues of the hyoid apparatus. (To begin these techniques, see p. 64.)

RESULT: The hyoid is related to tension in the jaw, TMJ, O-A Junction, and the neck and forelimbs. Releasing tension in the hyoid helps to release tension in these other areas as well.

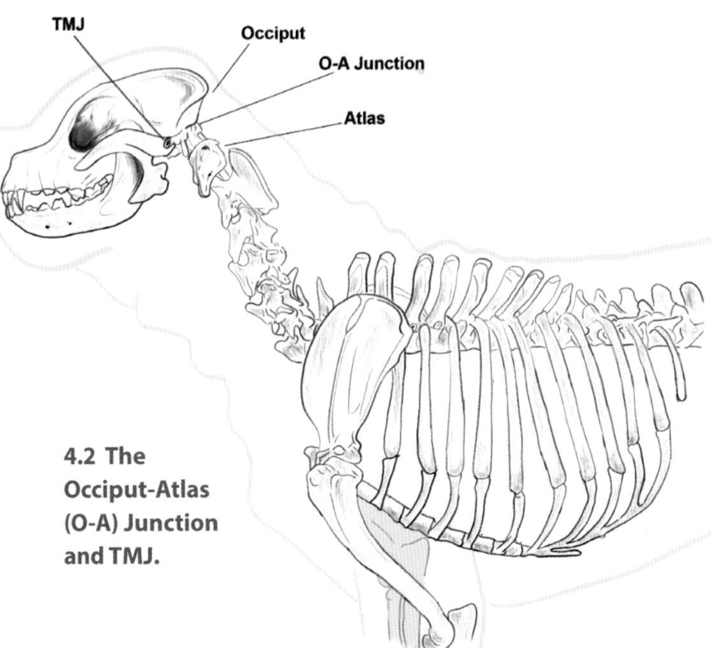

4.2 The Occiput-Atlas (O-A) Junction and TMJ.

> **FROM THE VET**
>
> ### How Many Vertebrae in a Neck?
>
> All mammals have seven cervical vertebrae, except manatees that have six, two-toed sloths with five to seven, and three-toed sloths that have eight to nine. Giraffes have only seven cervical vertebrae, but they're larger.
>
> Birds, amphibians, and reptiles have variable numbers of cervical vertebrae depending on the species. The number of thoracic, lumbar, sacral, and caudal vertebrae is variable among mammals.
>
> —*Dr. Robinett*

More Anatomy and the Effects of Releasing Tension

The Skeleton

The main parts of the dog's skeleton that you're concerned with in this chapter include the following:

- The *occiput* is that part of the head or skull that joins with the first vertebra of the neck (fig. 4.2). That bump at the very top of your dog's head is called the *occipital protuberance* (or "that bump on the top of his head").
- The *cervical vertebrae* are the seven vertebrae (plural) of the neck. They are labeled *C1 through C7.*

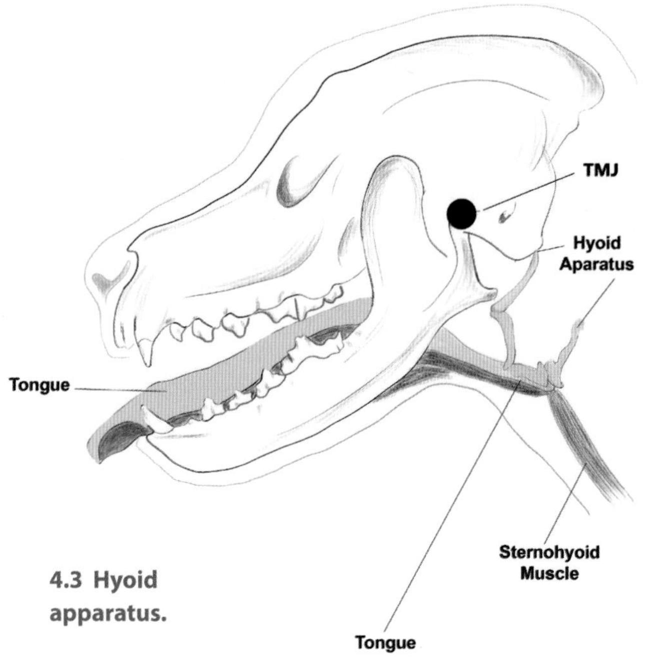

4.3 Hyoid apparatus.

FROM THE VET

Tension in the TMJ

Dogs that play ball a lot and carry balls around or dogs that chew on bones may be very tight at the TMJ points, and the jaw muscles will be very tight and tense. Dogs can also develop arthritic issues with the TMJ. These dogs may be sensitive on the TMJ points or may act like they don't like work over this area, so make sure to start with *Air Gap* or a very light touch. I always get big yawns and sometimes kisses from many of my patients after working in this area!

—Dr. Robinett

- The *atlas*, or C1, is the first vertebra of the neck.
- The *O-A Junction* is where the occiput joins with the atlas. This is an important junction in the dog.
- The *TMJ* is the *temporal mandibular joint*—three big words for where the jaw attaches to the noggin, or head (see fig. 4.2). The t*emporal* bone is the part of the skull just below the temple, the *mandible* is the jaw, and the *joint* is where they hinge or join together. (TMJ: smaller word, easier to understand!)
- The *hyoid apparatus:* This small but important assembly of bones and cartilaginous parts attached to the tongue and larynx, "hangs" from the skull between the two mandibles (fig. 4.3).

The function of the hyoid is to provide a flexible suspensory function to the tongue and larynx. It's attached to the temporal region of the skull, but also has muscles that go the other way and attach to the sternum.

The hyoid is important in that it's a delicate structure that can be damaged easily, but also it can be used to release tension in the TMJ, in the area of the O-A Junction, and in the area of the sternum and C7-T1 Junction through its muscular connections there.

Injuries or abnormalities of the hyoid apparatus can be caused by car accidents, dog bites, abusive use of training collars, and congenital abnormalities.

Muscles, Tendons, and Ligaments

There are muscles attached in the area of the O-A Junction that affect movement in the head and neck as well as in other areas of the dog (fig. 4.4). Some examples of these are the:

- *Brachiocephalic (brachiocephalicus)* or head-to-foreleg muscles. These are involved in moving the head from side to side, pulling the scapula forward, and bringing the foreleg forward.
- *Splenius capitis,* and major ligaments such as the *nuchal ligament,* attach in the area of the O-A Junction and run along the top and side of the dog's neck to attach at the other end to the thoracic spine between the shoulder blades, and to other muscles that move the forelimbs.
- To make matters even worse—or better, depending how you look at it—there are muscles and ligaments such as the *spinalis* and *longissimus dorsi* that continue from the shoulder area down the dog's back to the lower back and sacrum.
- The TMJ and muscles of the jaw and neck are involved with a lot more than just chewing and eating. There are other muscles that attach in this area such as the *sternocephalic* (sternum to head) and *sternohyoid* (sternum to hyoid) that run from

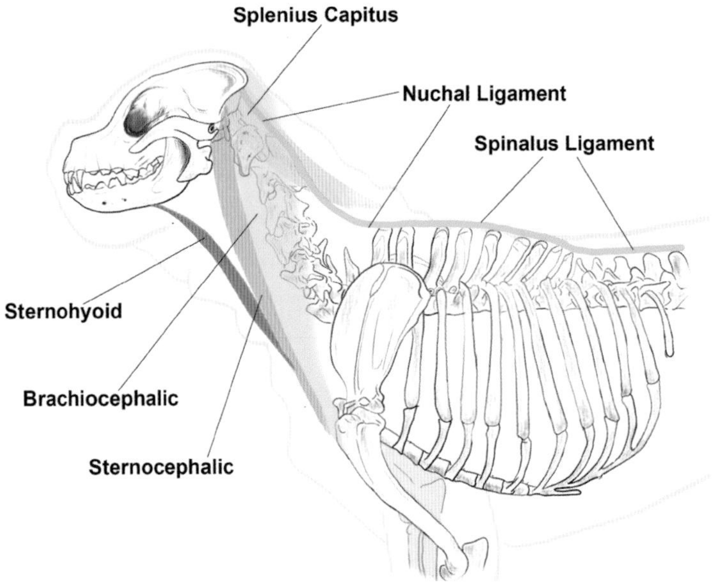

4.4 Ligaments and muscles of the head-neck junction.

Don't Let the Anatomy Get to You!

Remember not to get overwhelmed by the anatomy. While it's helpful to have a mental picture of how muscles and the skeleton work together (biomechanics) and how tension in one area can affect the rest of the body, it's important not to get too much into your head about which muscle is which and whether you're in the right place. While doing this work, "stay out of your head" and follow the dog's *Responses*. You have to be a little out of your mind to do this properly!

here down the neck and chest, attaching on the other end at the sternum.

- And that's not to mention nerves. It's through this O-A Junction that most nerves pass from the brain through the spinal column to the rest of the body. Consequently, tension in this area can affect what's going on in the rest of the body.

Biomechanics, Comfort, and Relaxation in the Body

Tension in the Head-Neck Junction can be uncomfortable for the dog and can affect behavior and movement. To get an idea of how important the O-A Junction is, think of times you yourself may have accumulated tension at the base of your skull and back of your neck through work, stress, or both. As humans, we're able to do something to relieve the tension, or at least communicate (complain) to someone that we need help. Your dog doesn't have that option, except maybe through unwanted or fearful behavior.

From a biomechanical standpoint, releasing tension in this area provides mobility to the head or occiput and the first two vertebrae of the neck: up-down, side-to-side, twist or rotate, and everything in between. Releasing tension in this area also starts the process of releasing tension in the:

- *Dorsal* muscles that run along the top of the spine and along the back to the pelvis, sacrum, and driving muscles of the hind end (see p. 97).
- *Ventral* muscles that run underneath the spine and along the belly to the groin, pelvis, sacrum, and driving muscles of the hind end. This ventral connection between the Head-Neck Junction and the hind end is via muscles and fascia that

FROM THE VET

Tension in the Occiput-Atlas Junction Affects the Whole Body

I find that dogs, just like people and other animals, carry and hold a lot of tension at the O-A Junction or upper neck. That muscular tightness or tension can continue all the way down the neck and into the shoulders. Tension at the upper neck can affect movement of the front legs. This muscular tension may even continue all the way down the back and cause stiffness or affect the gait with the hind legs as well. I often wonder if dogs and other animals get headaches because of this like people do. I did have a case of a Doberman Pinscher who had a severe cervical or neck problem. The owner reported that he hid in the closet and did not want to go outside, and seemed sensitive to light when his neck was hurting. I do think that dog did have headaches secondary to neck pain. He responded well to chiropractic, acupuncture, and the Masterson Method to relax the muscles and once his neck pain was controlled, he quit hiding in the closet.

—*Dr. Robinett*

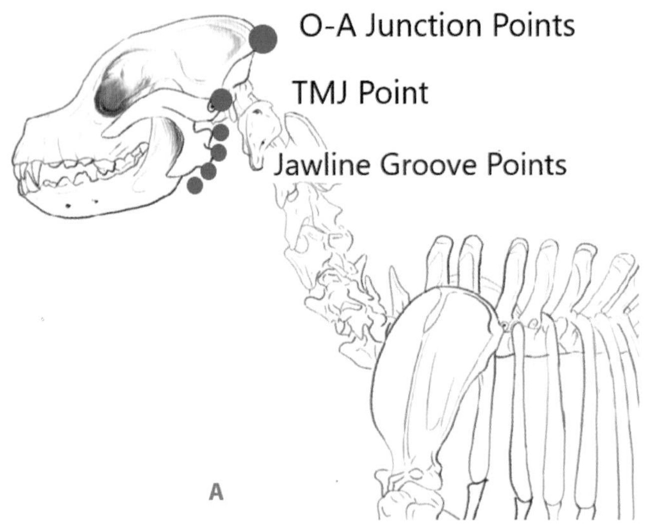

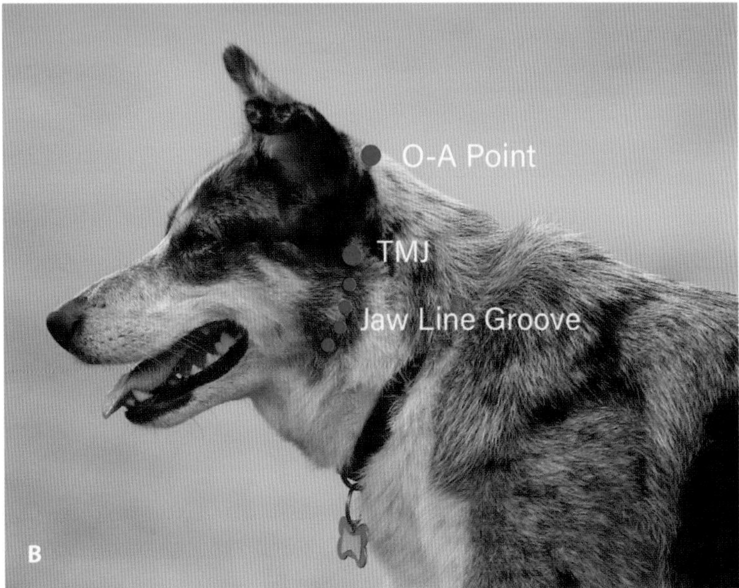

4.5 A & B TMJ and Jawline Groove Points.

run down the front of the neck to the chest and sternum (*brachiocephalic, sternocephalic, and sternohyoid*), and continue under the belly to the groin and hind end.

It's important to keep in mind the balance between the dorsal muscles and fascia versus the ventral muscles and fascia. It's also important to keep in mind the muscular interconnections in the dog's body in general. What's going on in one part of the body affects what's going on in other parts. Releasing tension in one area of the body can release tension in other areas. The O-A Junction is one of the key junctions that affect what's going on in the whole body.

Search, Response, Stay, Release

GOAL: To apply the process of *Search, Response, Stay, Release* to (figs. 4.5 A & B):

1 The connective tissue and muscles associated with the *TMJ.*

2 The muscles underneath the Head-Neck Junction in the area of the *jawline groove.*

3 The muscles in the area on top of the Head-Neck Junction—the *O-A Junction Point.*

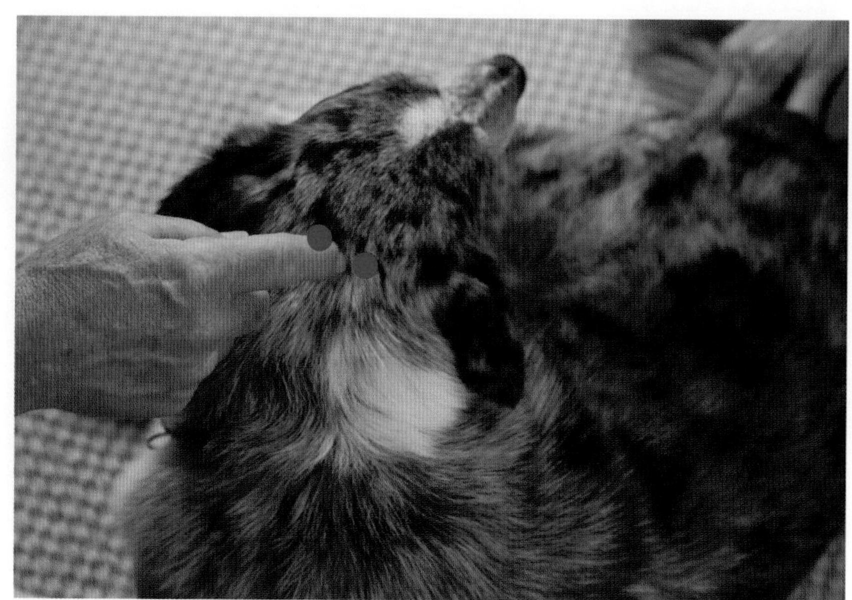

4.6 The O-A Junction Points, highlighted in red.

WHERE YOU WORK

TMJ Point

You *Search* in the area of the *TMJ* joint itself. To find the TMJ on yourself, put your finger just in front of the bottom of your ear and open and close your mouth. Right at the bottom of your ear, you'll feel where there is movement, and if you slide your fingertip just a tiny bit higher, you'll feel where there is no movement. Between them is the actual joint. On your dog it's in the same area—just below the dog's ear.

Once you've found the area of the TMJ, the easiest way to find the exact spot on your dog is to ask him—meaning, *Search* for the *eye blink*. When using *Air Gap* pressure (meaning no pressure), tension in the attachment of muscles and ligaments associated with the TMJ will show up as blinks from the dog.

Jawline Groove Points

The *Jawline Groove* is the groove between the mandible or jaw, and the front of the atlas or first vertebra of the neck. To find this groove, place your fingertips below the dog's ear in the area of the TMJ Point and run them down into the space between the back of the jaw and the neck. The *Jawline Groove Points* are generally found from the bottom of the TMJ Point to the base of the jaw.

The O-A Junction Points

The O-A Junction is between the top of the skull and the first vertebra of the neck. The main landmark that you're looking for is the bony bump at the back of the top of your dog's head. If you have a Lab, a Great Dane, or an Irish Setter, you won't be able to miss it. On other dogs you may have to feel for it.

The O-A Junction is just behind this bump, and the *Responses* that you're searching for are in the area behind and on each side of this bump (fig. 4.6). Your dog will tell you exactly where the tension is and where you need to *Stay* for a *Release*.

This work can be done with your dog standing, sitting, on your lap, or lying down.

Choose a place to begin: TMJ Point, Jawline Groove Points, or O-A Junction Points (see the following Quick Overview for the Jawline Groove Points as an example).

Scan to view Occiput-Atlas (O-A) Points video

Quick Overview: Step-by-Step

JAWLINE GROOVE POINTS

Here I am demonstrating Search, Response, Stay, Release on the Jawline Groove Points, as an example. The same steps apply in the areas of the TMJ and the O-A Junction.

Step 1. *Search*. Using the tip(s) of either one or two fingers, barely touching the hair, slowly (I said SLOWLY!) and gently search with your fingertip(s) in the area of the points (fig. 4.7 A). Your dog will tell you exactly where to stop when you get a...

Step 2. *Response*. Watch closely for a blink or other change of behavior, in this case a blink (fig. 4.7 B).

Step 3. *Stay*. Keep your finger over that spot, maintaining *Air Gap*. Resist the urge to move the finger, push, rub, or stroke. This may take one second or one minute. Be patient. Breathe and relax, until you get a...

Step 4. *Release,* such as licking and chewing or yawning (fig. 4.7 C).

When you are finished, you can either repeat the process on the opposite side or continue the process in one of the other areas on the same side.

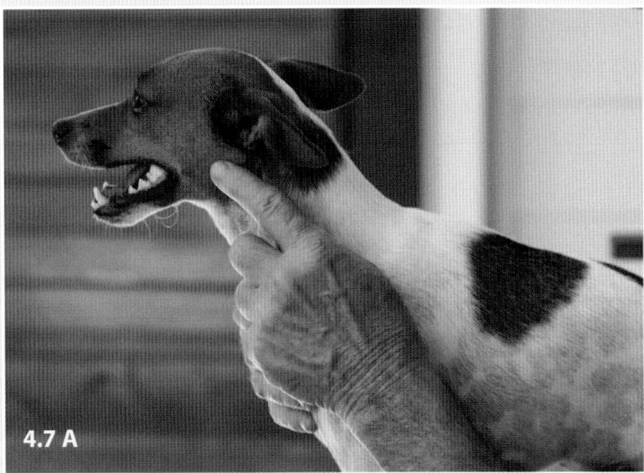

4.7 A

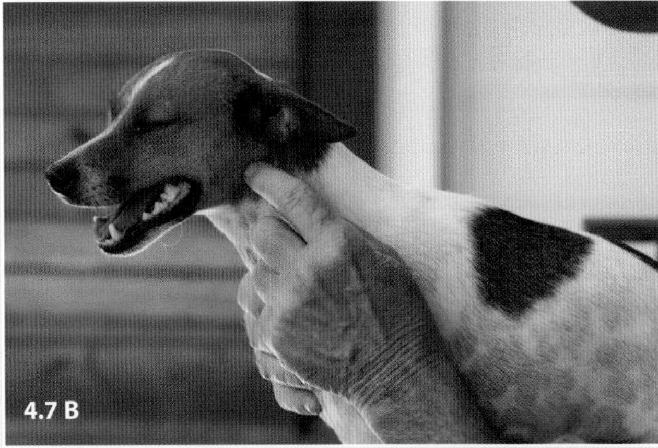

4.7 B

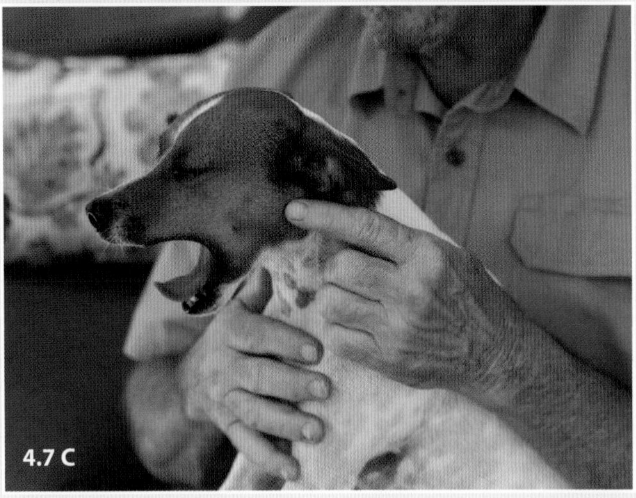

4.7 C

Tips

The Tips offered here and What Ifs that follow are basically the same whether using *SRSR* on the Bladder Meridian, the TMJ Point, the Head-Neck Junction, or on any other area of the body.

Start with your dog resting comfortably on your lap, or sitting or standing next to you. If he's a little restless you can pet or reassure him. Otherwise, wait until he's relaxed and somewhat "with you."

You may use one hand to reassure the dog or "ask" him to remain with you, but when you start searching for *Responses* with the fingers of the other hand, try not to have any pressure on the dog from the "asking" hand. You want the dog to feel what's going on with the searching hand and not to be distracted by any pressure from the "asking" hand.

When you get a *Response, Stay* with it until you get one of the *Release Responses*—or not. It might be a yawn, a lick and chew, a sigh, lying down, or fussiness, then relaxing. The larger the *Release Response,* the larger the amount of tension there is to let go.

When you get a *Release*, you can continue *Searching* or you can take your hand off and give the dog a chance to feel what's going on. If you don't get a *Response* or a *Release*, don't lose sleep over it. Just move on to another point.

Don't be too concerned about being on the exact location of a point. Your dog will tell you where it is. Not all points are in the exact same places on all dogs. To find them, *Search* in the area and your dog will tell you where to *Stay*. (You may have to get used to your dog telling *you* what to do for a change, but once you get used to that, everything will be fine.)

Remember that there may be more than one point or points of tension in the same area.

What Ifs?

- ***What if my dog becomes uncomfortable at some point?***

When your dog gets uncomfortable with what you're finding and wants to walk away, you can stop, or soften and ask him to stay with you a little longer, or you can let him wander off and wait for him to come back. If he insists on getting up and walking around, let him. He'll come back.

Keep in mind that if he's really uncomfortable and you make him stay with you, the part of his nervous system that blocks out tension will take over, and the part that releases tension will not work.

- ***What if the opposite happens? What if my dog starts out standing or sitting, then becomes so relaxed that he flops over or even goes to sleep?***

This can happen, especially when the dog starts releasing deeper tension. It's still possible to continue *SRSR* if the area is still accessible, as long as your dog doesn't fall asleep. When the dog is asleep, he can't feel or show you what's going on. In this case, you'll have to continue later when he's awake. (Besides, he might need a good nap right about now.)

Scan to view Head Up (Occiput-Atlas) Release video

Movement Techniques

Head Up (Occiput-Atlas) Release

GOAL: To get the dog to relax the weight of his head into your hand and ask for gentle movement of the junction in a relaxed state.

WHERE YOU WORK

The Occiput-Atlas Junction is the space between the top of the skull or occiput, and the top of the first vertebra or atlas (see fig. 4.2, p. 50). When the dog's head rests on something, the space between these two closes, shortening and relaxing the muscles in this area. The greater the relaxation of these muscles, the greater the release of tension.

With larger dogs, Head Up can be done in whatever position is comfortable for you, and (even more importantly) allows the dog to relax his head into your hand (figs. 4.8 A & B).

Quick Overview: Step-by-Step

HEAD UP (OCCIPUT-ATLAS) RELEASE

This Release works best when the dog is relaxed and sitting but can be done anytime the dog is relaxed.

Step 1. Position yourself sitting or kneeling next to your dog. You may also do this with your dog partially or fully on your lap.

Step 2. Place one hand gently on the dog's head or neck just behind the ears (fig. 4.9 A).

Step 3. Cup your other hand under the jaw or chin to support the weight of his head. You may rest your fingers over his nose to ask the dog to stay with you. Keep your arms and hands soft.

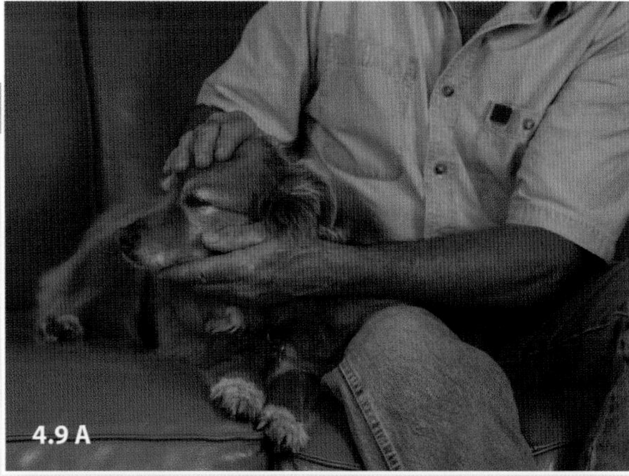

4.9 A

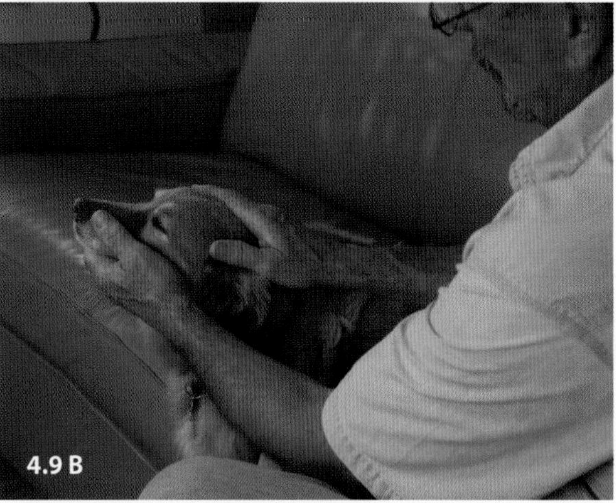

4.9 B

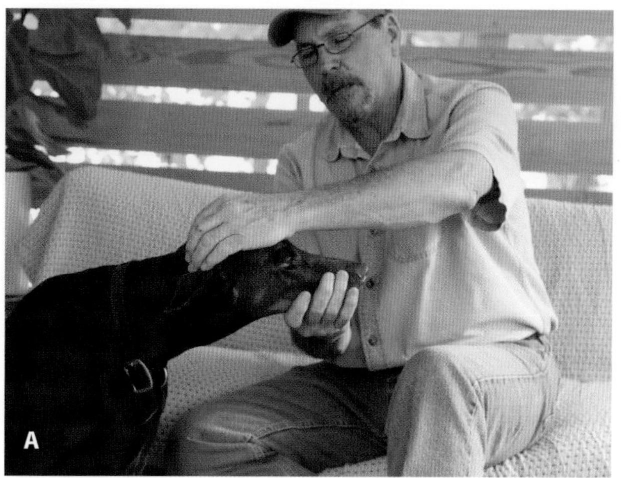
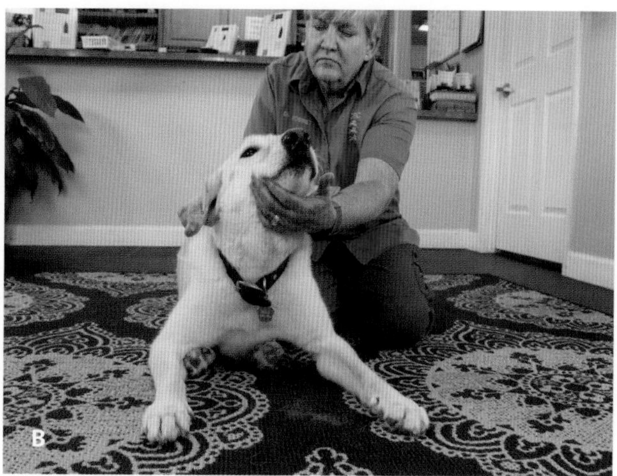

4.8 A & B Head Up (Occiput-Atlas) Release while sitting in front of the dog (A) and while sitting behind him (B).

Step 4. Wait for him to relax his head into your hand as much as possible. Keep both hands, arms, and shoulders completely relaxed. You should not be gripping the nose or putting pressure on his head. His head should be as relaxed as possible in your hand.

Step 5. Supporting the weight of the head as much as possible, slowly and gently raise your "nose hand." Watch for a blink as you do this (fig. 4.9 B). If you miss the blink or if the dog becomes uncomfortable as you lift, you're beyond the limit of his comfort range this. Soften and lower the nose until he blinks, or to a point where he appears to feel comfortable.

Step 6. When you've found that position, allow him to relax here even more.

Step 7. Gently remove your hands and give the dog time to feel any changes in the body and *Release* (fig. 4.9 C).

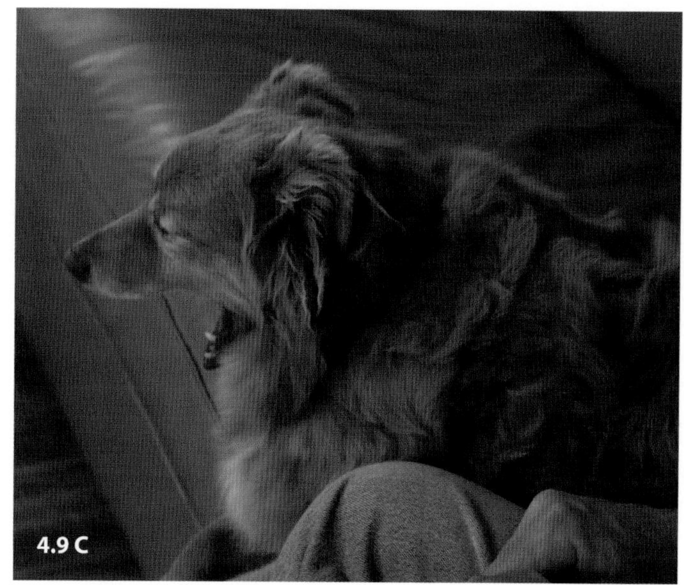

4.9 C

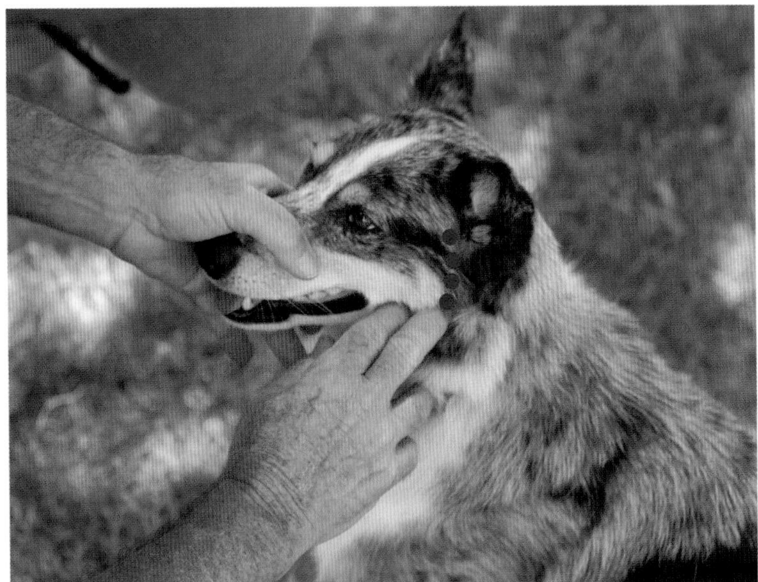

4.10 Jawline Groove Microflexion Points.

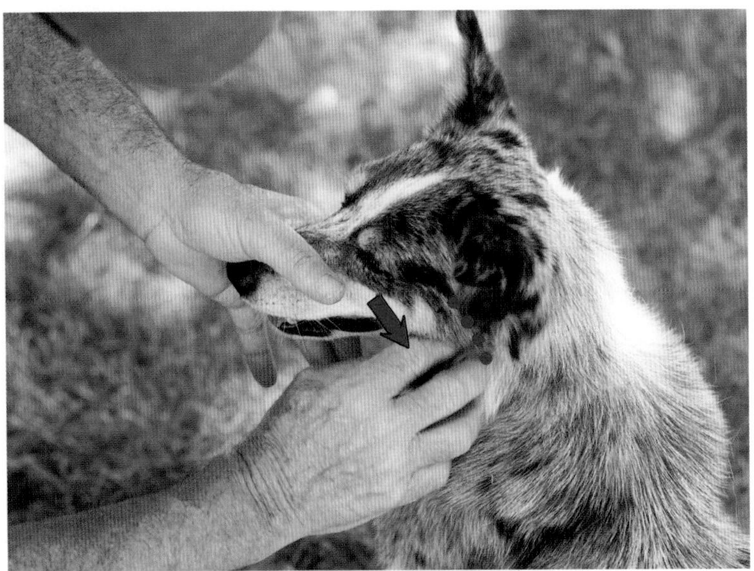

4.11 Lateral Cervical (Neck) Microflexion Points.

Tips

Start slow and small. The slower and smaller the movement, the more the dog relaxes into your hand, and the more tension your dog will be able to release.

Jawline Groove Microflexion and Lateral Cervical Microflexion

GOAL: To ask for gentle movement of the muscles, tendons, and ligaments between the neck, head, and jaw while they are in a relaxed state.

WHERE YOU WORK

The Jawline Groove is the space between the back of the skull and the front of the first cervical vertebra, the atlas (fig. 4.10). When the head is brought to the side in a relaxed state during *Jawline Groove Microflexion*, the space between these structures closes, shortening and relaxing the connective tissue and muscles here. Micro-wiggling further releases tension in the connective tissue and muscles.

As the dog's head is brought farther around in a relaxed state during *Lateral Cervical Microflexion*, the spaces between the cervical vertebrae close, shortening and relaxing the muscles in this area (fig. 4. 11).

"Wiggle" means a very tiny side-to-side micromovement, almost the same movement you would use with your fingers to ring a tiny bell. When micromovement in a relaxed state (wiggle) is added, this further releases tension in the connective tissue and muscles in the jawline groove and cervical vertebrae.

Quick Overview: Step-by-Step

JAWLINE GROOVE MICROFLEXION

Step 1. Position yourself sitting or kneeling next to your dog. You may also do this with your dog partially or fully on your lap.

Step 2. Place one hand gently on or under his nose, keeping your hands, arms, shoulders, and body completely relaxed. This is your "nose hand." Wait for him to relax his head into your nose hand as much as possible.

Note: You may allow your fingers to wrap softly (I said SOFTLY!) around the nose.

Step 3. Place the tip or back of your first or index finger of your other hand gently into the groove just below the ear and behind the jaw. This is your "groove finger."

Step 4. Bring his nose slightly toward you with the nose hand (see fig. 4.10).

Step 5. Keeping the tips of your groove finger resting in the groove, gently wiggle his nose side to side with the nose hand. Keep the hands soft and the movement small—more like a "micro-wiggle" (fig. 4.12 A).

Step 6. Soften both hands.

Step 7. Slide your groove finger slightly lower in the groove.

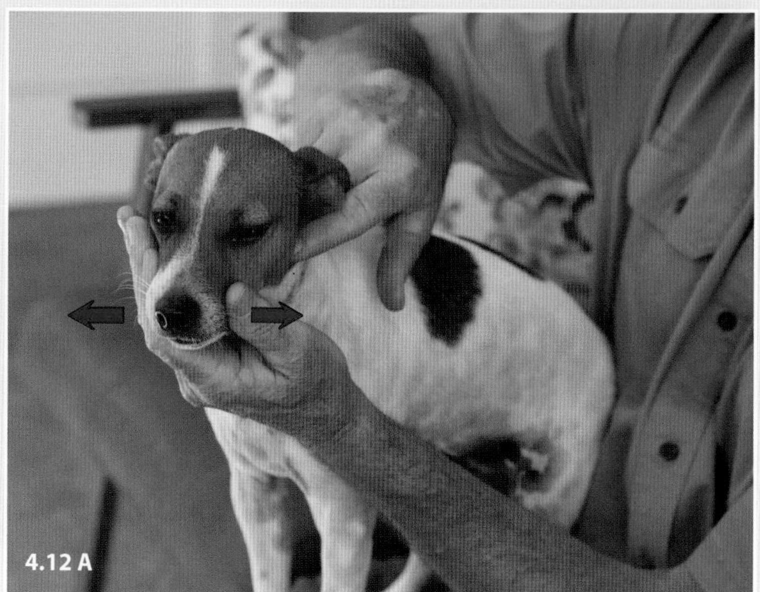
4.12 A

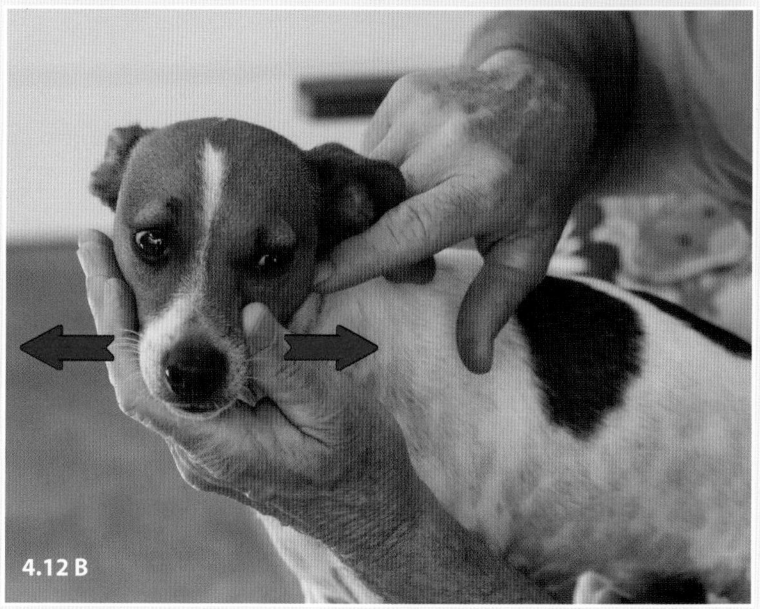
4.12 B

JAWLINE GROOVE MICROFLEXION (continued)

Step 8. Keeping your groove finger in the groove, gently bring his nose toward you and wiggle his nose two or three times. Remember, the dog's head and neck have to be relaxed (fig. 4.12 B).

Step 9. Soften both hands.

Step 10. Continue to repeat the wiggle farther down the groove. Gently remove your hands and give the dog time to feel any changes in the body ("see what the dog has to say").

These steps are the same with larger dogs, except that it may be easier to position yourself in front of, next to, or standing over your dog rather than having him on your lap (fig. 4.13 A). They are also the same with tiny dogs, except that you'll find that you may only need to use your fingers rather than your hands (fig. 4.13 B).

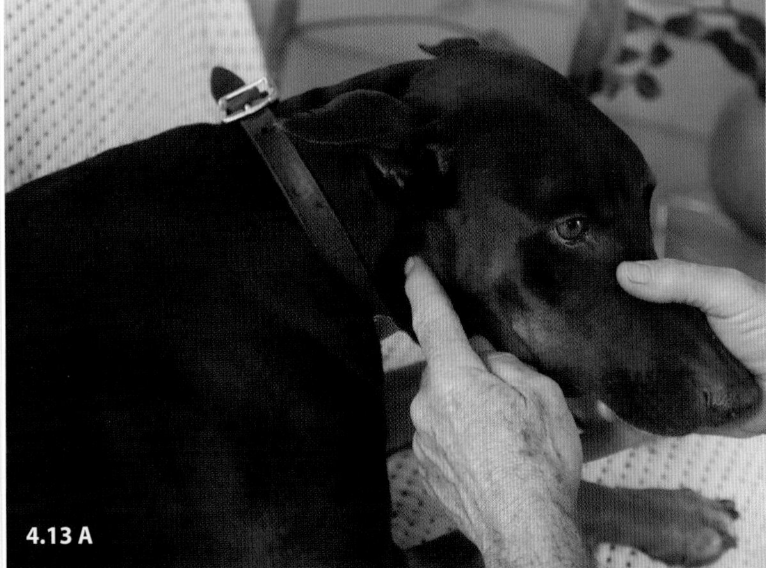

4.13 A

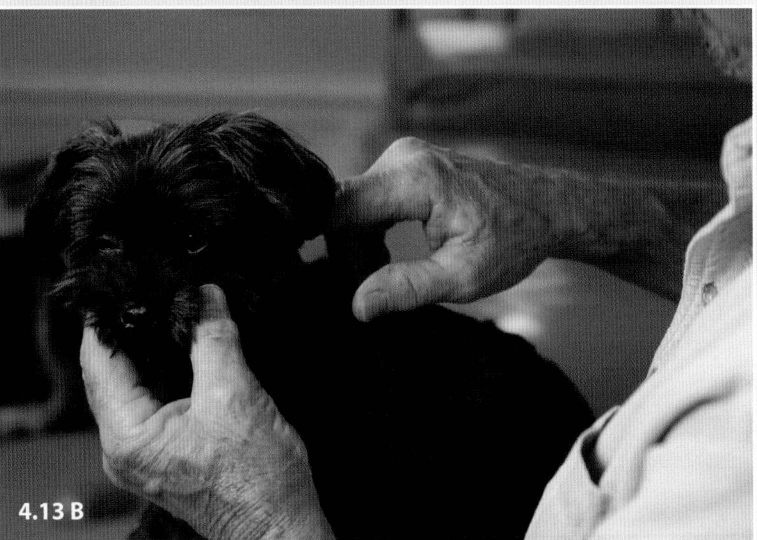

4.13 B

4.13 A & B Showing Jawline Groove Microflexion with a larger and smaller dog.

Quick Overview: Step-by-Step

LATERAL CERVICAL MICROFLEXION

Step 1. With your "nose hand" (and his nose) in the same position as for the previous technique, place your groove finger(s) slightly farther down the neck toward his shoulder. This hand is now the "neck hand." (Note: On a large dog this might be two or three inches. On a tiny dog, this might be half an inch.)

Step 2. Bring your dog's nose around the neck finger toward you and give the nose two or three gentle wiggles. Use almost no pressure with the neck finger. You are basically using the finger as a fulcrum for the "wiggle" (fig. 4.14 A).

Step 3. Soften both hands and slide your neck finger an inch farther down the neck toward his shoulder (see fig. 4.11–p. 60).

Step 4. Gently bring his nose around your neck finger a little farther toward the shoulder and wiggle it two or three times (fig. 4.14 B).

Step 5. Soften both hands and slide your neck finger an inch farther down the neck toward his shoulder.

Step 6. Gently bring his nose around a little farther toward you and wiggle it two or three times. You should have enough "neck room" to repeat this in three or four places between the jawline groove and the shoulder.

Step 7. Gently remove your hands and give the dog time to feel any changes in the body.

These steps are the same with larger dogs, except that it may be easier to position yourself next to, in front of, or standing over your dog, rather than having him on your lap (fig. 4.15).

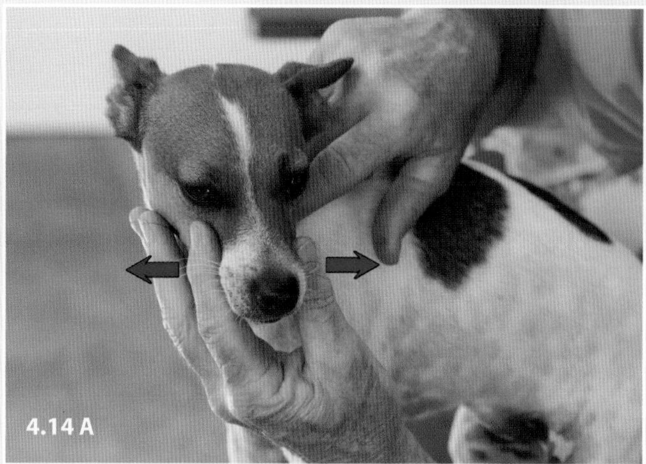

4.14 A

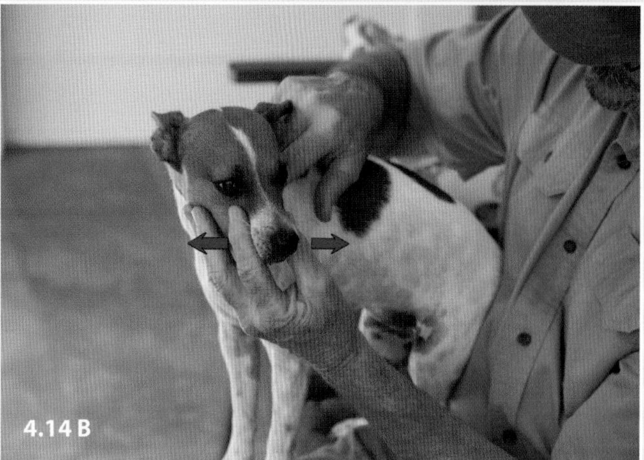

4.14 B

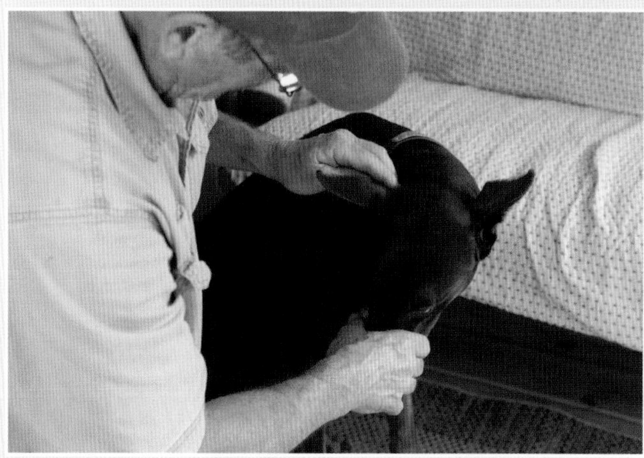

4.15 Showing Lateral Cervical Microflexion with a larger dog.

Scan to view Jawline Groove and Lateral Cervical Microflexion video

Tips

Keep both nose and groove/neck hands soft, with only *Egg Yolk* pressure under the groove/neck fingers. Their job is to act as a focus or "fulcrum" for the wiggle.

Keep the wiggles or micromovements "micro," especially in the *Jawline Groove*. The dog's body can internally brace against larger movements. The dog's muscles tend to relax with a "wiggle."

What Ifs?

- ***What if my dog braces or doesn't relax into my hand?***

The first thing to do is soften both hands. Often, we think we're soft, but the dog isn't feeling it. No matter how soft you think you might be, you should do regular "softness checks." While watching the dog's eyes, consciously soften your hands and arms. If the dog's eyes, ears, or body softens, that means you weren't soft enough before (figs. 4. 17 A & B).

Hold, Wait, and Melt Techniques

Hyoid Release

GOAL: Apply the process of *Hold, Wait, and Melt* to the muscles and connective tissues of the hyoid apparatus.

WHERE YOU WORK

The hyoid apparatus lies at the top of the throat between the two branches of the jaw, or mandibles

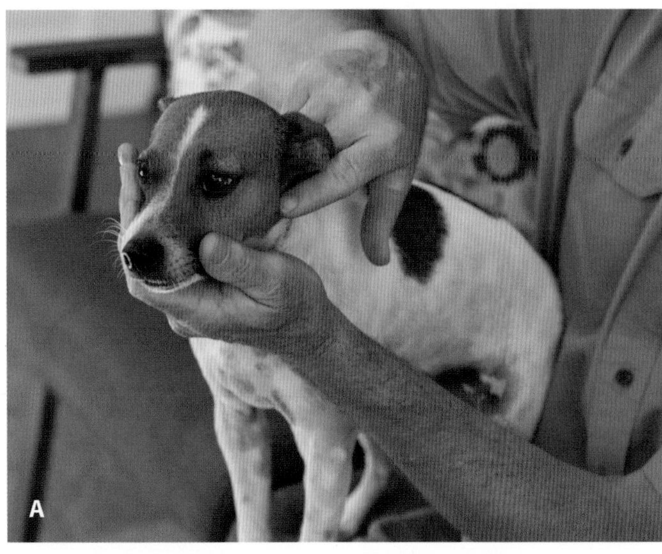

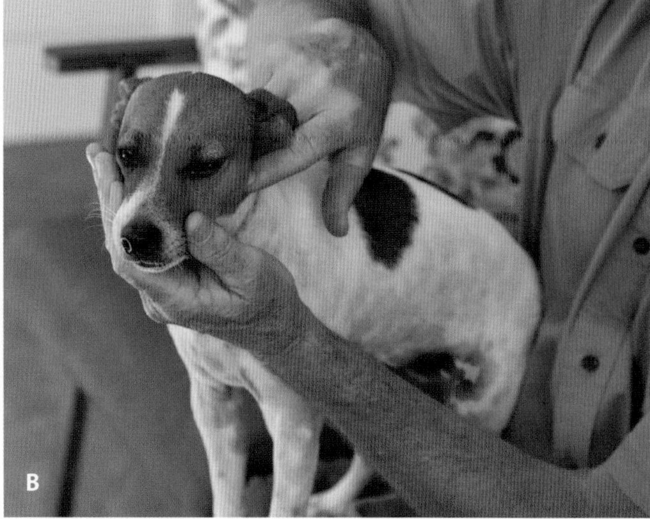

4.17 A & B Neck and eyes tense (A) and soft (B).

Quick Overview: Step-by-Step

THE HYOID RELEASE

Step 1. Position yourself sitting or kneeling and in front of or next to your dog. You can stand if your dog is on a table.

Step 2. Using the tips of two or three fingers of both hands, barely touching the surface of the skin place the fingertips in the space underneath either side of the jaw (fig. 4.17 A).

Step 3. Gently feel for a slight bump or bulge between the two mandibles (see fig. 4.3—p. 51). When you feel this bump, soften the fingers of both hands to Air Gap.

Step 4. Stay softly at Air Gap on this spot until you get a *Release*. Usually, a *Release* of some kind will occur within 10 to 30 seconds. Sometimes it will be subtle, such as turning the head away (fig. 4.17 B), lying down, or otherwise fidgeting. When your dog releases, he may want to lie down. If you don't get a *Release* within 30 seconds, soften your hands even more.

Note: After releasing the hyoid, you can check for movement by holding your fingertips on either side of the hyoid and, using no more than Egg Yolk pressure, gently move or wiggle the hyoid from side to side.

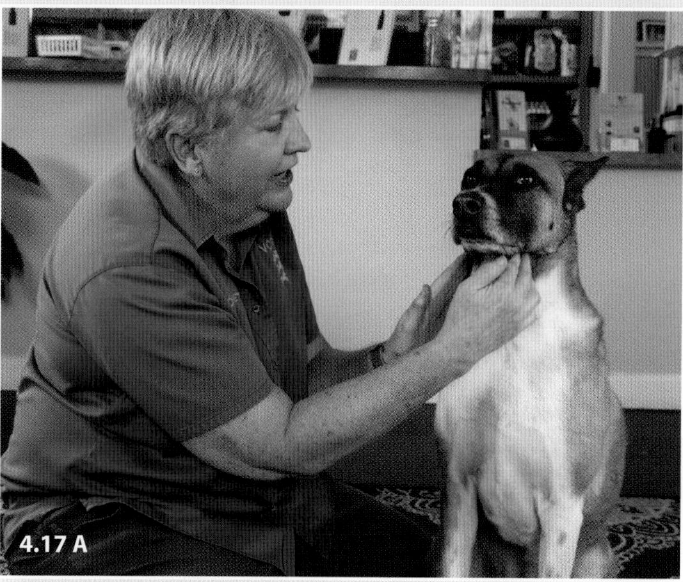
4.17 A

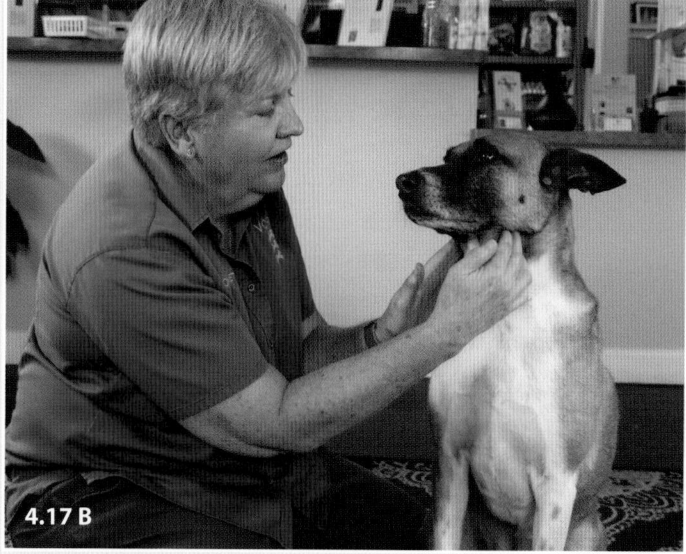
4.17 B

Scan to view Hyoid Release video

Scan to view Hyoid Movement Check video

FROM THE VET

The Importance of the Hyoid

Releasing the hyoid apparatus and keeping it moving freely enables the tongue to move more easily, aids in swallowing, assists with movement of the jaw and TMJ, and keeps the neck moving better because of the release of tension in muscles such as the sternohyoid that run along the neck between the hyoid and sternum (fig. 4.18).

—*Dr. Robinett*

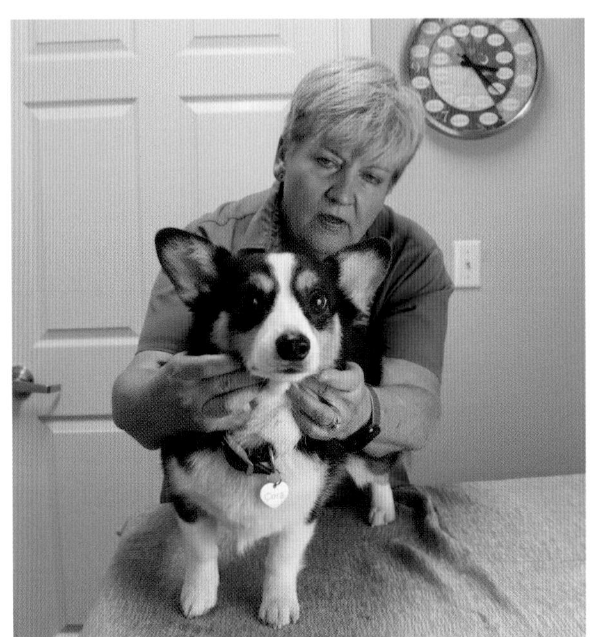

4.18 The hyoid lies underneath the jaw, between the two mandibles.

(see fig. 4.3—p. 51). It is the slight bump or bulge that is felt at the junction underneath the chin and the front of the neck.

What Ifs?

- ***What if I get no responses at all in this area?***

It may be there is no tension in this area, which is good. You may not be going softly enough, and the dog is guarding against the pressure, in which case you need to soften more.

- ***What if I feel that the hyoid is tight on one side and that it isn't moving as well as it should?***

In this case, it sometimes helps to move on to other areas that might help further loosen this area such as the TMJ Points, Jawline Groove, and Lateral Cervical Microflexion, and the Neck, Scapula, Trunk, and Sternum Pectoral Points (fig. 4.19).

Also, when you give your dog's nervous system time to "rest" and process releases, often you will come back later or the next day and find areas that you felt had not released are now softer.

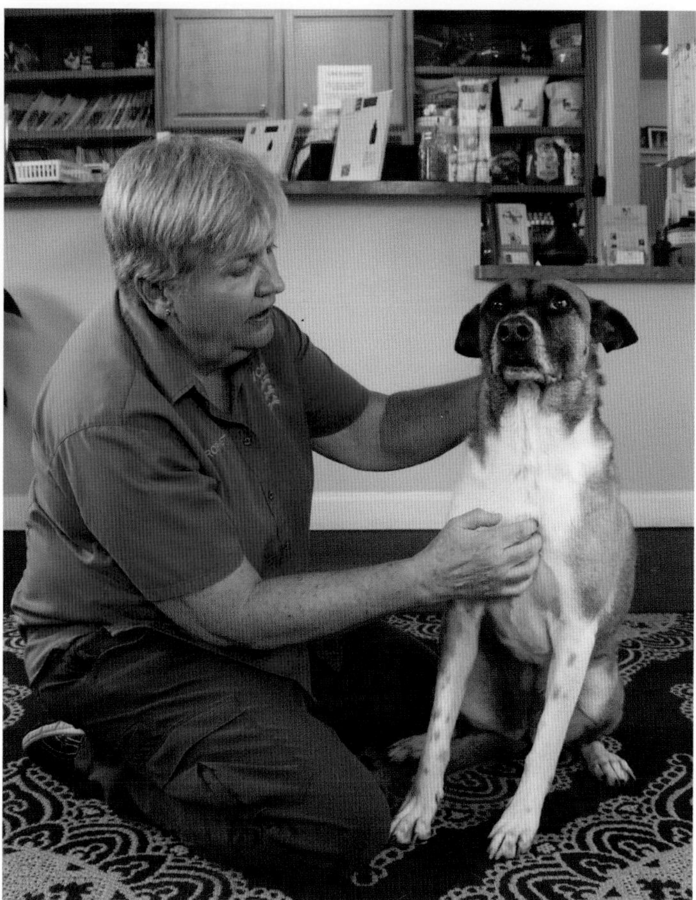

4.19 If you don't get a hyoid release, move on to other areas such as the sternum that are connected to and may help release tension in this area.

FROM THE VET

Be as Light as You Would with Yourself

You can feel the hyoid on yourself and practice the release on yourself before trying it on your dog. Feel with the fingertips of both hands under the back part of the chin and where the front part of the neck starts. The bulge under the skin is where the hyoid apparatus is located, which holds the larynx and upper part of the trachea in place. Gently place your fingers on either side of that bulge and push very gently to one side, then to the other. Very gently wiggle it from side to side, but barely move it. If it does not want to move to a certain side or feels "stuck" on one side, wait and hold until it releases, and then try the gentle side-to-side motion. Your neck should feel more relaxed after the release if your hyoid was not moving well. Remember how this felt on yourself and how light your contact should be when working on your dog.

—Dr. Robinett

5

CHAPTER 5

The Neck-Trunk (C7-T1) Junction and Forelimbs

This chapter discusses the various areas of the Neck-Trunk (C7-T1) Junction and the forelimbs that accumulate tension, and offers exercises to release tension in these areas using the three categories of techniques that I outlined in Part One:

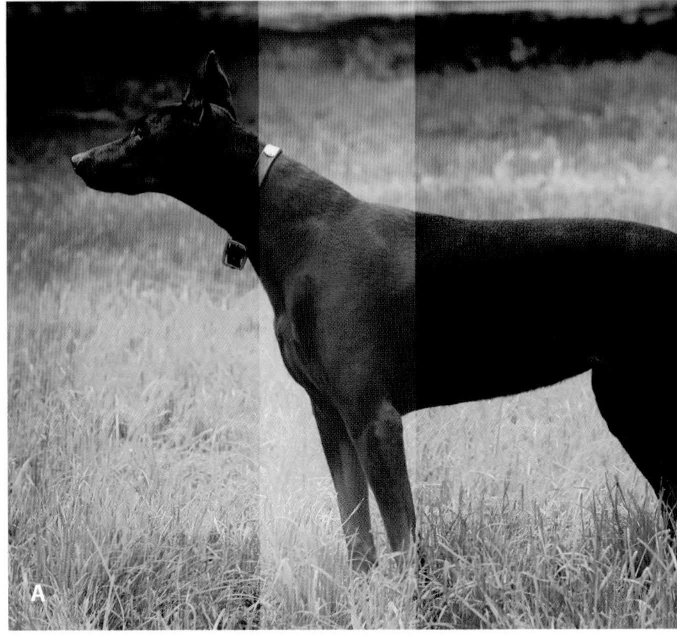

A

Search, Response, Stay, Release (SRSR), page 4; *Movement Techniques,* page 5; *Hold, Wait, and Melt Techniques (HWM),* page 6.

Search, Response, Stay, Release

Scapula Trunk Points, Sternum and Pectoral Points, Lower Forelimb Points

GOAL: To apply the process of *Search, Response, Stay, Release* to muscles that attach the forelimbs to the trunk; connective tissue of the vertebral junction of the neck and trunk (C7-T1); and connective tissue of the forelimbs themselves. (To begin these techniques, see p. 73.)

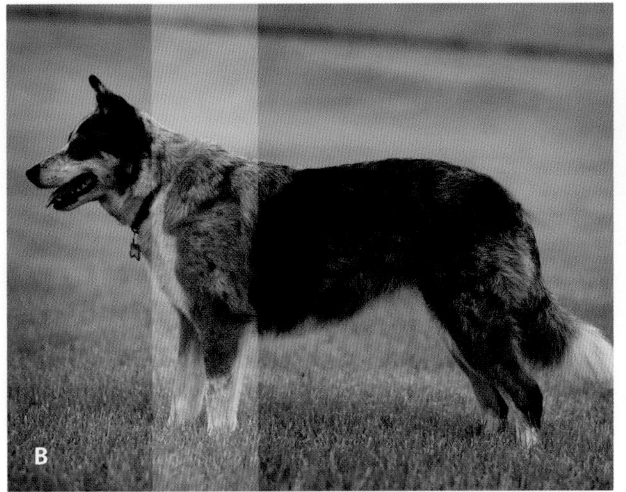

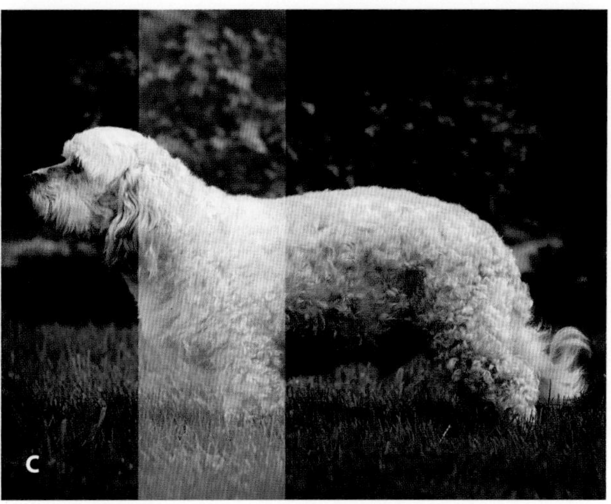

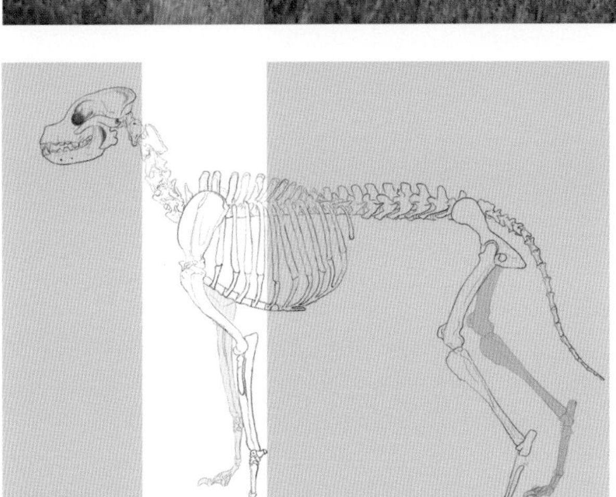

5.1 A–D The Neck-Trunk Junction and forelimbs.

RESULT: *Search, Response, Stay, Release* releases tension in the deeper muscles and connective tissues of the area on which you are working. This results in improved elasticity and suppleness in these muscles and prepares this junction for the *Movement Techniques* that follow. It also makes your dog feel really good!

Movement Techniques

Scapula and Forelimb Movements, Lower Forelimb Movements

GOAL: To search for responses while moving the scapula and upper and lower forelimb through specific ranges of motion in a relaxed state. (To begin these techniques, see p. 76.)

RESULT: Movement in a relaxed state releases tension in the muscles, tendons, and ligaments associated with these structures and restores natural movement and suspension to them. It also prepares the C7-T1 Junction for the *Hold, Wait, and Melt Techniques* that follow.

Hold, Wait, and Melt Techniques

C7-T1 Release

GOAL: To apply the process of *Hold, Wait, and Melt* to the muscles and connective tissues underneath the scapula and around the C7-T1 Junction. (To begin these techniques, see p. 93.)

RESULT: Releases tension in the connective tissues and restores movement to the C7-T1 Junction. Restoring movement to this junction allows muscles in other areas of the body associated with this junction to relax.

More Anatomy and the Effects of Releasing Tension

The Skeleton

The main parts of the spine you're concerned with in this chapter are the *cervical spine, the thoracic spine,* and where the last *cervical vertebra* (C7) joins the first *thoracic vertebra* (T1). This is what we call the Neck-Trunk or C7-T1 Junction (fig. 5.2 A). Other skeletal parts you're concerned with in this chapter are as follows (fig. 5.2 B):

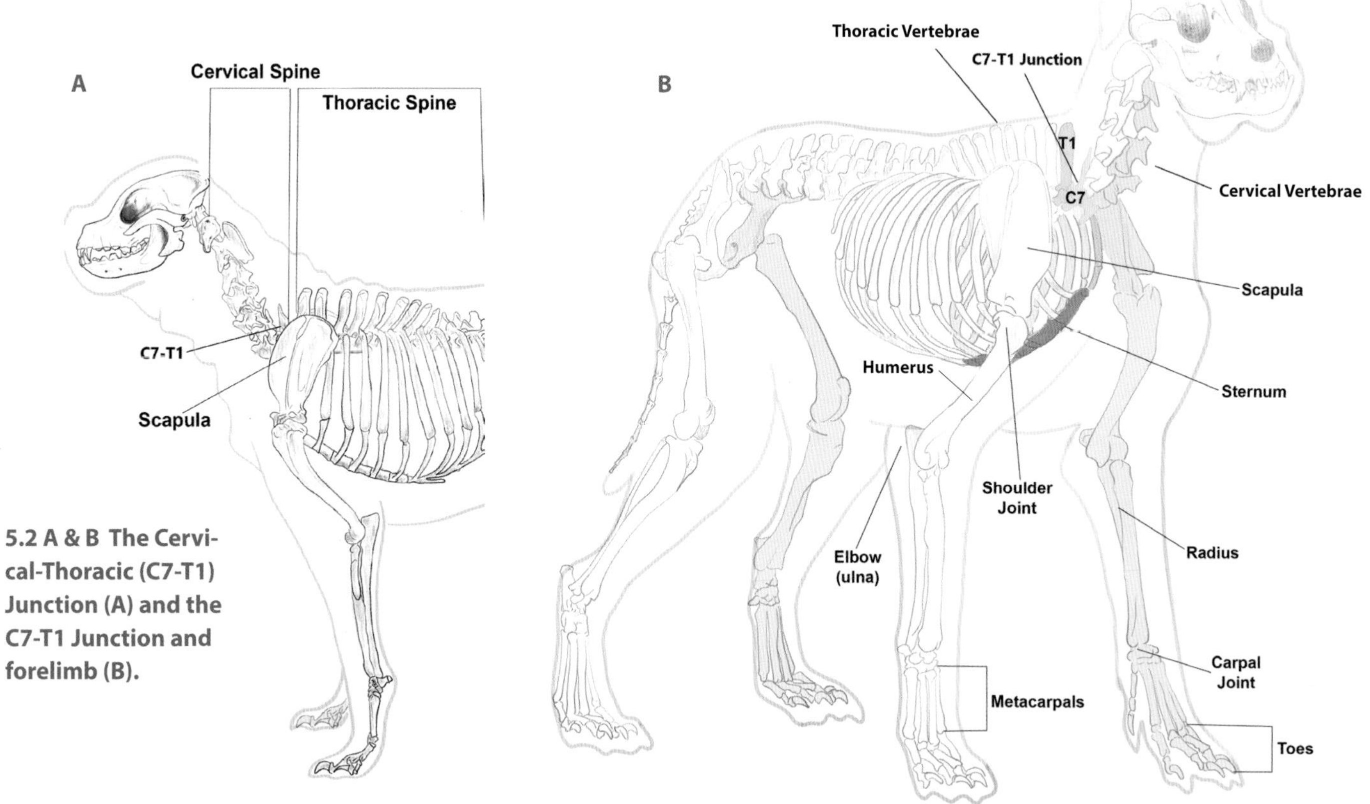

5.2 A & B The Cervical-Thoracic (C7-T1) Junction (A) and the C7-T1 Junction and forelimb (B).

- The *sternum* is where the first nine ribs of the trunk join at their lower ends. The sternum is important in that muscles that attach here also connect to the Head-Neck Junction, hyoid, and TMJ, and via the abdominal-ventral train of muscles and fascia, to the groin muscles and hind end.
- The *scapula* (shoulder blade) is a flat bone attached to the trunk via a strong network of muscle and fascia. As you can see in the illustrations on page 70, the two *scapulae* cover the area of the C7-T1 Junction.
- The *humerus* is the next bone of the forelimb. It's a short (but necessary) bone.
- The *shoulder joint* is the joint between the scapula and the humerus. It is the first actual joint of the forelimb.
- The *radius* (no, not the name of a Roman emperor) is the next bone down. This would be the forearm in a human.
- The *ulna* (no, not the name of a Swedish actress) is attached and runs parallel to the radius. The *olecranon process* is that pointy bone at the back of the *elbow,* which is the next joint down.
- The *carpus* or *carpal joint* is equivalent to the wrist on a human. It's at the lower end of the radius. It's a complex of smaller joints attached to the four *metacarpals* that extend into the dog's paw and toes.
- The carpal, metacarpal, and toe joints are supported by tendons and ligaments that act as front-end shock absorbers, especially when bearing weight during the dog's movement.

Now let's take a look at some of the muscles and connective tissues of this junction.

Muscles, Tendons, and Ligaments

As with the rest of the body, many muscles of the Neck-Trunk C7-T1 Junction are multitaskers. They both *stabilize* and *move* the skeleton. They support the head and neck as well as the shoulders and trunk. They move the forelimbs as well as move and bend the head and neck. They are strong and multilayered, and many lie underneath the scapula.

Muscles associated with this junction also have connections to other parts of the body. As you saw in the previous chapter, many muscles of the head and upper neck have attachments to the C7-T1 Junction. The muscles of the forelimbs and neck work together to create movement in the front end.

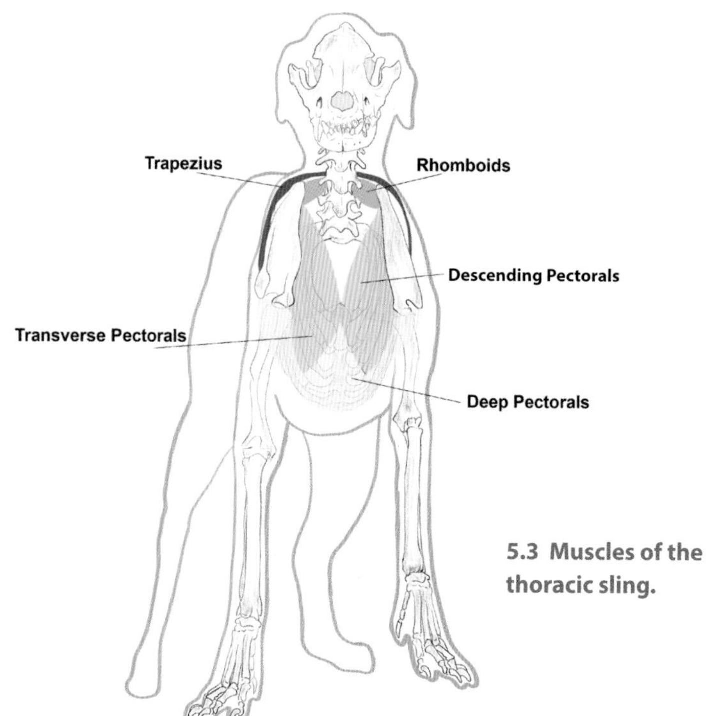

5.3 Muscles of the thoracic sling.

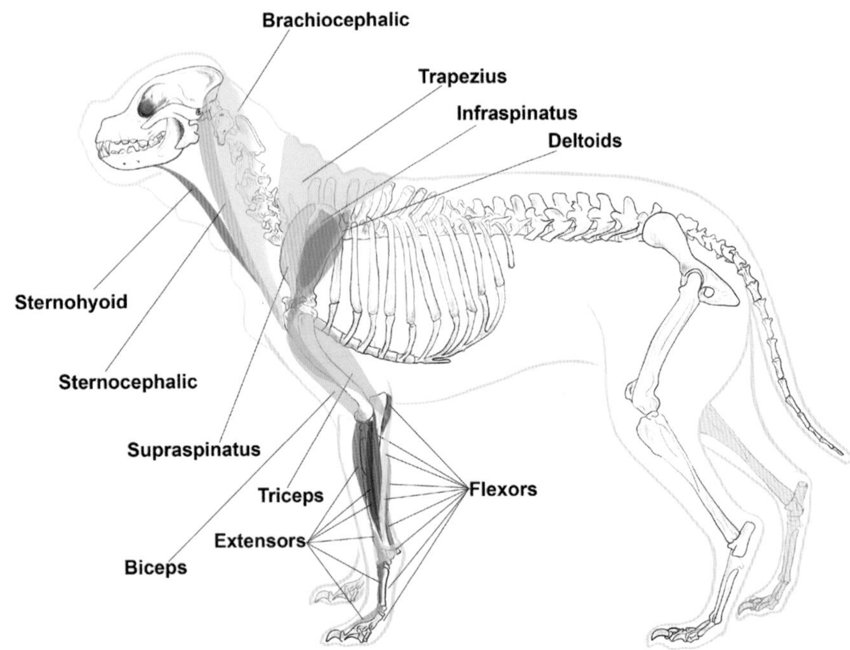

5.4 Muscles of the Neck-Trunk Junction and forelimb.

Importance of the Thoracic Sling

The muscular attachment of the scapula to the trunk allows for the range of motion, speed, and flexibility that the dog relies on to survive. Imagine the speed and agility of a pack of ravenous canines, careening through the aisles of your local supermarket to be the first to the dog food section! And in the wild, it's even more critical.

An interesting feature of the dog's forelimb is that there is no joint that attaches the scapula to the trunk. Unlike a human, who has a clavicle or collarbone that connects the forelimb to the body, a dog does not have a collarbone. The shoulder blade is attached to the trunk by muscles, fascia, and connective tissue (fig. 5.3). This is often referred to as the "thoracic sling." Many of these muscles are involved in movement, and many attach to the cervical spine and the area of the Head-Neck Junction.

Some of these muscles are the *pectoral* (chest) muscles that attach along each side of the sternum at one end and on the inside of the forelimb at the other. They are involved in both movement *and* stabilization of the forelimb. They are part of the thoracic sling that supports the trunk between the forelimbs.

Wait, there's more (fig. 5.4)! The *trapezius* muscle lies on top of the neck and shoulder. There is a front half and a back half (both in yellow in the illustration). The front half is the *cervical* part that attaches on top of the neck, and the back half is the *thoracic* part that attaches to the top of the trunk between the shoulder blades. Both parts also attach onto the scapula and are involved in both stabilizing the scapula and lifting and drawing the leg forward.

The *supraspinatus* and *infraspinatus* muscles are involved in movement and support of the scapula. The *supraspinatus,* along with other muscles, extends the shoulder joint to bring the leg forward. When the leg is planted, its partner the *infraspinatus* flexes the shoulder joint to bring the leg back, pushing the dog forward.

The *tricep* muscle originates on the back edge

FROM THE VET

Helping with Congenital Joint Problems

Elbow dysplasia is a congenital problem and can need surgery to correct when young to prevent a lifetime of discomfort and pain. Using *Head-Neck Junction*, *Neck Trunk Junction*, and *Scapula and Forelimb Movement Techniques* can help to *Release* tension associated with this problem and keep your dog more comfortable, flexible, and moving better.

—*Dr. Robinett*

of the *scapula* and inserts on the *olecranon* at the point of the elbow. It opens or extends the elbow and flexes the shoulder joint.

The *extensor* muscles on the forelimb open the elbow and carpus (wrist) of the leg to extend or reach the leg forward, while *flexor* muscles close these joints to pull the leg back when the foot is planted on the ground, propelling—or at least easing—the body of the dog forward.

Equally important are muscles that work with the head and neck to create both movement and stability in the front end. For example:

The *brachiocephalic* (arm-to-head) muscle originates at the base of the head near the atlas at the top end and inserts on the humerus of the forelimb at the bottom. It has two basic functions: 1) When the head and neck are fixed, it brings the foreleg forward, and 2) when the leg is fixed, it brings the neck down and the head forward.

The *sternocephalic* (sternum-to-head) muscle originates on the sternum and inserts on the temporal bone of the head. Its function is to move the head and neck from side to side.

The *sternohyoid* (sternum-to-hyoid) muscle originates on the sternum and inserts on the hyoid. One of its functions is to move the tongue. As the various muscles and areas of the dog work together to perform different functions, tension in the muscles in one area can create tension and affect the function and comfort of muscles in other areas. It's your job to help release that tension and keep them balanced.

Search, Response, Stay, Release

GOAL: To apply the process of *Search, Response, Stay, Release* to:

1 The muscles and connective tissues that attach the scapula to the trunk.

Foreleg Discomfort

Compensation for any kind of foreleg discomfort will show up as tension in the Neck-Trunk (C7-T1) Junction. This can also create increased tension in the muscles connecting the front end to the hind end, such as the *longissimus dorsi* and the *iliocostal* muscles, leading eventually to discomfort and overall stiffness in the body.

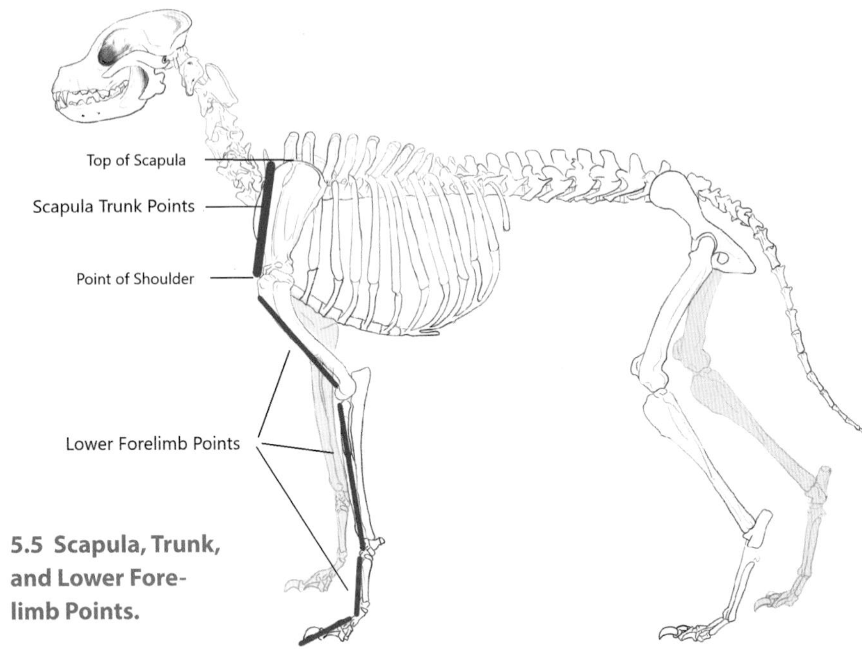

5.5 Scapula, Trunk, and Lower Forelimb Points.

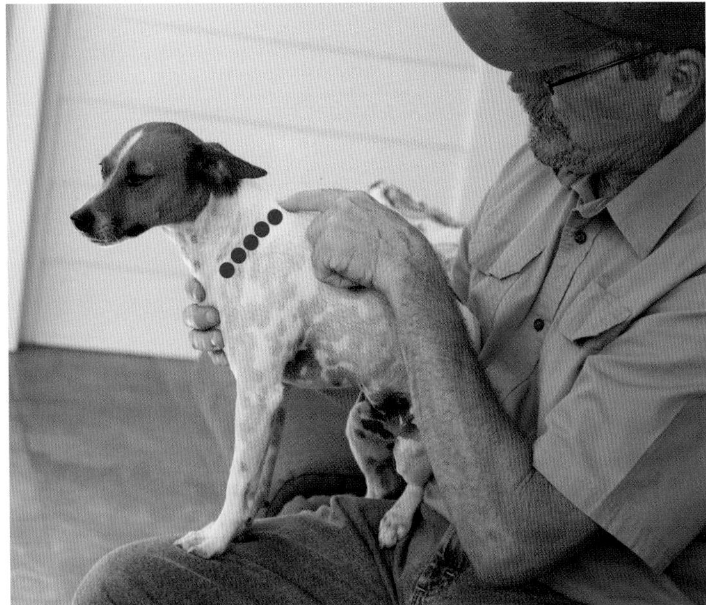

5.6 The top of the scapula to the point of the shoulder and shoulder joint.

2 The muscles and connective tissue of the vertebral junction of the neck and trunk (C7-T1).

3 The muscles, tendons, and ligaments of the forelimb itself.

WHERE YOU WORK

Scapula Trunk Points

(thoracic sling, cervical traps, supra and infraspinatus, brachiocephalic)

To find the scapula, feel for the two bones next to each other where the topline of the back meets the topline of the neck. These are the tops of the two shoulder blades (scapula).

Follow the front of the scapula down to the point of the shoulder. This is the shoulder joint, where the first bone of the forelimb—the humerus—joins the scapula (figs. 5.5 and 5.6).

Sternum and Pectoral Points

(thoracic sling, pectorals, brachiocephalic, sternocephalic, sternohyoid)

To find the sternum, run your fingers from the front of the base of the neck down the middle of the dog's chest. You'll feel a bump or protuberance in the middle of the chest directly between the two points of the shoulder. This bump is the top or point of the sternum. The bony part below is the rest of the sternum (figs. 5.7 and 5.8 A–C).

The pectorals are short muscles that attach along each side of the sternum at one end, and on the inside of the forelimb at the other (see fig. 5.3, p. 71).

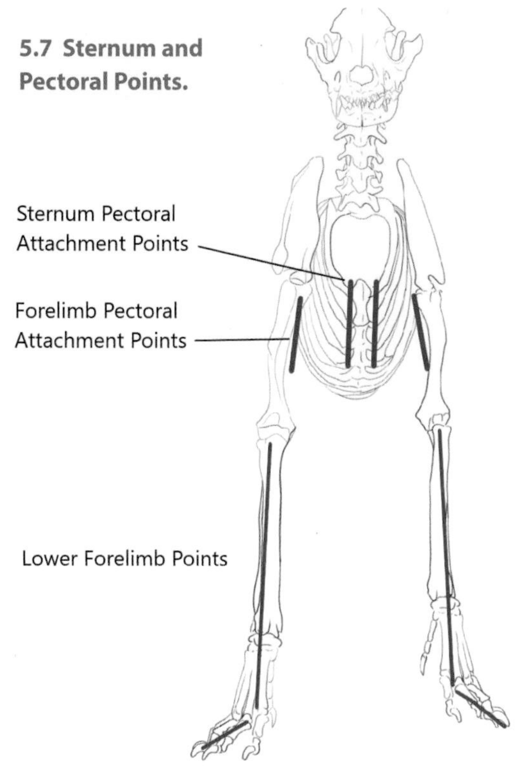

5.7 Sternum and Pectoral Points.

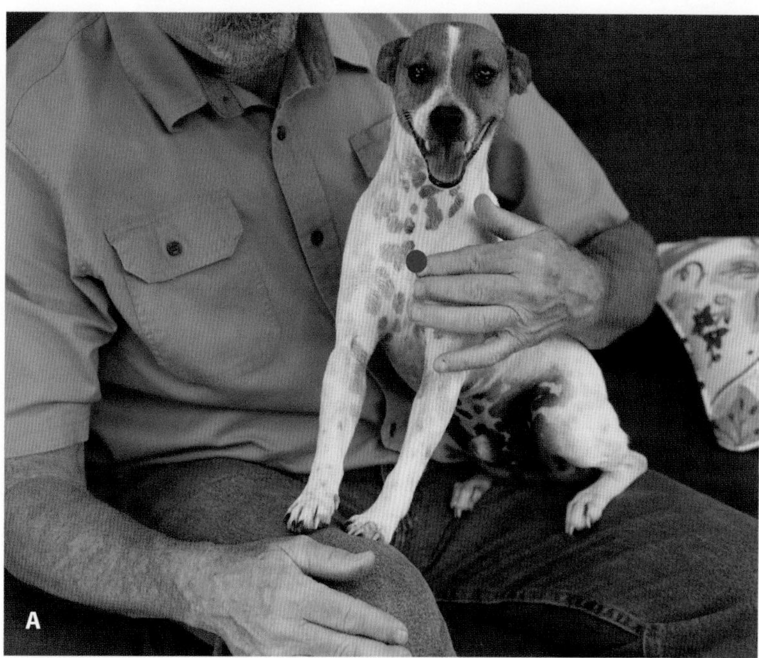

5.8 A–C The point of the sternum (A). For the sternum-pectoral attachments, search along each side of it (B). For the forelimb-pectoral attachments, search from inside the point of the shoulder down to inside the elbow (C).

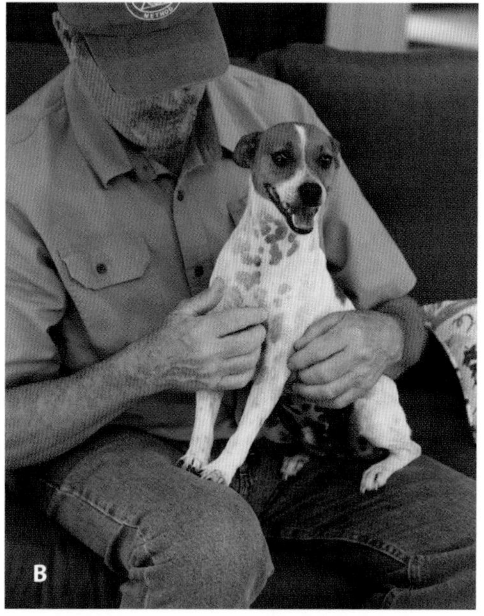

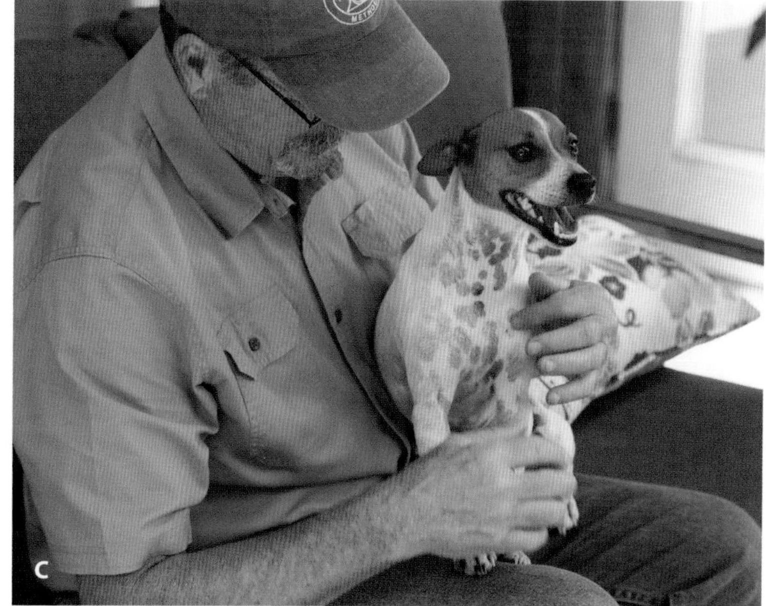

Scan to view Scapula, Trunk, Sternum, and Pectoral Points video

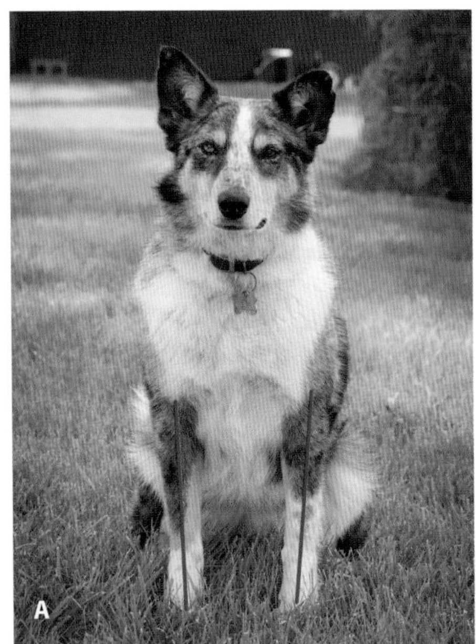

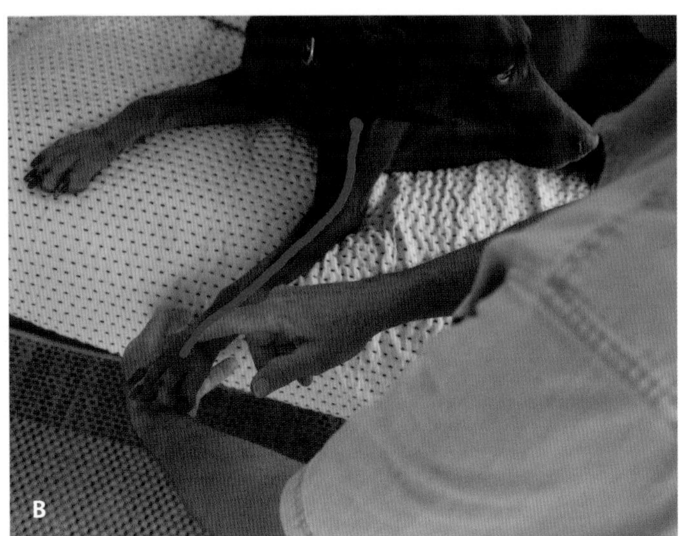

5.9 A & B The lower forelimb points (A). Start at the point of shoulder and go to the tips of the toes (B).

How to Know If You're in the Right Place

The space between the forelimb and the sternum can be small, making it difficult to determine whether you're precisely on the attachment at the sternum end of the pectoral muscle or the attachment at the forelimb end of the pectoral muscle.

There's a trick to making it less difficult: *Don't worry about it!* Your intention makes a difference. That's why it's helpful to have just a basic mental picture of what you're working on.

- If your intention is to *Search* on the sternum end of the pectorals, that's where the dog will feel it.
- If your intention is to *Search* on the forelimb end of the pectorals, that's where the dog will feel it.
- If your intention is to *Search* in the area between the forelimb and the sternum, that's where the dog will feel it.

Your dog's *Responses* will tell you. When he's responding, you're in the right place. Doubt the doubt.

Lower Forelimb Points

(shoulder joint, elbow, carpus, toes, extensors and flexors, metacarpal tendons and ligaments)

To find these points, trace a line from the point of the shoulder down the front of the leg to the metacarpals, paw, and toes (figs. 5.9 A & B). These points are very sensitive. If you use any pressure at all, your dog won't show you any *Responses*. *Search* by barely touching the tips of your fingertips to the hairs.

Choose a place to begin: Scapula Trunk Points, Sternum and Pectoral Points, or Lower Forelimb Points (see the following Quick Overview for the Sternum and Pectoral Points as an example).

Quick Overview: Step-by-Step

STERNUM AND PECTORAL POINTS

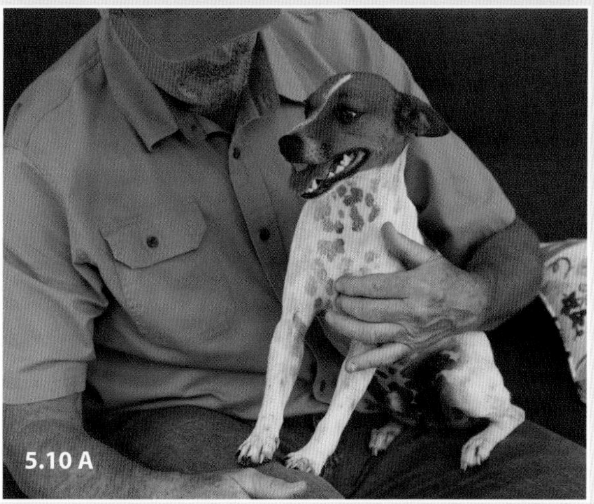

5.10 A

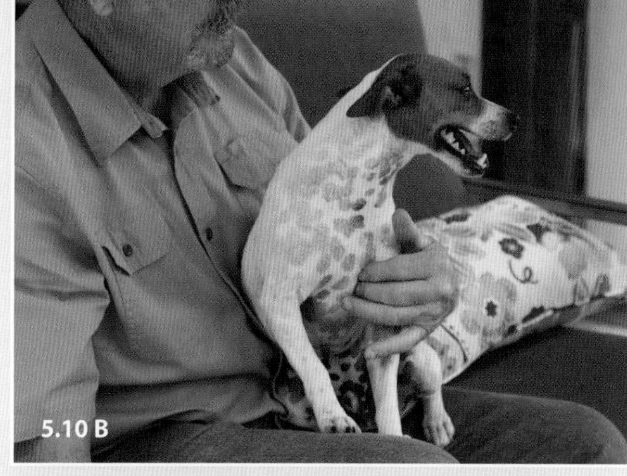

5.10 B

Step 1. *Search*. Using the tip of either one or two fingers, barely touching the hair, slowly (I said SLOWLY) and gently *Search* with your fingertip(s) in the area of the points (fig. 5.10 A). Your dog will tell you exactly where to stop when you get a…

Step 2. *Response.* Watch closely for a blink or other change of behavior—in this case, *looking away* (fig. 5.10 B).

Step 3. *Stay*. Keep your finger over that spot, maintaining Air Gap. Resist the urge to move the finger, push, rub, or stroke. This may take one second or one minute. Be patient. Breathe and relax, until you get a…

Step 4. *Release*, such as licking and chewing or yawning.

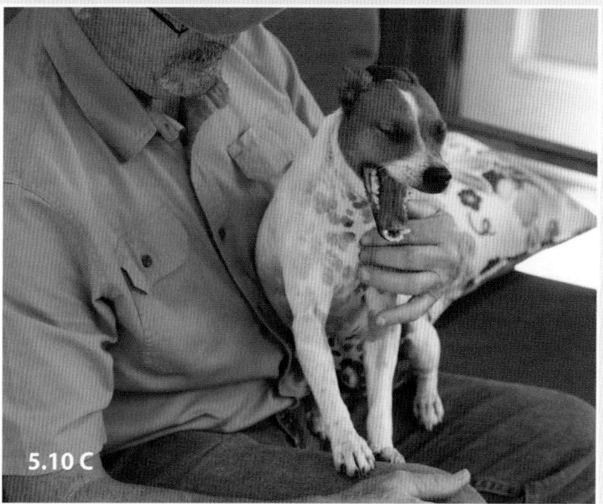

5.10 C

When you are finished, you can either repeat the process on the opposite side or continue the process in one of the other areas on the same side (fig. 5.10 C).

Case Study

DIFFERENT TYPES OF RESPONSES

Notice while *Searching* that your dog's *Response* may not always be a blink but can be any noticeable shift in behavior such as looking away or suddenly looking uncomfortable (figs. 5.11 B and E). This is a sign that the dog is feeling something and you should try *Staying* there to see what happens.

Notice also that the *Release* may not always be accompanied by a lick or a chew or a sneeze or a yawn. After *Staying* on the spot, you may get another shift in behavior such as suddenly relaxing or lying down. This is sometimes the *Release* (figs. 5.11 C and F).

For example, Izzy was guarded during the session and didn't want to show outward signs that she was feeling anything. If you're patient, stay light with your touch, follow the subtle signs, and trust that it's working, your dog will reward you—or rather you'll reward your dog—with a release of tension that she's been holding and guarding. This was her particular pattern of *Responses* that day.

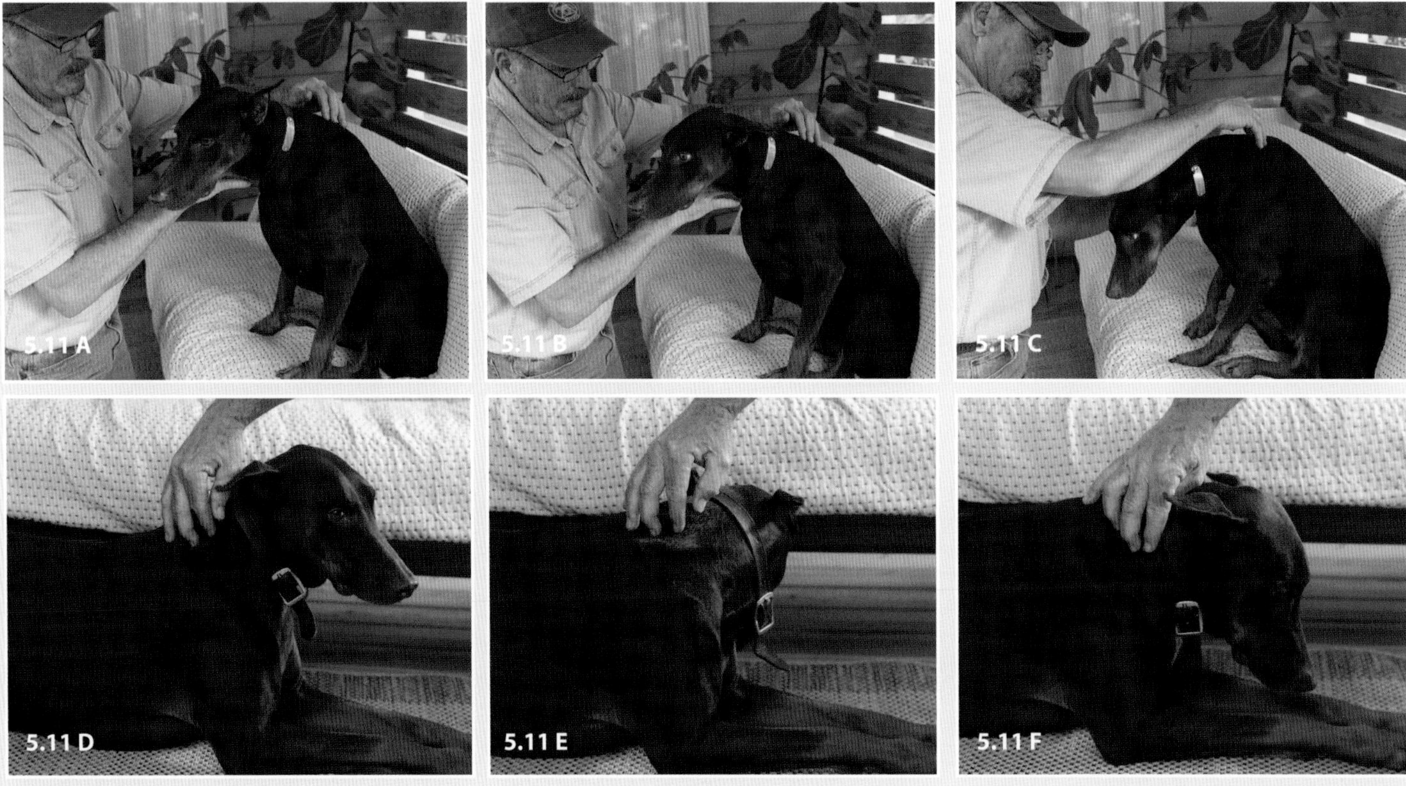

5.11 A 5.11 B 5.11 C

5.11 D 5.11 E 5.11 F

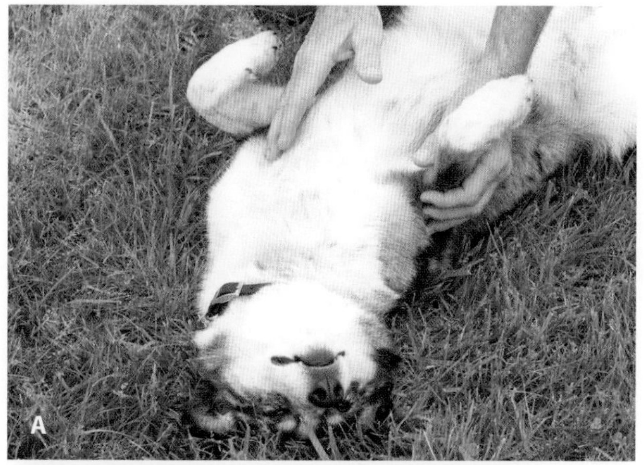

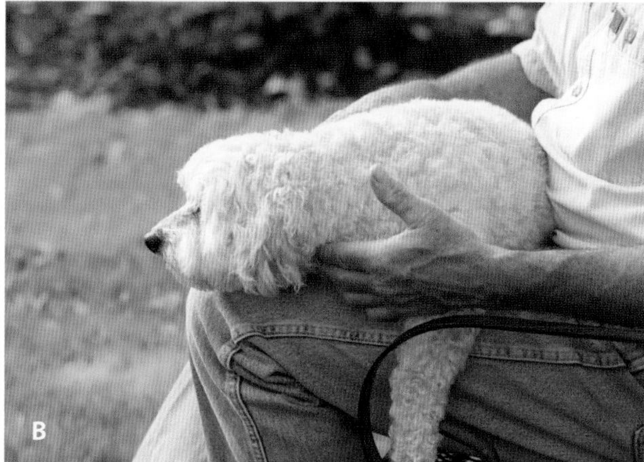

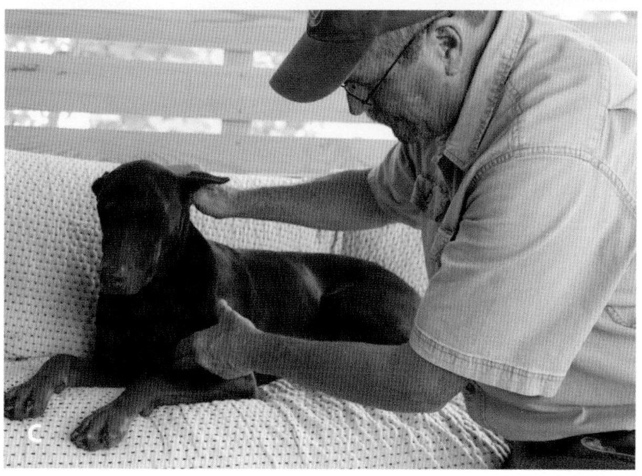

Tips

As you can see, these *Search, Response, Stay, Release* points can be done with your dog–and you—in various positions (figs. 5.12 A–C). Basically, wherever he—and you, to some degree—are comfortable.

Movement Techniques

GOAL: *Movement Techniques* look for *Responses* while moving the scapula and upper and lower forelimbs through specific ranges of motion in a relaxed state.

There are different ways you can position yourself and the dog to do these Techniques. The three most common are:

- With you facing the dog and working with the leg on the *near side*.
- With the dog sitting or standing and you working with the leg on the *opposite side*.
- With the dog lying on his side, and you working with the leg on the *upward-facing side*.

It's often easier when working with larger dogs to face the dog and work with the leg on the *near side*.

5.12 A–C Working with *Search, Response, Stay, Release* on the ground (A), on your lap (B), and on the couch (C).

SCAPULA AND FORELIMB MOVEMENTS—*NEAR SIDE*

(Shown facing the dog and working with the leg on the near side.)

Step 1. Sit or kneel facing your dog. Position yourself in close so you're not pulling the dog off balance when you lift the leg.

Step 2. Place one hand under the dog's elbow. This is the "elbow hand." Lifting under the elbow encourages him to slightly extend and relax the leg.

Step 3. Place your other hand under the forelimb above the wrist. This is the "forelimb hand."

Step 4. Soften both hands. Gently lift upward with both hands just enough to allow the dog's leg to relax into your hand. This is the *neutral* position (fig. 5.13). Remember, if the dog tenses or starts to pull his leg away, soften and yield.

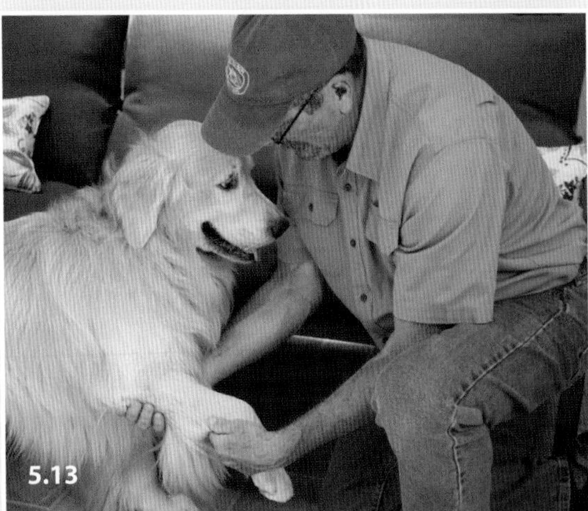

5.13

Scapula Raise and Lower—Near Side

Step 1. When you feel the leg is as relaxed as possible (neutral position), slowly take the weight of the elbow and scapula *upward* with the elbow hand so the scapula slides gently upward along the dog's trunk (fig. 5.14 A). Watch his eye for a blink. When you see a blink, pause at that position for just a second. A blink is a sign that he's feeling something. On a large dog, you would be lifting less than an inch.

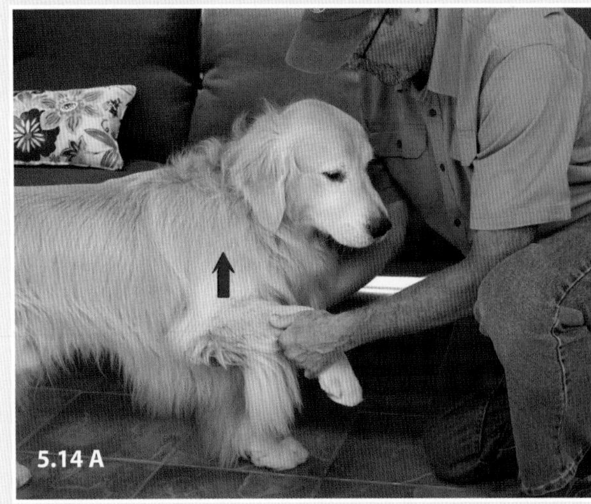

5.14 A

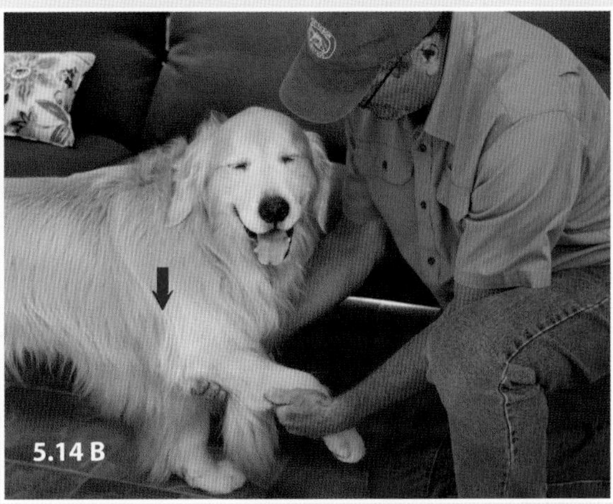
5.14 B

Step 2. Slowly lower the elbow and scapula to the neutral position while supporting the weight of the leg, watching for a *blink* (fig. 5.14 B).

Step 3. With the dog's leg relaxed in the *neutral* position, slowly lower your hands, allowing the scapula to drop an inch.

Step 4. When the dog is comfortable with this, continue to slowly raise and lower the scapula, gently increasing the range of motion as you search for *blinks*.

Forelimb Forward, Back, and Lateral—Near Side

Step 1. With your hands in the same position and the leg relaxed in the *neutral* position, gently extend the leg *forward*. Remember to support the weight of the leg as much as you can. Use the elbow hand to bring the elbow forward to straighten the leg. The dog should be relaxing the scapula and leg forward as you watch for the blink. Don't pull. It's not a stretch (fig. 5.15 A).

Step 2. Gently bring the leg and scapula *back* toward the hind end of the dog. Watch for the blink.

Note: It's sometimes easier to face the other direction when bringing the leg to the side or back. Find the position that's easiest for you and the dog (fig. 5.15 B).

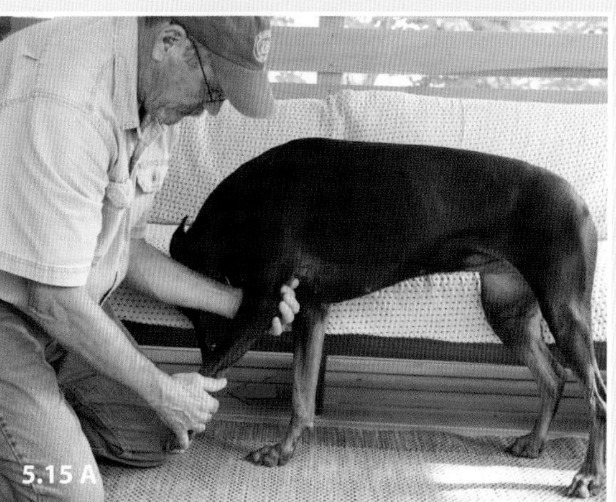
5.15 A

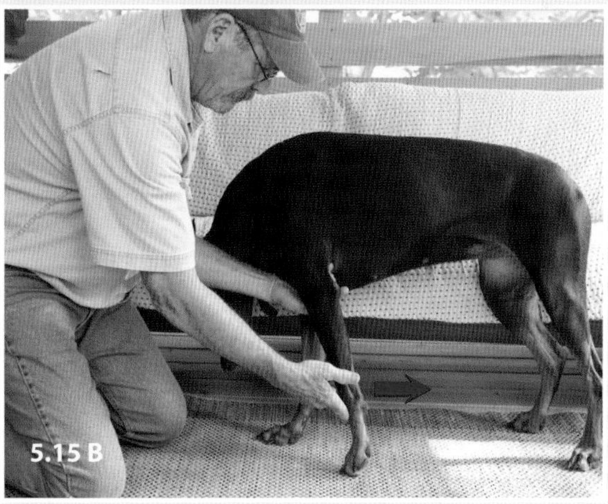
5.15 B

Scan to view Scapula Raise and Lower video

SCAPULA AND FORELIMB MOVEMENTS (continued)

Scan to view Forelimb Forward, Back, and Lateral video

Step 3. With one hand inside the elbow and the other inside the lower limb, gently bring the leg *laterally*, or out to the side (fig. 5.15 C). Remember, this is not a stretch, it is a movement in a state of relaxation. Support the weight of the leg as much as you can and watch for the blink.

Set the leg down and see what the dog "has to say." If he needs to move, walk around, yawn, or stretch, let him. When you are finished on this side, you can repeat the process on the opposite side or move on to another area altogether.

Remember the "No Thumbs" Rule (see p. 15) when handling the leg. This will eliminate the tendency to grab or pull on the forelimb.

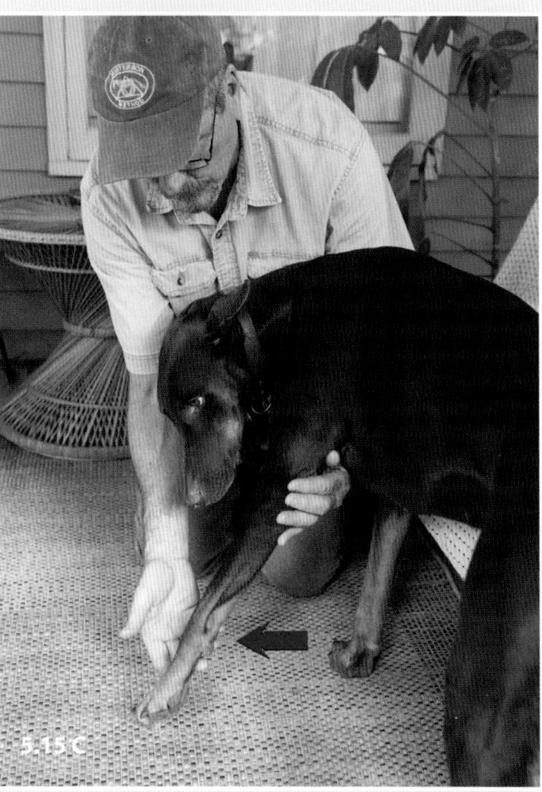

5.15 C

SCAPULA AND FORELIMB MOVEMENTS—*OPPOSITE SIDE*

(Shown working with the leg on the opposite side.)

Here, the steps are the same, except that you sit next to the dog or with the dog on your lap, reaching over and around him to work with the opposite leg. Let's start with the right leg (fig. 5.16).

Step 1. Position yourself next to your dog's left shoulder, or with your dog sitting on your lap facing forward. It's okay to have your body in contact with the dog's.

Step 2. Reach over the top of the dog with your right arm and cup your right hand under the dog's right elbow (elbow hand).

Step 3. Reach around the front of the dog with your left arm and use your left hand to support the dog's forelimb above the wrist (forelimb hand).

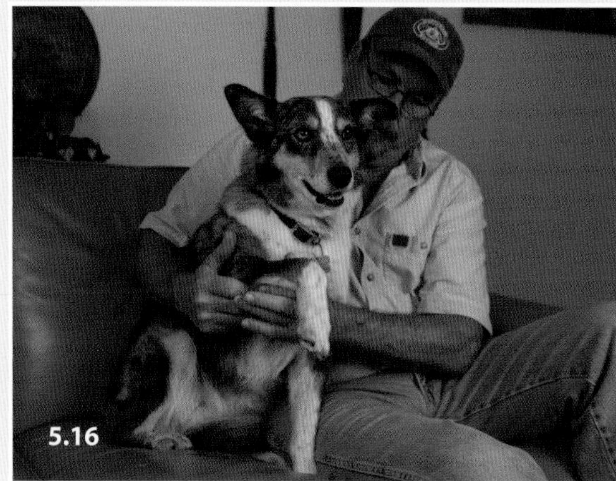

5.16

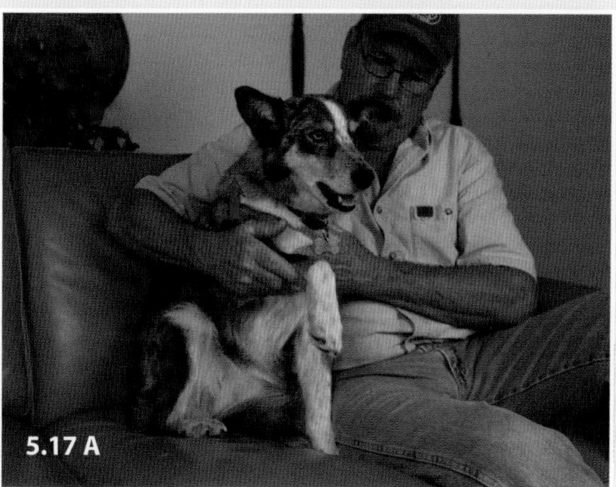

5.17 A

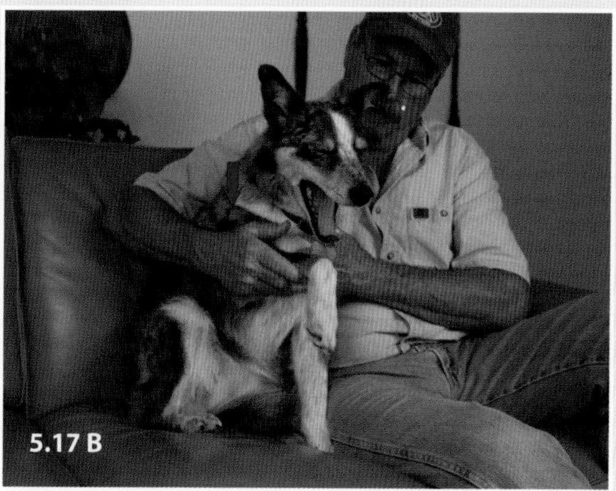

5.17 B

Step 4. Soften both hands and allow the dog's elbow to relax into your elbow hand. You can encourage the dog to relax by gently lifting upward on the elbow until you feel some weight in your hand (neutral position).

Scapula Raise and Lower—Opposite Side

Step 1. When you feel the leg is as relaxed as possible (neutral position), slowly take the weight of the elbow and scapula upward with the elbow hand so the scapula slides gently upward along the dog's trunk (fig. 5.17 A).

Step 2. Slowly lower the elbow and scapula to the neutral position while supporting the weight of the leg, watching for a blink, or in this case, a *Release Response* (fig. 5.17 B).

If the dog is comfortable, you can continue to slowly raise and lower the scapula.

Forelimb Forward, Back, and Lateral—Opposite Side

Step 1. With your hands in the same position, once the leg is relaxed, gently extend the leg forward. Remember to support the weight of the leg as much as you can (fig. 5.18 A).

Step 2. Next, gently bring the leg toward the hind end of the dog. You may wrap the fingers of your

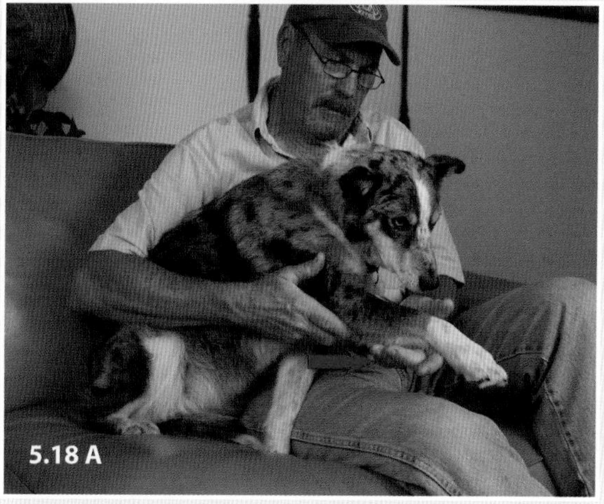

5.18 A

SCAPULA AND FORELIMB MOVEMENTS (continued)

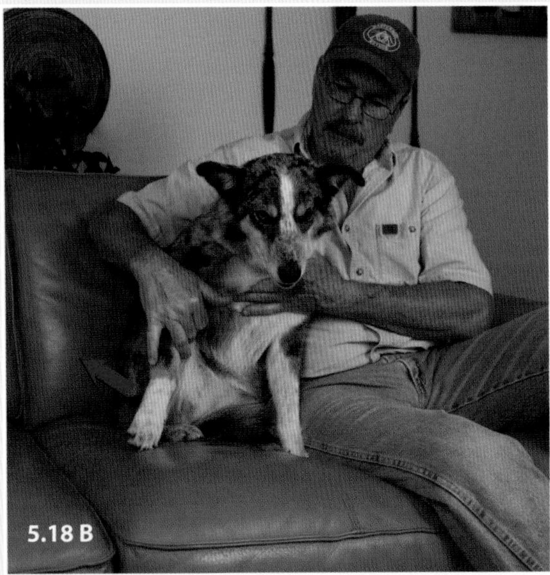

5.18 B

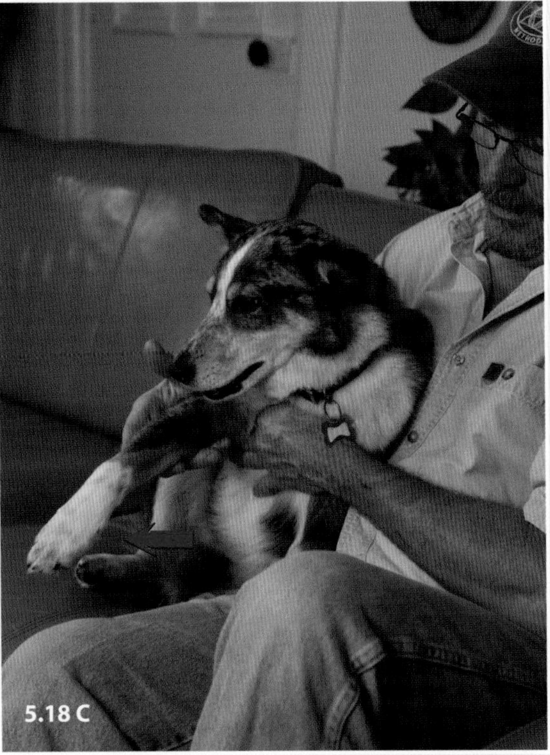

5.18 C

elbow hand around the front of the elbow to help bring the leg back (fig. 5.18 B).

Step 3. Supporting the weight of the leg, gently bring the leg lateral, or out to the side. Remember, this is not a stretch. Again, the blink will tell you where to pause and hold for a second (fig. 5.18 C).

Be Especially Gentle with Older Dogs

An older dog's scapula may have more stiffness and less range of motion. Start the movement more gently and limit the movement. Feel your way through it. As the dog relaxes, you can ask for more. If he tenses, ask for less.

And remember, NO THUMBS when handling legs!

SCAPULA AND FORELIMB MOVEMENTS—*DOG LYING DOWN*

(Shown working with the dog lying down.)

This is essentially the same as working with the leg on the same or near side, except that he is lying on his side. To give the scapula room to move, the dog must be lying flat on his side.

Step 1. Position yourself sitting or kneeling at his front end.

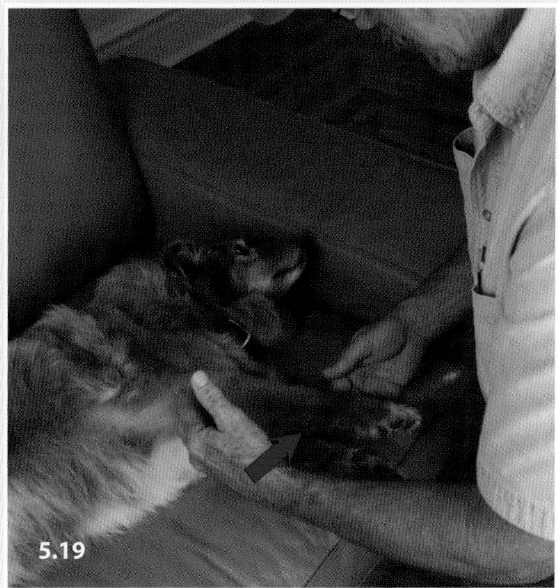

5.19

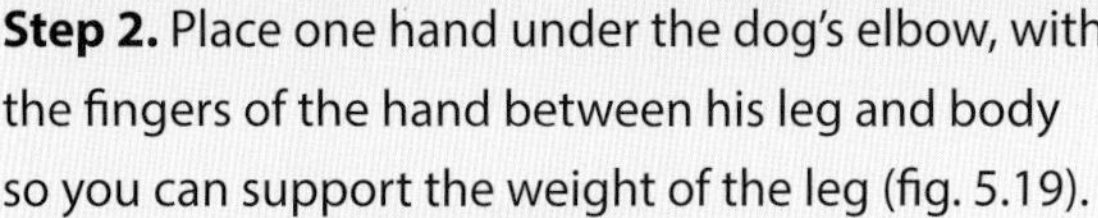

Step 2. Place one hand under the dog's elbow, with the fingers of the hand between his leg and body so you can support the weight of the leg (fig. 5.19).

Step 3. Gently place the other hand around the forearm above the wrist (no thumbs).

Step 4. Soften both hands and gently take the weight of the forelimb (neutral position).

Scapula Raise and Lower—Dog Lying Down

Step 1. When you feel the leg is as relaxed as possible (neutral position), use both hands to slowly slide the elbow and scapula upward so the scapula gently slides along the dog's trunk, watching for blinks (fig. 5.20).

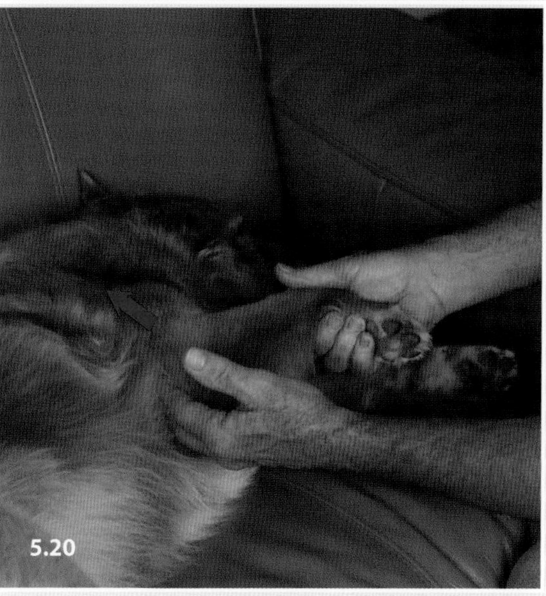

5.20

Step 2. Slowly lower the elbow and scapula to the neutral position while supporting the weight of the leg. If the dog is comfortable with this, you can continue to slowly raise and lower the scapula.

Forelimb Forward, Back, and Lateral—Dog Lying Down

Step 1. With one hand under the elbow and the other under the lower forelimb, gently extend the leg forward (fig. 5.21 A).

Step 2. With one hand under the elbow and the other under the forelimb, gently bring the leg back (fig. 5.21 B).

Step 3. Use both hands to gently bring the leg out to the side away from the dog. Keep the leg relaxed

SCAPULA AND FORELIMB MOVEMENTS (continued)

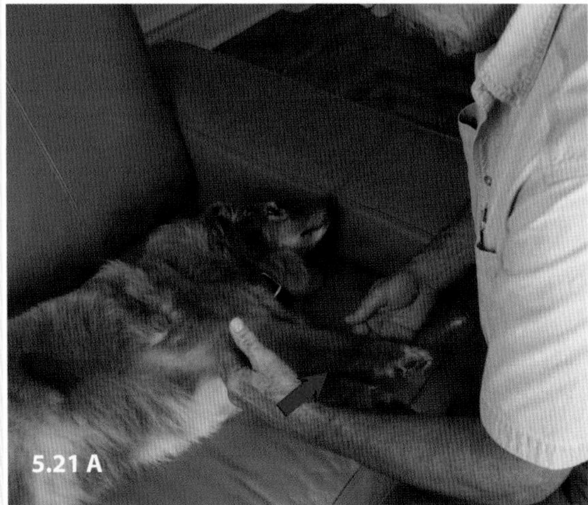
5.21 A

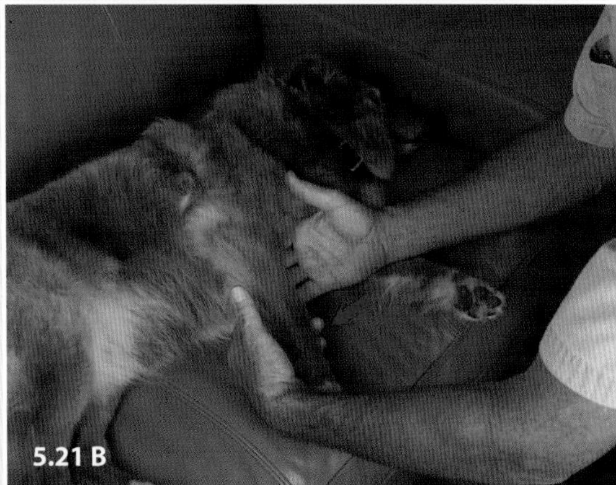
5.21 B

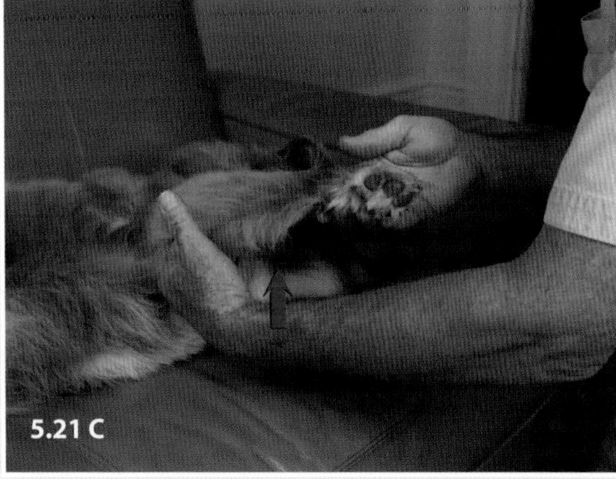
5.21 C

by supporting its weight as much as you can. Again, the blink will tell you where to pause and hold for a second (fig. 5.21 C).

Working with Tiny Dogs

Note that when working with tiny dogs, the scapula and forelimb movements are the same except, of course, much smaller. You'll often end up using your fingers instead of your hands (fig. 5.22).

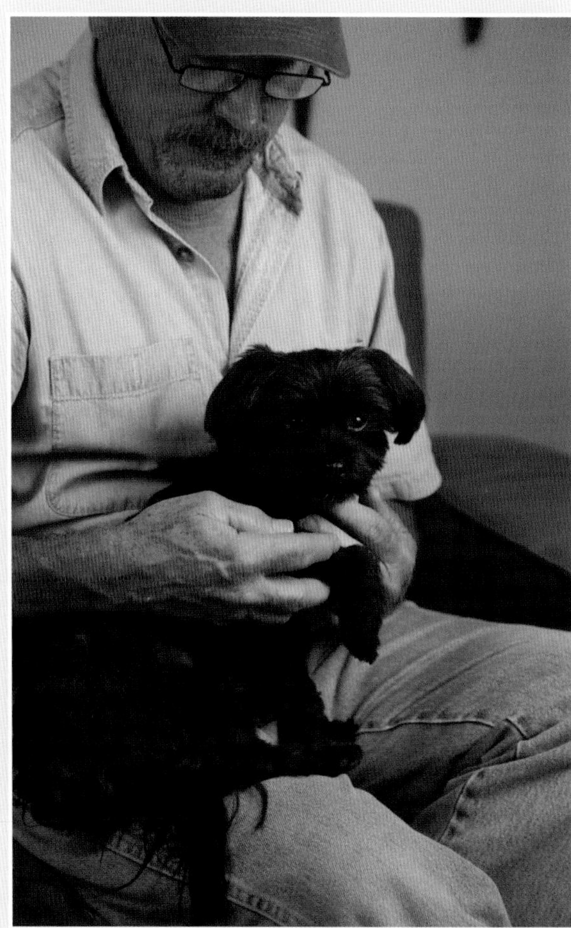

5.22 Gently bring the leg out to the side (lateral) with your fingers.

Body Language

Many dogs are uncomfortable having their front legs or paws grabbed or even held. It could be that their legs have been pulled on when trying to get away in the past, they could have sore front paws, or they might just not like their paws being handled. Be very soft and gentle when first asking for the legs, and be ready to soften and yield immediately if the dog pulls away (figs. 5.23 A & B). And remember, no grabbing!

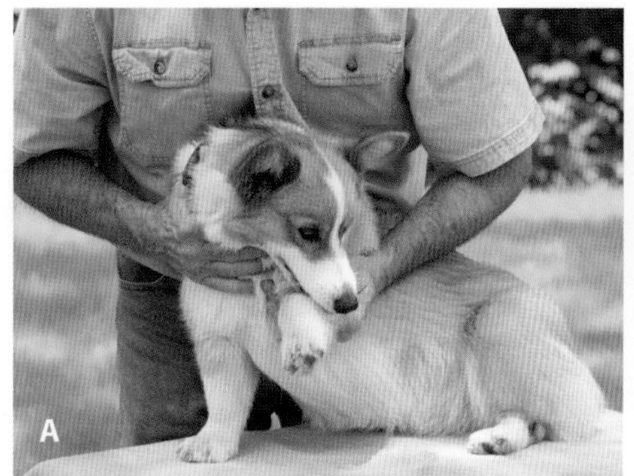

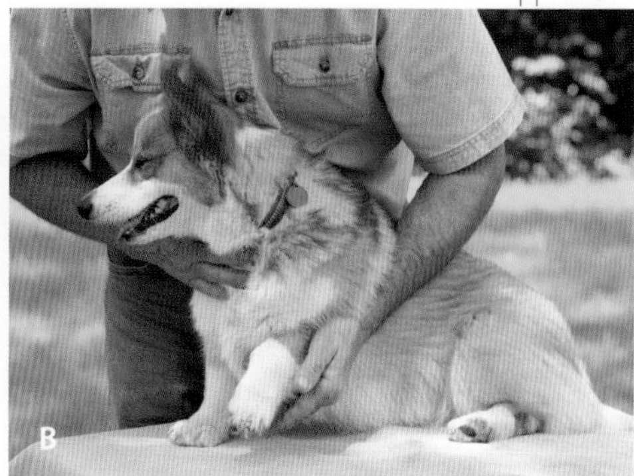

5.23 A & B A worried dog (A) and a trusting, happy dog (B).

Some dogs are intimidated when faced with someone directly in front of them. Remember, they don't know what you're doing when you first approach them with this, and they may be more afraid than you think. Adjust accordingly.

On the other hand, many dogs are uneasy with an unfamiliar person unless they are facing each other. The dogs want to keep an eye on the human at all times. This often happens with dogs who are uncomfortable in their hind end when you are working on them. They want to see what you're up to.

The important thing is that you pay attention to what the dog is saying about his comfort level by paying attention to his body language (figs. 5.23 C–F).

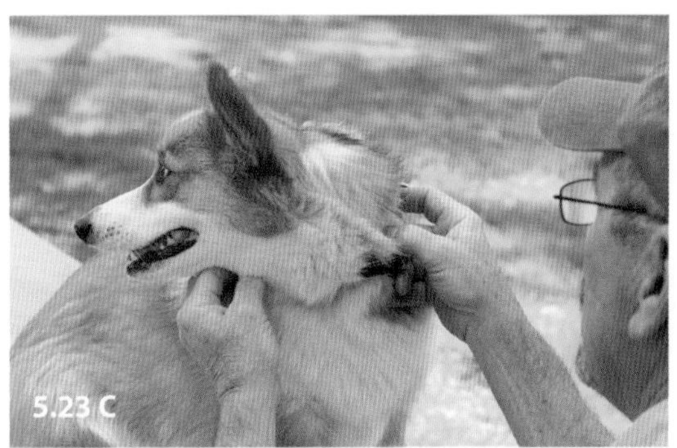

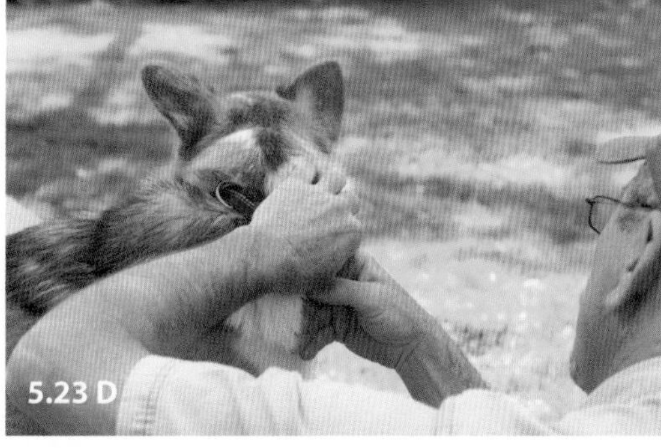

5.24 C–F The dog saying, "Face way too close" (C), "Still too close" (D), "A little better…but still too close" (E), and, "Thank you. Now I can relax" (F).

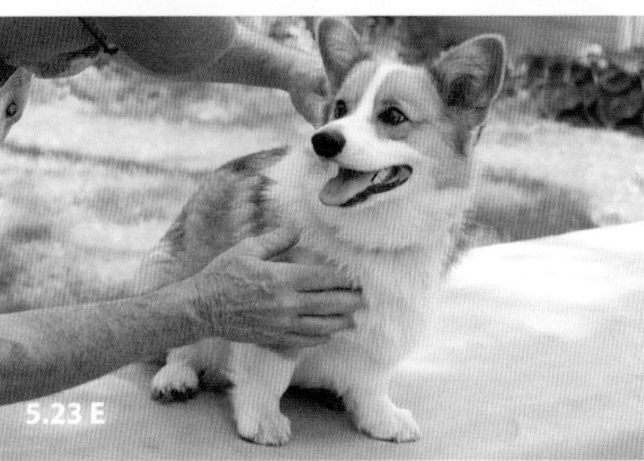

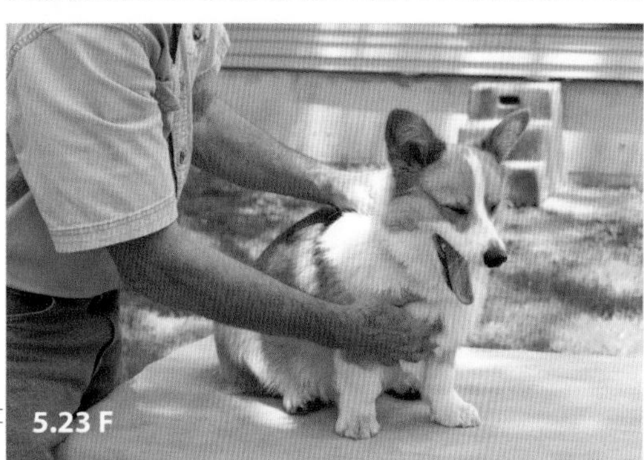

Quick Overview: Step-by-Step

LOWER FORELIMB MOVEMENT

LOWER FORELIMB MOVEMENT—*NEAR SIDE*

(Shown facing the dog and working with the leg on the near side.)

Step 1. Sit, kneel, or stand facing the dog. Position yourself in close so you're not pulling the dog off balance when you lift the leg.

Step 2. Place one hand under the dog's elbow to lift the leg, and the other under the wrist or paw to support the leg. Lifting under the elbow encourages him to slightly extend and relax the leg (neutral position).

Remember, if the dog tenses or starts to pull his leg away, soften and yield (fig. 5.24).

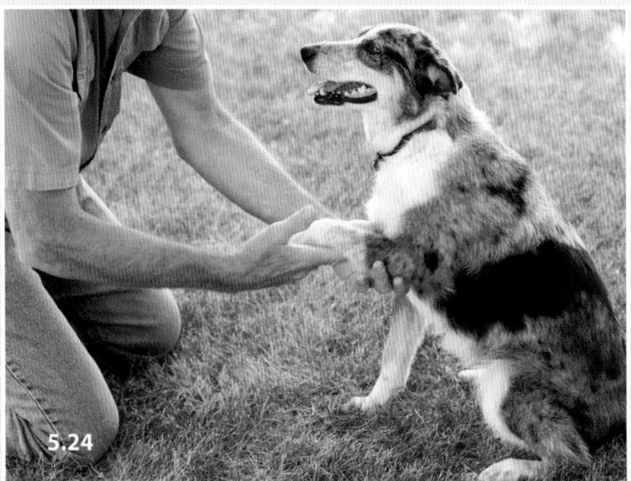

5.24

Metacarpal Movement (Flexors and Extensors)—Near Side

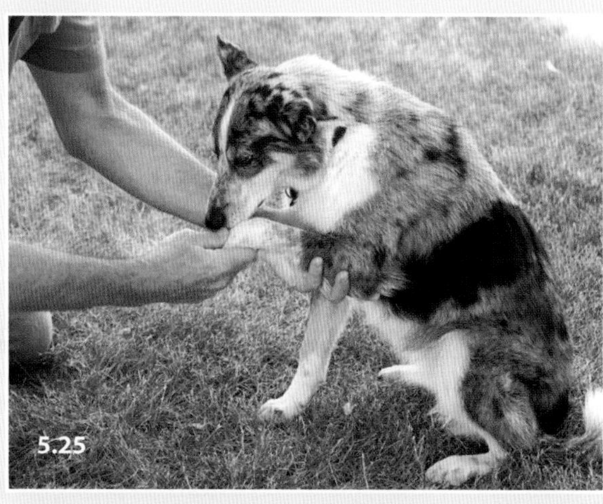

5.25

Step 1. Place the thumb of your paw hand on top of the wrist or carpal joint, as shown.

Step 2. When the leg is as relaxed as possible, slowly move the wrist through a gentle range of up-and-down and circular movements with the paw hand (fig. 5.25). Watch for the blink.

Step 3. When you get a blink, gently move the wrist through that point in the movement, continuing to watch for the blink.

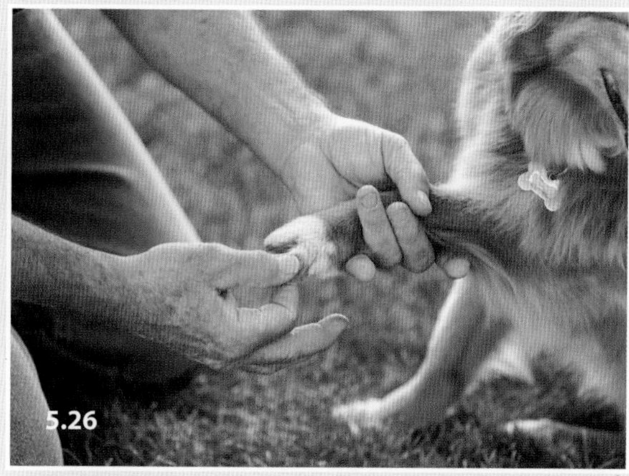

5.26

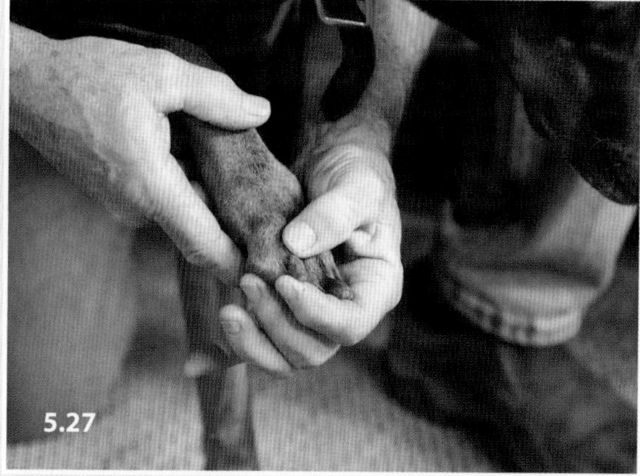

5.27

Toe Micromovement (Flexors and Extensors)—Near Side

Step 1. While continuing to support the leg with the leg hand, gently slide the thumb and fingers of the paw hand down to the toes (fig. 5.26).

Step 2. Using *very soft* fingers, gently wiggle each of the toes and toenails through a tiny range of motion, continuing to watch for the blinks.

Set the leg down and see what the dog "has to say." If he needs to move, walk around, yawn, or stretch, let him.

LOWER FORELIMB MOVEMENT—*OPPOSITE SIDE*

(Working with the leg on the opposite side.)

Here the steps are the same, except you'll be kneeling next to the dog or sitting with the dog on your lap, reaching around and under the dog to work with the opposite leg. Let's start with the left leg.

Step 1. Position yourself next to your dog's left shoulder or with your dog sitting on your lap facing forward.

Step 2. Reach over the top of the dog with your right arm and cup your right hand under the dog's (opposite) elbow.

Step 3. Reach around the front of the dog with your left arm and use your left hand to support the dog's foreleg under the wrist or paw (fig. 5.27).

Step 4. Soften both hands and allow the dog's elbow to relax into your leg hand (neutral position).

Metacarpal Movement—Opposite Side

Step 1. Place the thumb of your paw hand on top of the wrist or carpal joint, as shown.

Step 2. When the leg is as relaxed as possible,

LOWER FORELIMB MOVEMENT (continued)

Scan to view Lower Forelimb Movements video

slowly move the wrist through a gentle range of up-and-down and circular movements with the paw hand (fig. 5.28). Watch for the blink.

Step 3. When you get a blink, gently move the wrist through that point in the movement, continuing to watch for the blink.

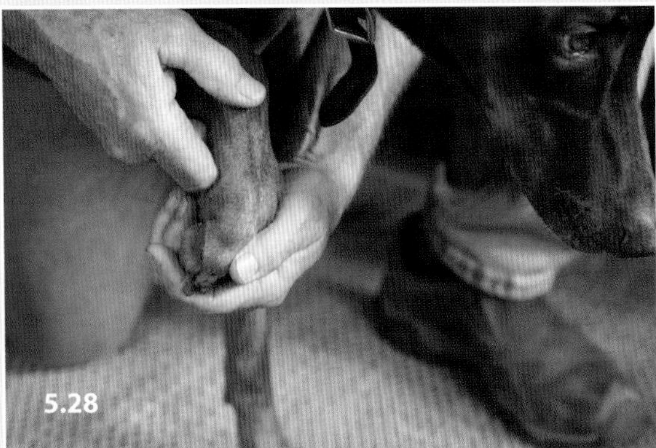

5.28

Toe Micromovement—Opposite Side

Step 1. While continuing to support the leg with the leg hand, gently slide the thumb and fingers of the paw hand down to the toes.

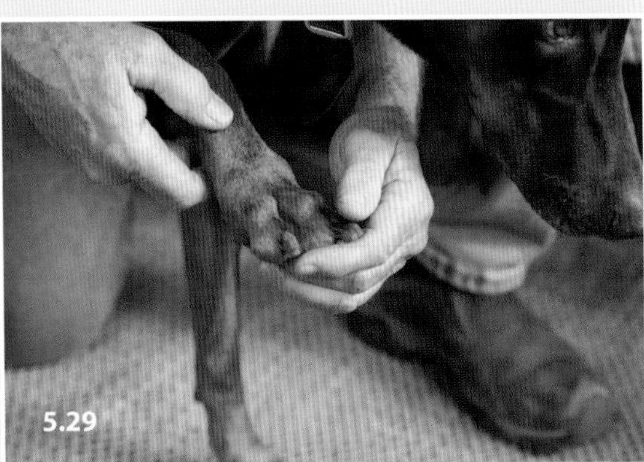

5.29

Step 2. Using very soft fingers, gently wiggle each of the toes and toenails through a tiny range of motion, continuing to watch for the blinks (fig. 5.29).

Working with Tiny Dogs

The metacarpal and toe movements with tiny dogs are the same, except, of course, much tinier. You'll usually end up using one hand for the movements and one hand to hold the dog (figs. 5.30 A & B). (Yes, we know she's cute!)

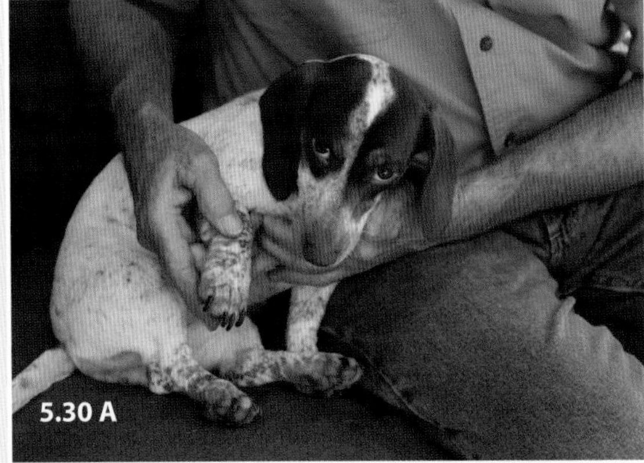

5.30 A

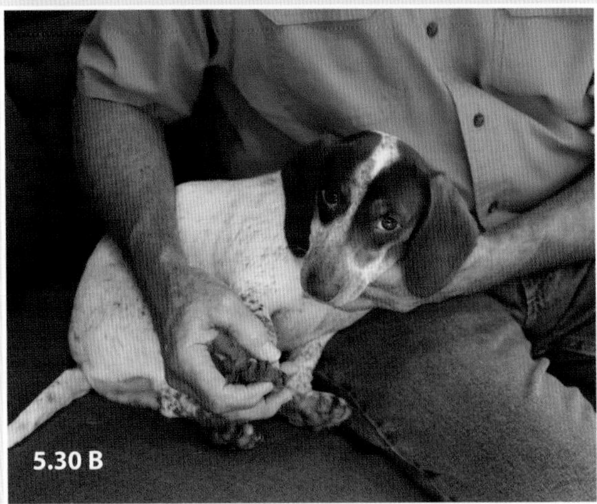

5.30 B

5.30 A & B Tiny metacarpals (A) and tiny toes (B).

More Body Language

You'd be surprised how sensitive and tender your dog's paws and toes can be. They're small; they have a lot of joints, tendons, and ligaments; they support the entire weight of the dog; and dogs use them a lot (figs. 5.31 A–E).

Note: Keeping the toenails trimmed, and releasing tension in the forelimbs regularly, will go a long way toward keeping your puppy's paws happy.

And pay attention to what your dog tells you with his body language!

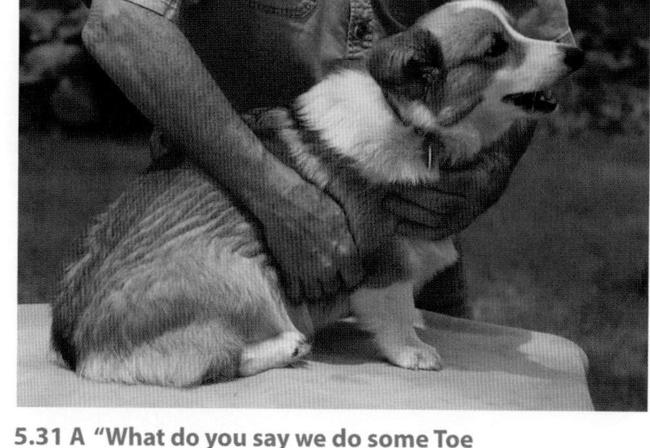

5.31 A "What do you say we do some Toe Micromovements?"

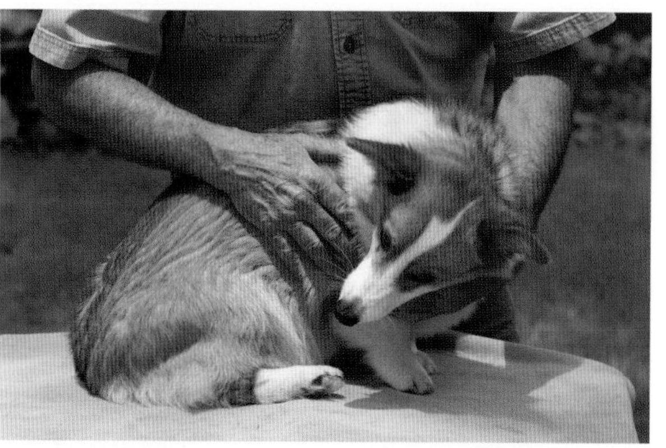

5.31 B "Let's not."

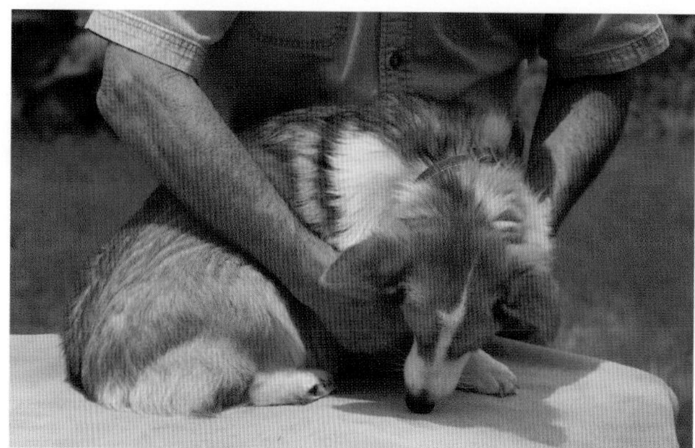

5.31 C "Come on. It'll be fine."

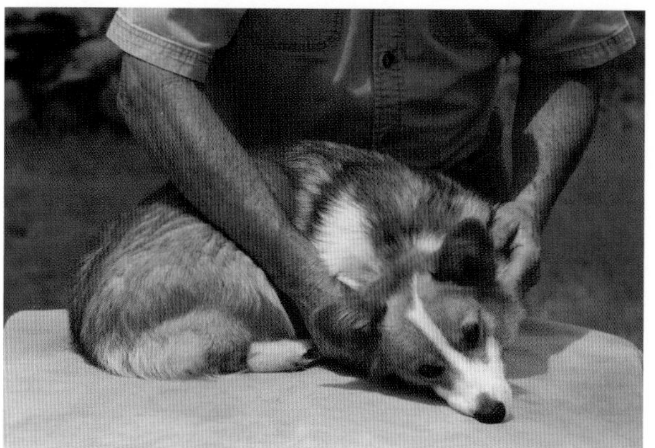

5.31 D "Nope."

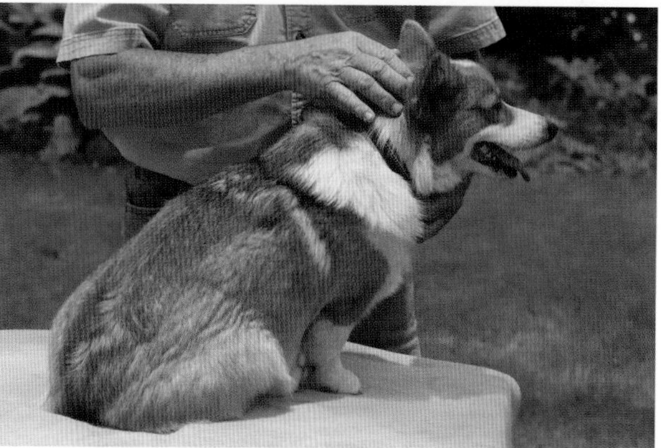

5.31 E "Got it. Let's do something else."

LOWER FORELIMB MOVEMENT—*DOG LYING DOWN*

(Working with the dog lying on his side, and you working with the leg that is on the upward-facing side.)

Let's start with the right leg and the dog lying on his *right* side.

Step 1. Position yourself sitting or kneeling at his front foot.

Step 2. Place your left hand under the dog's forelimb above the wrist.

Step 3. Gently place your right hand around the paw just below the wrist.

Step 4. Place the thumb of your right hand on top of the wrist or carpal joint, as shown (fig. 5.32).

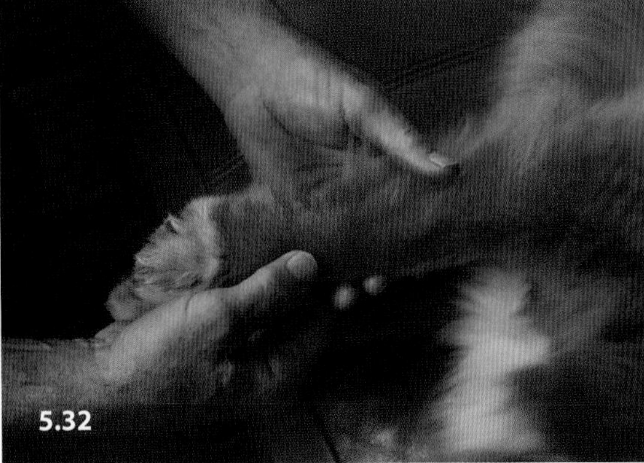

5.32

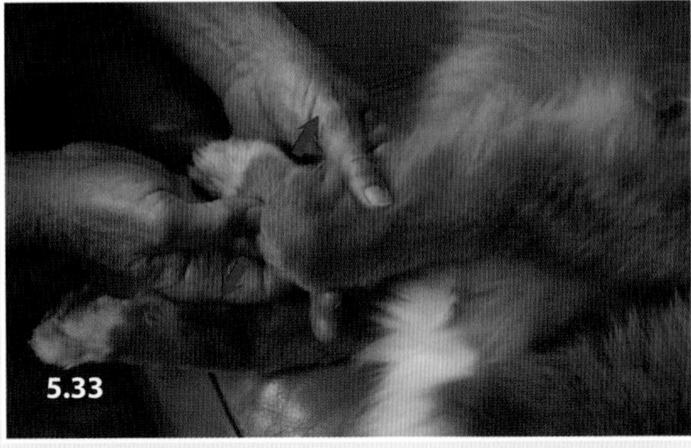

5.33

Metacarpal Movement—Dog Lying Down

Step 1. Slowly move the wrist through a gentle range of up-and-down and circular movements while watching for the blink (fig. 5.33).

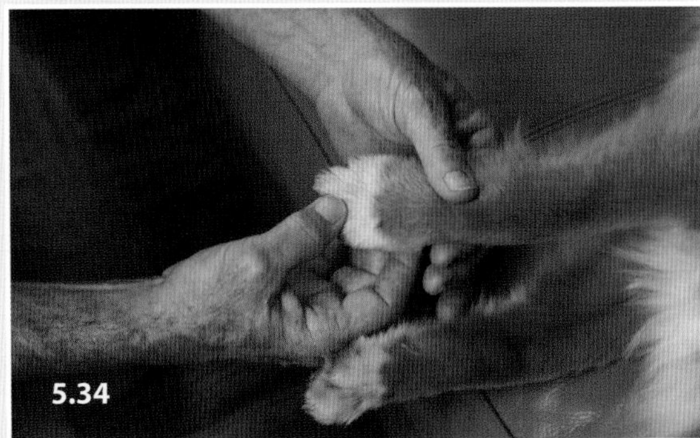

5.34

Toe Micromovement—Dog Lying Down

Step 1. Continuing to support the leg with the leg hand, gently slide the thumb and fingers of the paw hand down to the toes.

Step 2. Using *very soft* fingers, gently wiggle each of the toes and toenails through a tiny range of motion, continuing to watch for the blinks (fig. 5.34).

Movement Techniques While a Dog Is Sleeping

While there can be some benefit to doing Movement Techniques while the dog is sleeping, you'll get the best results doing these while the dog is awake and aware, and he can tell you where tension has accumulated and his nervous system can release it.

Tips

Take a deep breath before starting. When you start out tense, the dog will start out tense also.

Soften your hands, arms, and shoulders before starting any movement. Your muscles and the dog's must be as relaxed as possible.

Watch your dog's eyes. The movement should be slow enough so you can read a blink, or any other *Responses*, as you're going through the movement. The visual *Response* means the dog is feeling something at that point in the movement that he would not normally feel when moving the leg on his own.

Be aware of tensing up in the dog before it happens. The movement must be slow enough so you can feel it before the dog even *starts* to think about tensing (see QR code to a helpful video on this on p. 16).

Remember, the *Movement Techniques* are not stretches, they're *movement through a range of motion* while the limb is in a relaxed state.

Hold, Wait, and Melt Techniques

GOAL: Apply the process of *Hold, Wait, and Melt* to the muscles and connective tissue of the C7-T1 Junction.

WHERE YOU WORK

The C7-T1 Junction is where the lowest cervical (neck) vertebra meets the first thoracic (trunk) vertebra (see figs. 5.2 A & B—p. 70). You access it just under the front of the scapula, on each side of the neck. This can be done with the dog standing but is easier if done while the dog is relaxed and sitting, or even lying down (if not asleep). It can be done with the dog facing you, or with you positioned at the side of the dog, facing forward.

Why Do Smaller Dogs Respond More Quickly?

You'll notice that smaller dogs and younger dogs often respond and release much more quickly than larger or older dogs. There's a reason for this.... We just don't know what it is, but there is one.

Quick Overview: Step-by-Step

C7-T1 RELEASE

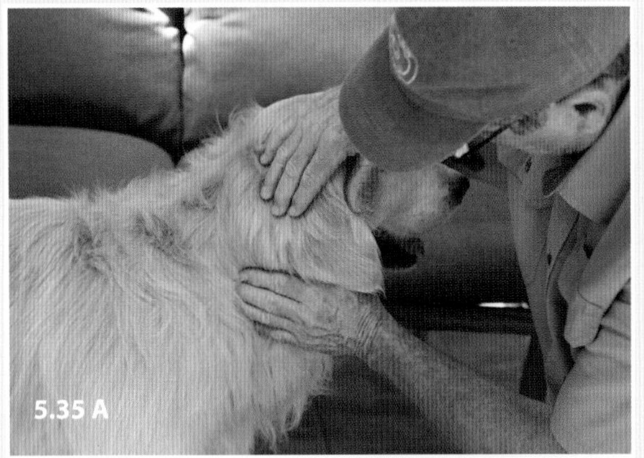
5.35 A

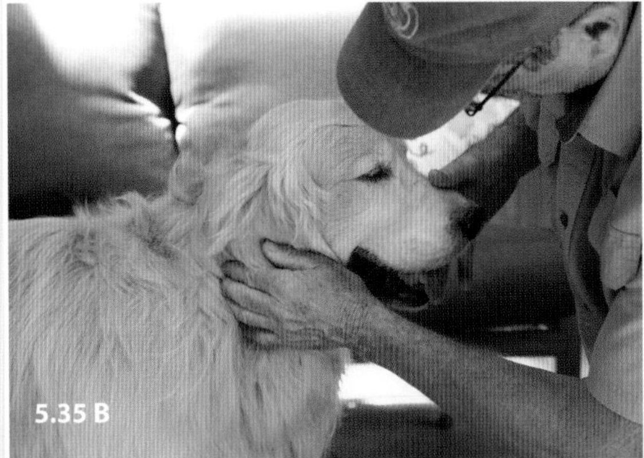
5.35 B

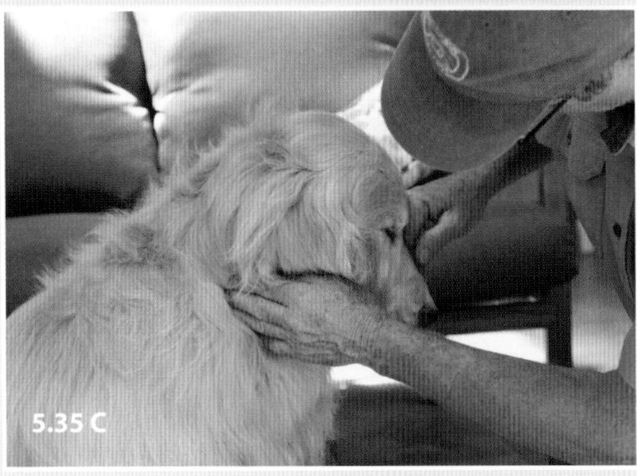
5.35 C

C7-T1 RELEASE—*FACING DOG*

(Let's start with you facing the dog, on the right side.)

Step 1. Position yourself with your dog facing you on the right side, or behind the dog facing forward on the right side.

Step 2. Place the palm of your left hand on the side of the dog's neck with the fingers just in front of the scapula. Using the edge of the last two fingers (fourth and pinky) of your right hand, find the groove where the front of the scapula meets the dog's neck and trunk. C7-T1 is underneath this (fig. 5.35 A).

Step 3. With your other hand, bring his nose slightly toward you to relax the muscles on this side of the neck (fig. 5.35 B).

Step 4. Gently add *Egg Yolk* pressure with the tips of these fingers against the neck in this groove just under the front of the scapula (fig. 5.35 C). Pay close attention to the dog's *Responses*. If you get a blink or subtle *Response*, hold at that subtle level of "pressure." It should be no more than *Egg Yolk*.

Step 5. Gently hold, breathe, and wait.

Step 6. Soften internally and *very slightly* soften the neck hand. When the dog *Releases* he will give you some sign such as licking, yawning, sighing, or lying down (fig. 5.35 D).

Step 7. Release and return to earth.

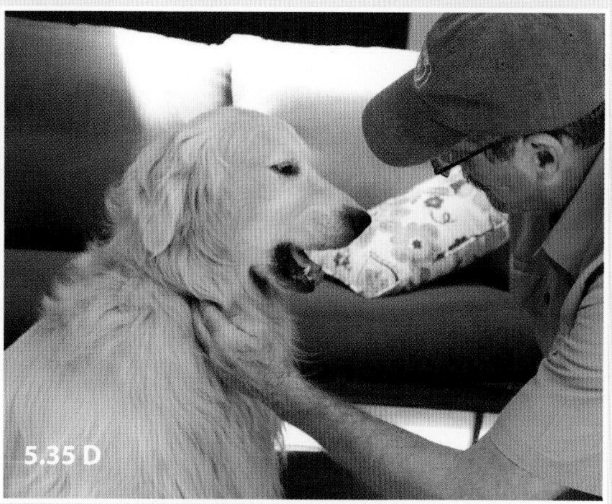

5.35 D

Scan to view C7-T1 Release video

C7-T1 RELEASE— *FACING FORWARD*

(Positioned at the side of your dog, facing forward.)

Step 1. Position yourself at the side of your dog, facing forward.

Step 2. Place the fingertips of your right hand just in front of the scapula on the right side. Find the groove where the front of the scapula meets the dog's neck and trunk—C7-T1 (fig. 5.36 A).

Step 3. With your other hand, bring his nose slightly to the right to relax the muscles on the right side of the neck.

Step 4. Gently add *Egg Yolk* pressure to the groove just under the front of the scapula. Watch for a change in behavior such as a blink or fidget.

Step 5. Gently hold and wait.

Step 6. Soften internally and *very slightly* soften the neck hand.

Step 7. Watch for some sign of *Release* such as licking, yawning, sighing, or, as in this case, lying down (fig. 5.36 B).

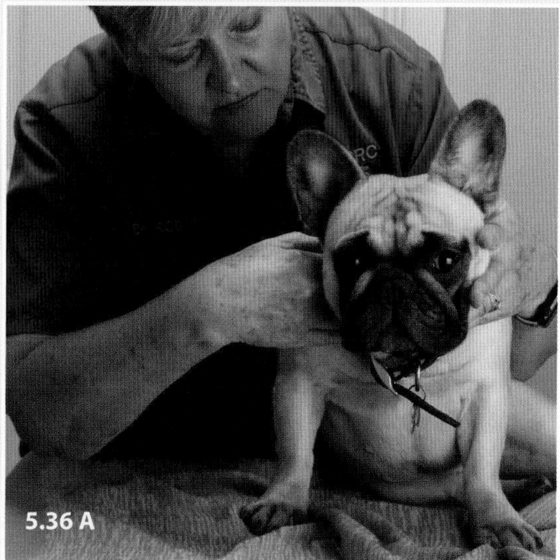

5.36 A

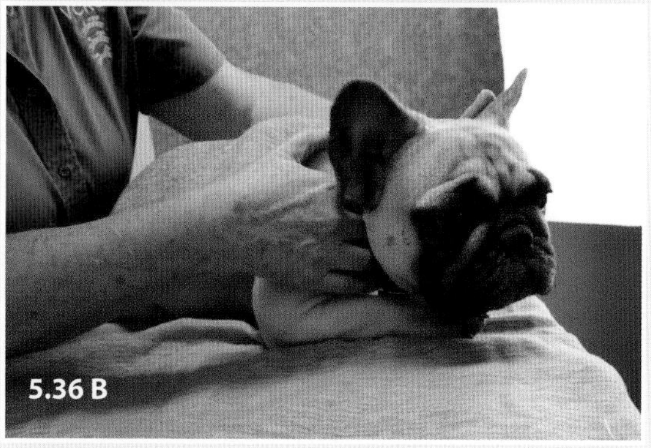

5.36 B

Tips

Remember, you're releasing tension in the muscles and connective tissue of the C7-T1 (Neck-Trunk) Junction underneath the scapula. This is a subtle technique that uses subtle levels of pressure to:

- Bring the dog's awareness to tension in this Junction in a way that he will not become uncomfortable.
- Keep the dog's awareness on it long enough for the nervous system to feel it and *Release* it.

Taking a breath and softening internally during the process helps the dog's nervous system—and yours—"let go."

It's important to use very light pressure and to hold, soften, and wait. If you use force, it won't work. You're allowing the dog's nervous system to do the releasing.

When Your Dog Won't Stay Up

If you have a squiggly dog (for example, Nellie), the C7-T1 Release can also be done while the dog is lying on the floor or ground, with your fingers resting just under the front of the scapula (figs. 5.37 A & B).

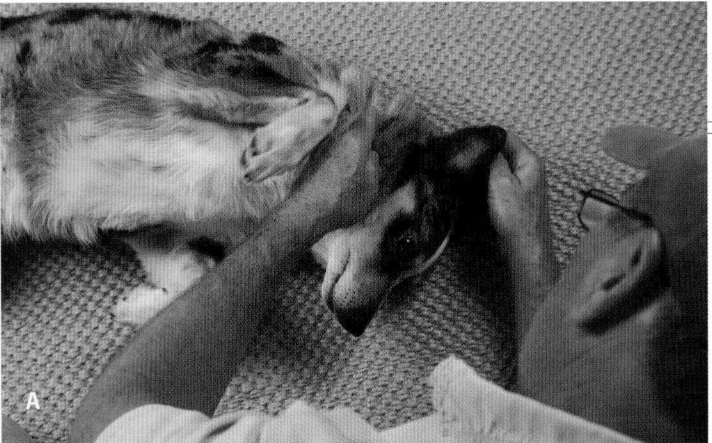

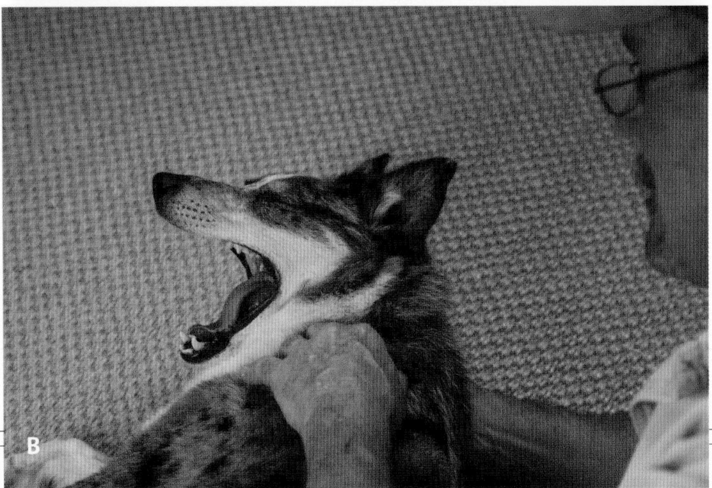

5.37 A & B Rest your fingers just under the front of the scapula (A) and soften (B).

6

CHAPTER 6

The Hind End (Lumbosacral-Pelvic) Junction and Hind Limbs

This chapter discusses the various areas of the Hind End (Lumbosacral-Pelvic) Junction and the hind limbs that accumulate tension, and offers exercises to release tension in these areas using the three categories of techniques that I outlined in Part One: *Search, Response, Stay, Release (SRSR)*, page 4; *Movement Techniques*, page 5; *Hold, Wait, and Melt Techniques (HWM)*, page 6.

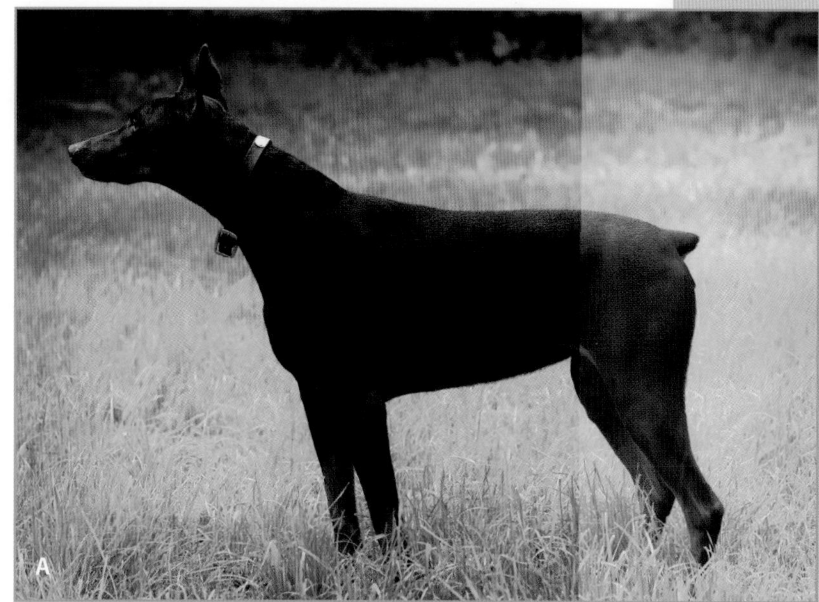

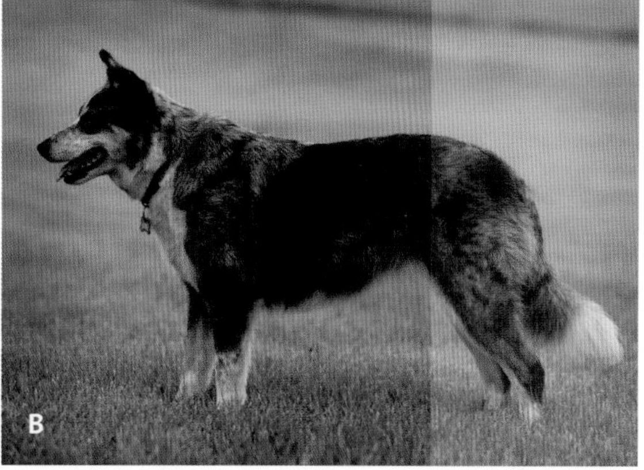

6.1 A & B The Hind End (Lumbosacral-Pelvic) Junction and the hind limbs.

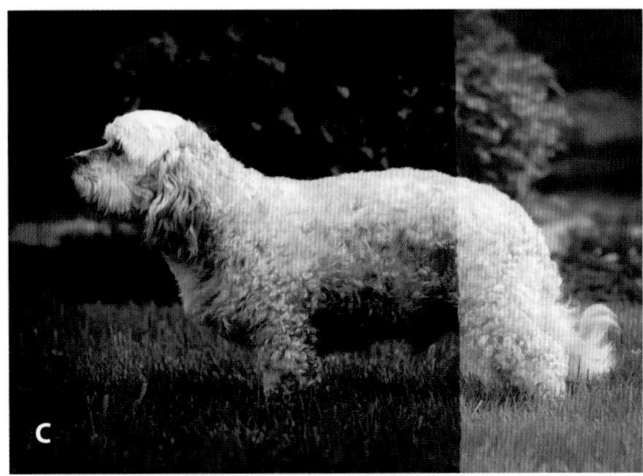

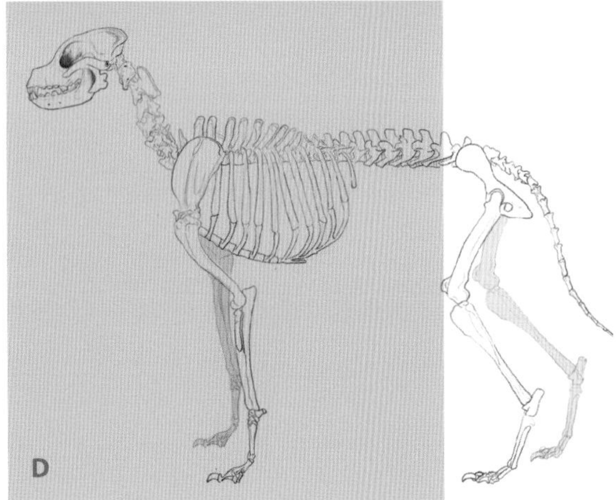

6.1 C & D The Hind End (Lumbosacral-Pelvic) Junction and the hind limbs.

Search, Response, Stay, Release

Lumbosacral-Pelvic Junction Points and Hind-Limb Points

GOAL: To apply the process of *Search, Response, Stay, Release (SRSR)* to key muscles, tendons, and ligaments of the Lumbosacral-Pelvic Junction and the hind limbs. (To begin these techniques, see p. 105.)

RESULT: *SRSR* releases tension in the deeper muscles and connective tissues of the Lumbosacral-Pelvic Junction. This results in improved elasticity and suppleness in these muscles and prepares this junction for the *Movement Techniques* that follow. This work also makes your dog feel very good!

Movement Techniques

Hind Limb and Lower Hind Limb Movement

GOAL: To search for responses while moving joints of the hip, stifle, and hock, and the lower limb, through specific ranges of motion in a relaxed state. This includes lateral and medial (inward and outward) movement of the hip joint, and flexion and extension (opening and closing) of the hip joint, stifle, and hock, as well as metatarsal movement and toe micromovement. (To begin these techniques, see p. 111.)

RESULT: Movement in a relaxed state releases tension in muscles, tendons, and ligaments associated with these structures, and restores natural movement to them.

Hold, Wait, and Melt Techniques

Sacrum Float and Pelvic Release

GOAL: To apply *Hold, Wait, and Melt Techniques* to the muscles and connective tissues of the sacrum, pelvis, sacroiliac joints, and Lumbosacral-Pelvic Junction. (To begin these techniques, see p. 123.)

RESULT: Releases tension and torque and restores movement to these joints and junctions. Restoring movement also allows muscles of the hind end and limbs connected to or associated with this junction to relax and release.

More Anatomy and the Effects of Releasing Tension

The Lumbosacral-Pelvic Junction is important in that forces exerted by the powerful muscles of the hind limbs transfer into the body through this junction.

When tension or unilateral tension (torque or twist) is put on this junction, muscles associated with it spasm and tighten to protect it. This affects movement and comfort in the rest of the body and can eventually lead to muscle, tendon, and ligament injuries, and joint diseases such as arthritis and dysplasia. Plus, it doesn't feel very good when the dog gets older.

The muscles, tendons, and ligaments of the limbs themselves accumulate tension. Tension, and especially uneven tension in these muscles, puts torque on joints, leading to joint and ligament problems. Releasing tension regularly in these muscles and connective tissues can help prevent joint and ligament disease and injuries.

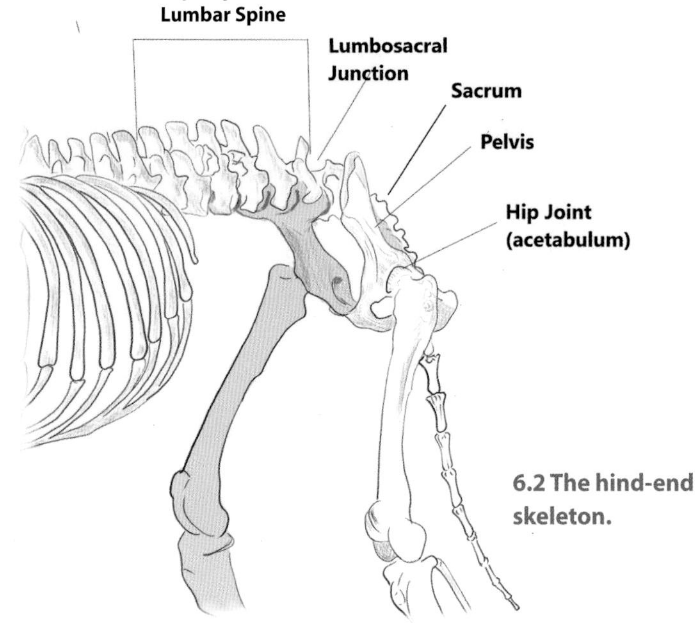

6.2 The hind-end skeleton.

The Skeleton

The main parts of the spine you are concerned with here are:

- *The lumbar spine*, the *sacrum*, and where they join together—the *Lumbosacral Junction* (fig. 6.2).
- The *sacrum*, the *pelvis* (*ilium*), and where they join together—the *Sacroiliac Joint*.
- Where the *femur* (thigh bone) and the *pelvis* join together—the *Hip Joint*.

We also have the bones and joints of the hind limb (fig. 6.3):

- *Femur*
- *Stifle joint*
- *Tibia*

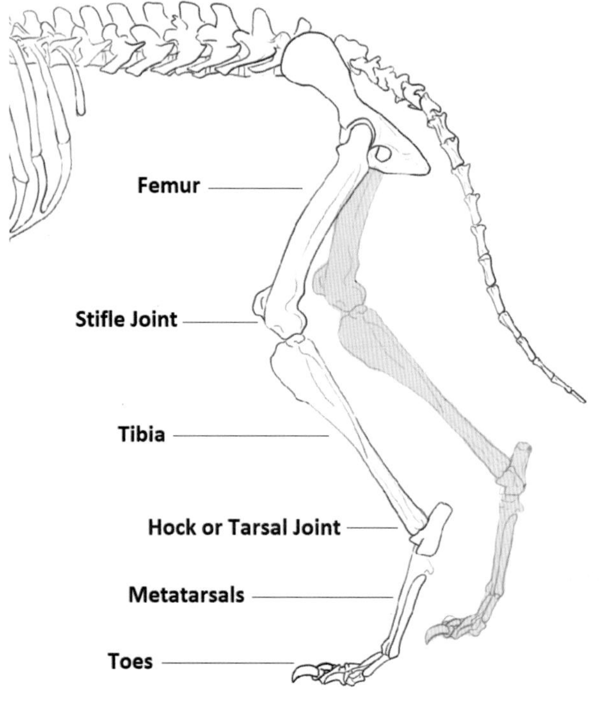

6.3 Hind-limb bones.

- *Hock joint*
- *Four metatarsals*
- And below that, the *paw* and *toes*

The hock, metatarsal, and toe joints are supported by tendons and act as shock absorbers during the weight-bearing phase of the dog's movement.

The pelvis is the largest bone of the hind end. It is the main structure to which both hind limbs attach, connecting the entire hind end to the spine.

There are three main parts to the pelvis (fig. 6.4):

The *ilium (pl, ilia)* is the largest and uppermost of the three main parts of each side of the pelvis. It is the part that attaches each side (branch) of the pelvis to the sacrum at the *Sacroiliac Joint*. The front edge of each *ilium* is called the *iliac crest.*

The *ischium (pl, ischia)* is the lowest and most rearward part of each side of the pelvis. The ischia are the two "butt-bones" of the dog—the bony parts you feel when the dog sits down abruptly on your lap. Ligaments and hamstring muscles attach at the ischium that stabilize the Sacroiliac Joint, and also drive the dog forward.

The *pubic symphysis (PS)* is located in the center between the two butt bones (ischia) below the tail. Groin muscles that *adduct* (bring the leg inward) and rotate the leg attach at the pubic symphysis. These and other muscles that attach to the pelvis can put unilateral or one-sided tension on the pubic symphysis.

Another important feature of the pelvis is the *acetabulum* (hip joint). The hip joint is a ball-and-socket type of joint where the head of the femur (ball) fits into the acetabulum (socket) of the pelvis. This ball-and-socket arrangement allows for a huge range of motion and flexibility, giving the leg the ability to reach inward, outward, forward, and back, and to twist or rotate.

Muscles, Tendons, and Ligaments

Muscles work in groups to perform different functions. Many muscles are multitaskers, meaning they work together with other muscles to perform different tasks.

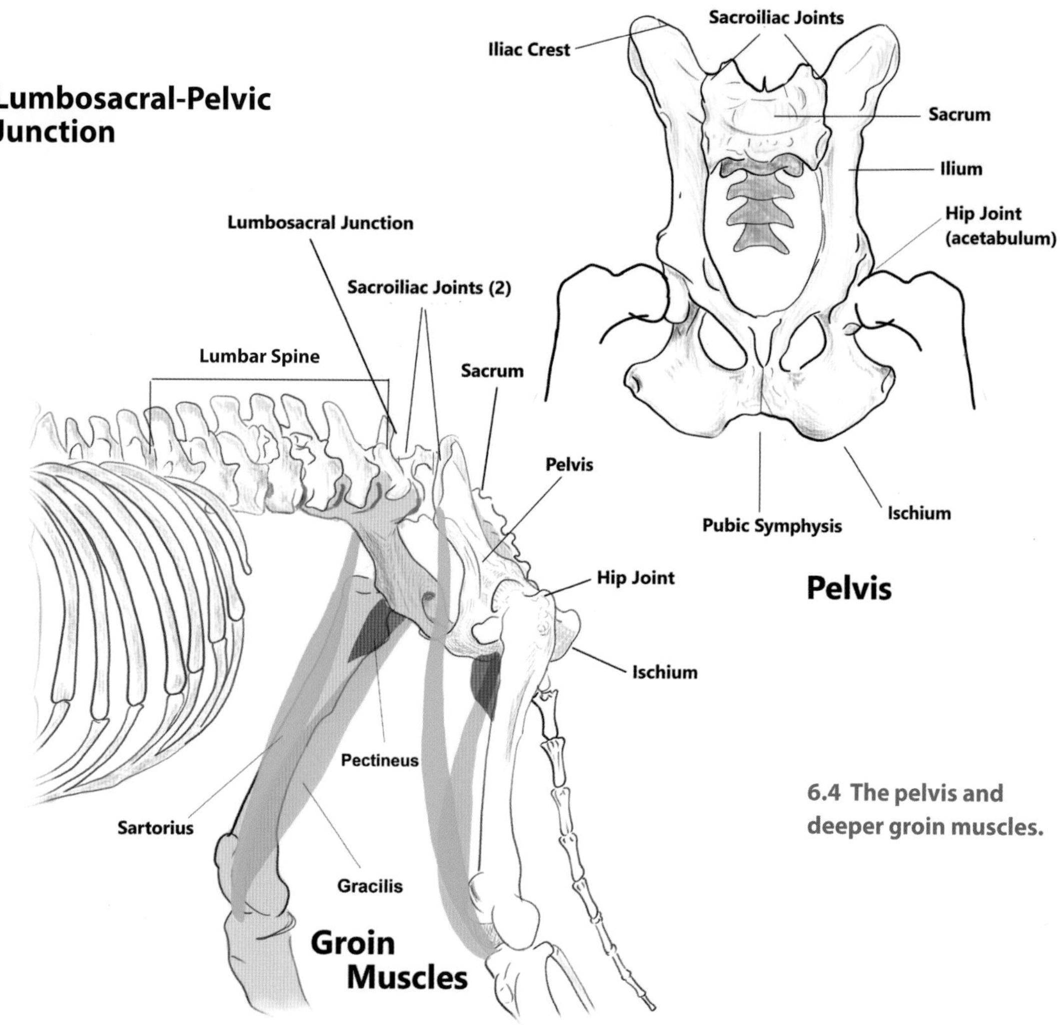

6.4 The pelvis and deeper groin muscles.

For example, there are muscles that move the hind limb (fig. 6.5). Many of these also support and stabilize the hip joint where the hind limb joins the pelvis. Releasing tension in these muscles improves range of motion in the hip joint, the stifle, and the lower limb.

There are muscles that flex the Lumbosacral Junction and lower back, allowing the hind end to come underneath the dog for greater length of stride when running. These muscles also support and stabilize the Lumbosacral Junction.

Interconnection

Keep in mind that the muscles and ligaments described in this chapter are involved in driving the dog forward (or sideways, backward, and upward),

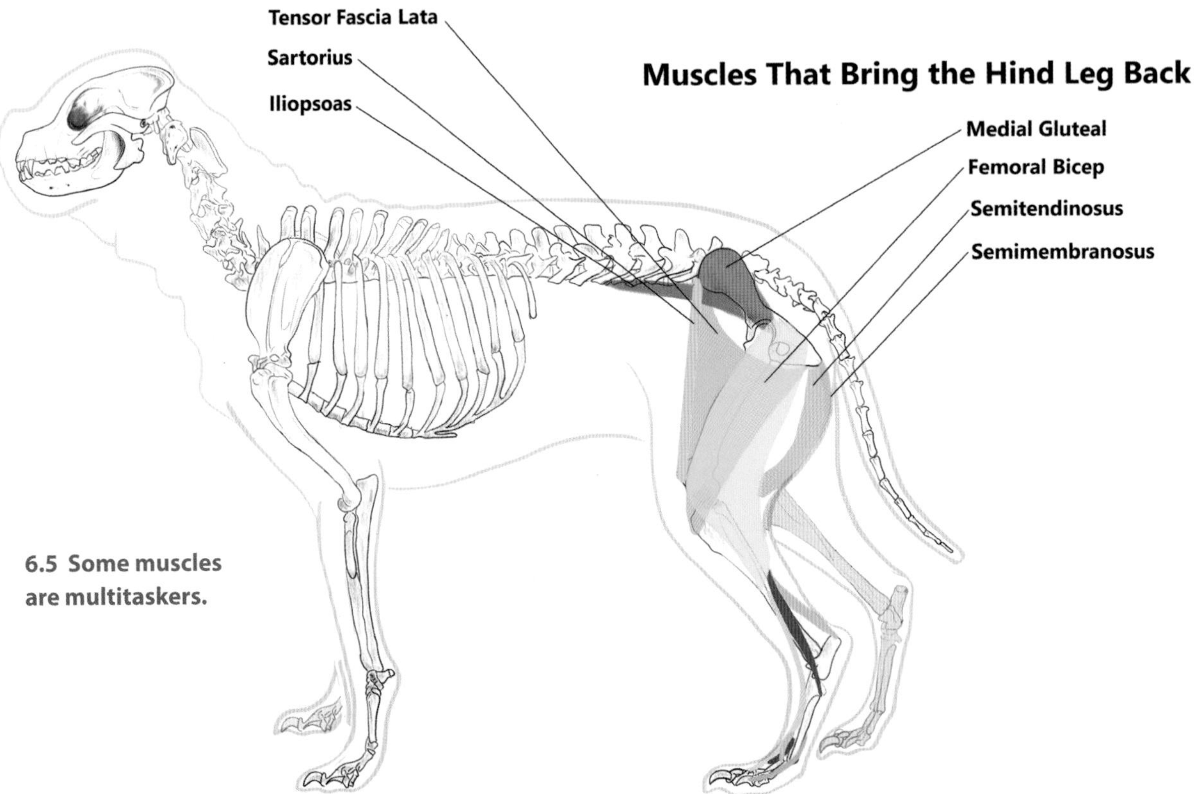

6.5 Some muscles are multitaskers.

in stabilizing the skeletal joints and junctions, or both. When tension builds in these muscles through repetitive motion or overexertion, it can put tension and torque (twist) on the hip joints, the sacroiliac joints, and the lower back and Lumbosacral Junction.

When these joints and junctions become torqued, not only do the muscles around them spasm or tighten to protect them, but continual tension in these muscles can lead to hip, sacroiliac, and lower-back issues. This explains, for example, why back pain in the dog is often associated with hip issues.

Compensation

The dog will compensate for pain or discomfort in one area by over-using another area. Compensation for an issue in one area leads to possible problems in other areas eventually. Releasing tension in a muscle doesn't just keep that muscle happy and healthy, but keeps all the muscles, joints, and junctions associated with it in other parts of the body happy and healthy.

You'll notice that older dogs often have hard, overdeveloped muscles in the lumbar (lower) back (even if they haven't spent their lives jumping for frisbees). An older dog with arthritis in an elbow or elbows, for example, will shift weight from the front end to the hind end and develop excessive tension in the muscles of the lower back. Releasing this tension as it builds will make your dog more comfortable in the lower back, and possibly prevent the lower back from becoming a problem. He'll also appreciate you for it.

Healthy Muscles Improve Movement and Prevent Injuries

While releasing tension in the muscles of the hind limb improves range of motion in the hip joint, the stifle, and the Lumbosacral Junction, even more importantly,, keeping these muscles healthy and supple also helps to prevent and manage hip, lower back, and stifle injuries and disease.

Muscles That Move the Hind Limb

Let's try to break some of these down into the basic functions that they perform.

Muscles That Bring the Hind Limb Forward

The *tensor fascia lata* (TFL) flexes the hip joint and extends the stifle. Working with other muscles, this movement would, for example, extend the entire leg forward. The TFL also abducts (brings out) the hind limb.

The *sartorius* muscle flexes the hip joint and flexes the stifle. When working with other muscles, this movement, for example, lifts the foot off the ground to be in a position to bring the leg forward. The *sartorius* also extends and supports the stifle when the dog is standing.

The *psoas* group of muscles (*psoas minor, major,* and *iliacus)* are important core as well as gymnastic muscles. They bring the hind limb forward and bring the hind end underneath the dog when running for greater length of stride. They also stabilize the Lumbosacral Junction. They attach underneath the *thoracic* and *lumbar spine* at one end, and the inside the *femur* at the other.

Muscles That Extend the Hind Limb Back (and Drive the Dog Forward)

The *medial gluteal* is the largest driving muscle of the hind end. It attaches at the *iliac crest* on one end, and goes over the top of the pelvis and attaches to a lever at the head of the femur at the hip joint on the other. When it contracts, it pulls the leg back, which drives the dog forward.

Muscles in the *hamstring group* also bring the limb back to push the dog forward. The *femoral bicep* is a large muscle that lies on the outside of the thigh. It extends the hip and hock, and both extends and flexes the stifle, depending on which part of the muscles is being used (multitasking) to drive the dog forward.

The *semitendinosus* and *semimembranosus* muscles extend the hip and hock backward, which moves the dog forward. These muscles attach at the *ischium* on one end, and inside the lower hind limb on the other.

Groin Muscles

Groin muscles such as the *gracilis* and even deeper *pectineus* are important. They attach at the pubic symphysis on one end, and inside the femur at the other.

These muscles adduct (bring the leg inward) and are also involved in driving the dog forward. Unilateral or one-sided tension in these and any muscles that attach to the pelvis can put torque or twist on the pubic symphysis, and consequently on the entire Lumbosacral-Pelvic Junction. Keeping these muscles from becoming excessively tight goes a long way toward keeping the dog's hind end healthy and happy.

FROM THE VET

Special Mention—The Stifle

The dog's stifle (analogous to the human knee) is a hard-working and fragile link in the hind limb. Unlike the ball-and-socket type of joint found in the hip, the stifle is a hinge type of joint designed to move in only a backward and forward motion. Injuries can occur here when twisting forces are applied. Important connective tissues are the many *cruciate, collateral,* and *patellar* (kneecap) *ligaments.* The *cranial cruciate ligament* is especially fragile and prone to injury.

Careful conditioning provides muscular support to help reduce the risk of injury—keeping the muscles, tendons, and ligaments flexible, supple, and balanced as they are being conditioned helps.

—*Dr. Robinett*

What Do Mathematics and Kidnapping Have in Common?

How do you remember *adductor* versus *abductor*? An *adductor* adds (*brings in*) the limb toward the body. An *abductor* abducts (*kidnaps*) the limb, taking it away from the body.

Muscles and Ligaments That Connect the Hind Limb to the Pelvis and the Pelvis to the Sacrum

The *hip joint* (where the hind limb connects to the pelvis) is stressed by the major driving muscles and muscles involved in moving the hind limb as the transfer of energy from the hind limb transfers to the pelvis. Releasing tension not only improves range of motion but helps to prevent and manage hip issues and to release tension on the sacrum and lower back.

The *sacroiliac joints* (where the pelvis connects to the sacrum) are also referred to as the *Sacropelvic Junction*. There are two basic sets of ligaments that connect the *pelvis* to the *sacrum:* the *sacroiliac ligaments* and the *sacrotuberus ligament.* These two

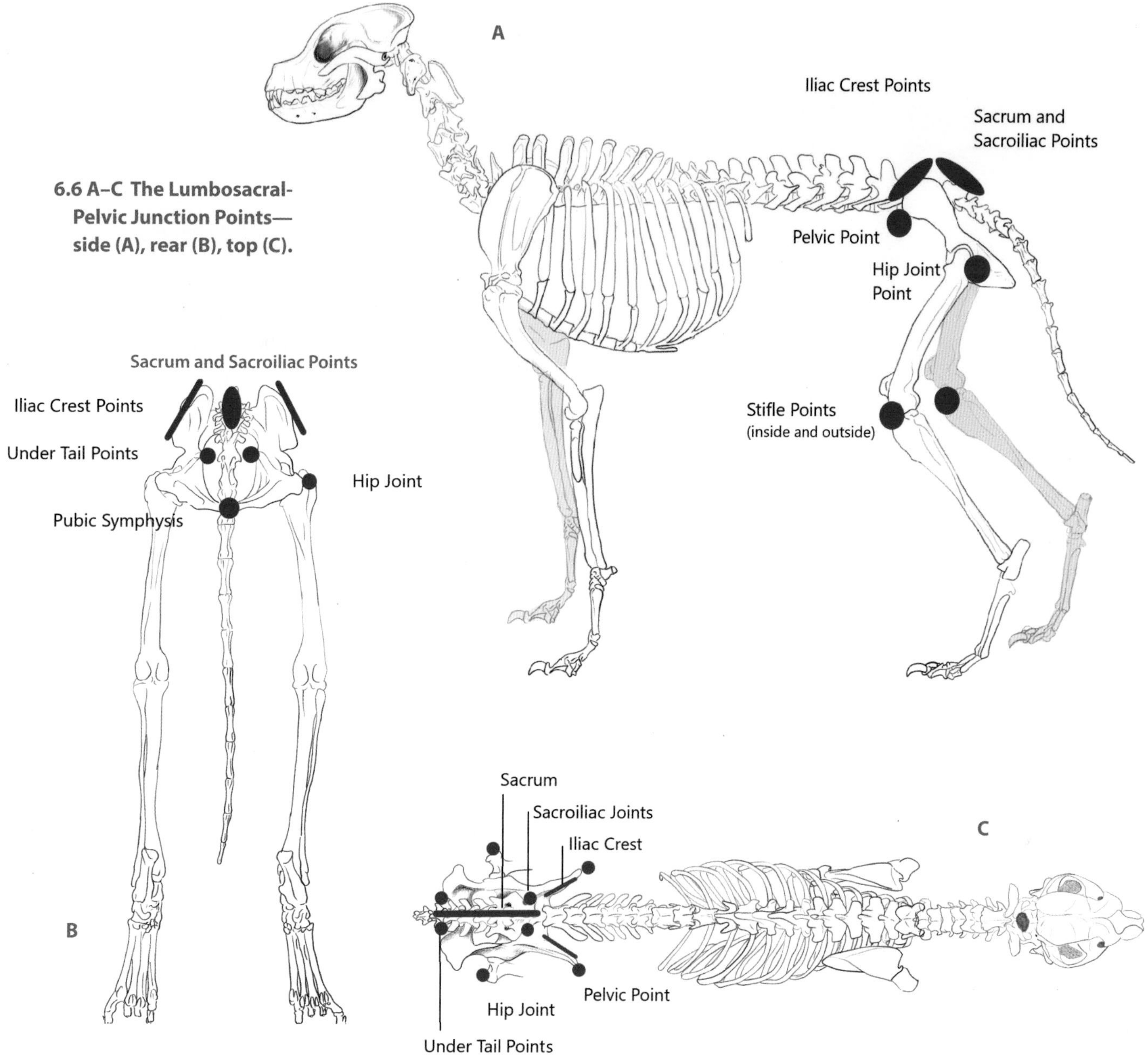

6.6 A–C The Lumbosacral-Pelvic Junction Points—side (A), rear (B), top (C).

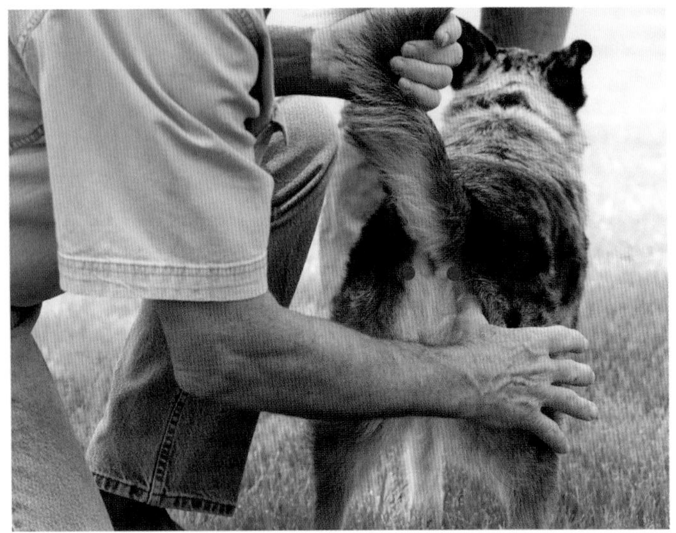

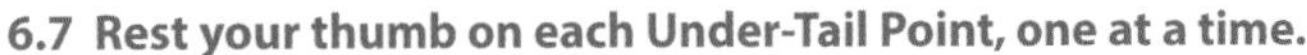

6.7 **Rest your thumb on each Under-Tail Point, one at a time.**

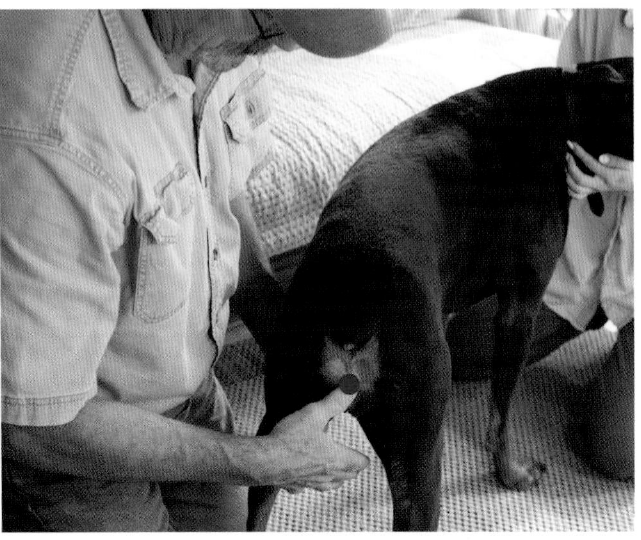

6.8 **The Pubic Symphysis Point.**

sets of ligaments stabilize the *sacroiliac joint*. Releasing tension on these ligaments helps to decrease torque on the *sacroiliac joint*.

You'll find more about the effects of tension on the *Lumbosacral Junction* in the next chapter (p. 128). Enough homework for now.

Search, Response, Stay, Release

GOAL: To apply the process of *SRSR* to:

- Muscles that put tension on the Lumbosacral-Pelvic Junction.
- Muscles, tendons, and ligaments of the hind limb itself.

WHERE YOU WORK

Lumbosacral-Pelvic Junction Points

Under-Tail Points (*sacrotuberous ligament, semitendinosus* and *semimembranosus,* and *femoral biceps)*—These points release tension in muscles that pull on the sacrum and put torque on the sacroiliac joints (fig. 6.7).

> **Useful Fact**
>
> The *sacrotuberus ligament* is absent in the cat. That's because cats are SPECIAL!

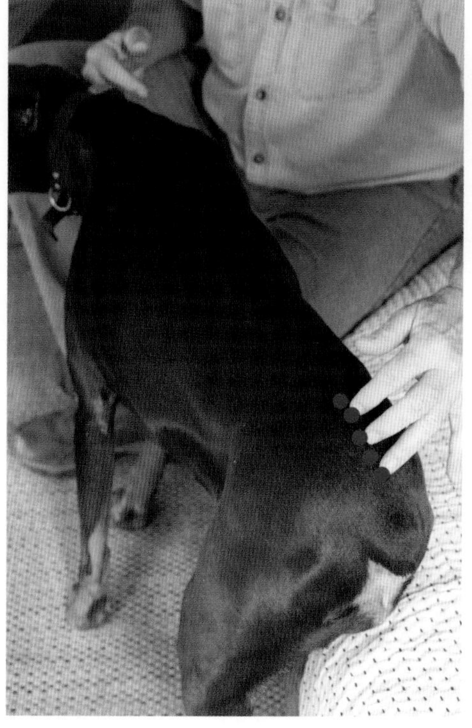

6.9 The Sacrum and Sacroiliac Points.

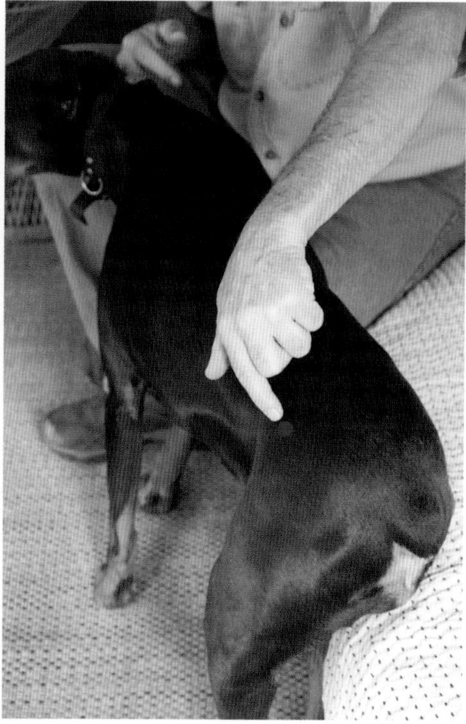

6.10 The Pelvic Point.

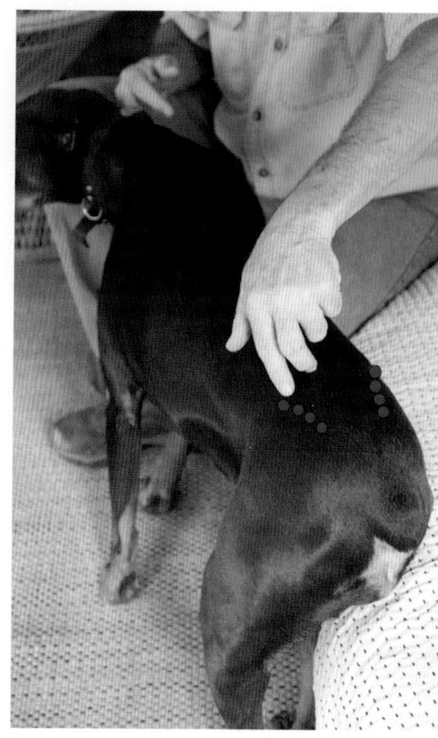

6.11 The Iliac Crest Points.

Pubic Symphysis (PS) Point (*pectineus, gracilis, adductors*)—The *pubic symphysis* is a bony part that joins the two wings of the pelvis and is located between the two *ischia* (butt bones) below the tail—underneath the plumbing outlets (fig. 6.8). Unilateral tension that puts torque or twist on the pelvis can be released with this point.

Sacrum and Sacroiliac Points (*sacroiliac ligaments, medial gluteals*)—These are on a line that runs down the top of the sacrum (fig. 6.9). These points help to release tension in muscles that put torque on the *sacrum* and *sacroiliac joints*.

Pelvic Point (*tensor fascia lata, sartorius*)—The Pelvic Point is on the bony protuberance on the outside edge of the pelvis or *tuber coxa* (fig. 6.10).

Iliac Crest Points (*medial gluteals*)—These lie along the front edge of the ilia of the pelvis, on both sides (fig. 6.11).

Groin Points (*pectineus, gracilis, adductors, psoas,* and *iliopsoas*)—The Groin Points are inside the thigh from the *Stifle Point* up into the crease of the groin, on both sides (fig. 6.12).

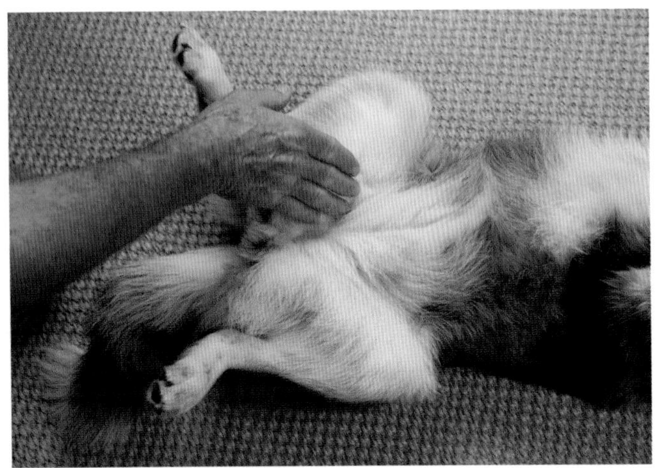

6.12 The right Groin Points.

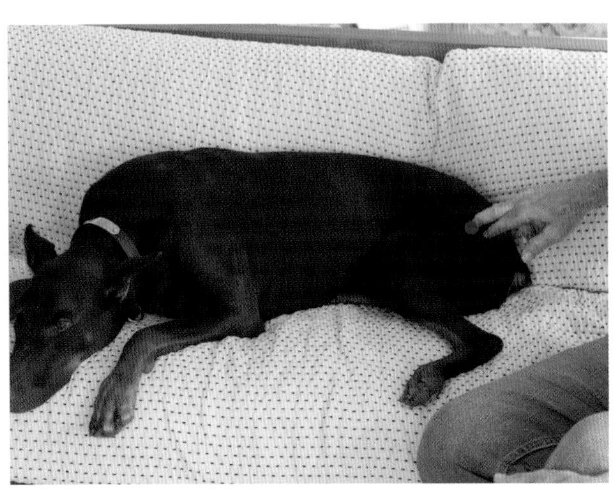

6.14 The Hip Joint Point.

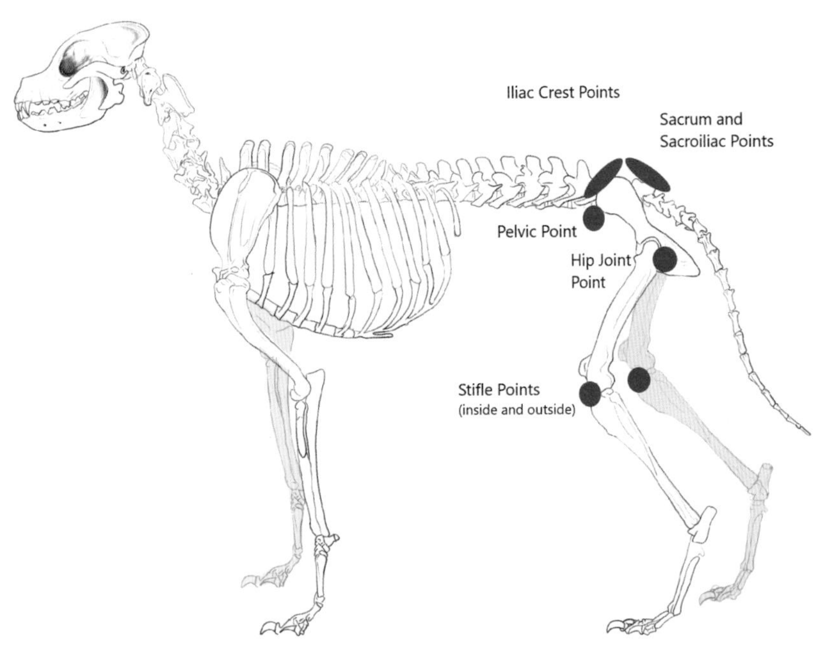

6.13 The Groin and Hind Limb Points.

Hind-Limb Points

Hip Joint Point (*medial gluteals*)—The actual *hip joint* isn't easy to feel, but if you start by searching in the area shown in the illustration (fig. 6.14), your dog will tell you exactly where he is holding tension in the hip joint.

Stifle Points (*quads, stifle,* and *patellar ligaments*)—Feel for the bony part of the dog's knee (or stifle). The *Stifle Points* are just inside and outside of that bony protuberance (figs. 6.15 A & B).

Lower Hind Limb Points (*extensors* and *flexors*)—These points are anywhere from the front of the hock down, on the front and both sides of the metatarsals, and on the paw (fig. 6.16). These points are very sensitive. If you use any pressure at all, your dog won't show responses. Search by barely touching the tips of your fingertips to the hairs.

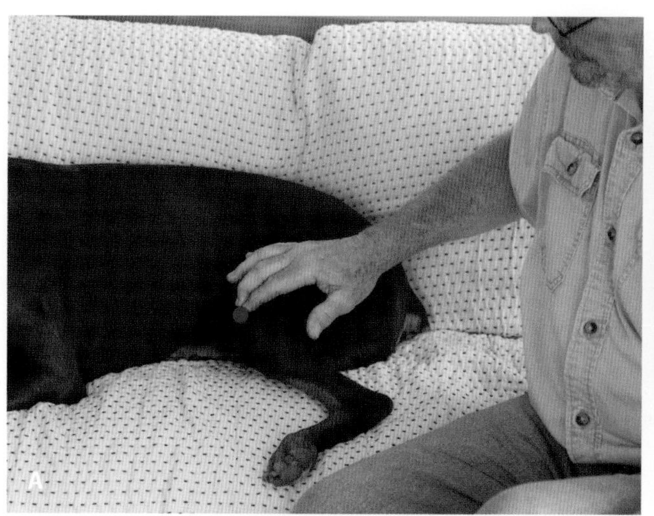

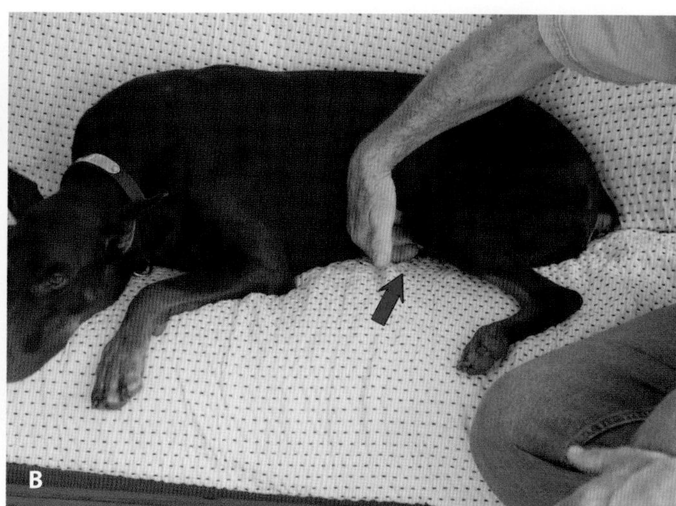

6.15 A & B The outside (A) and inside (B) Stifle Points.

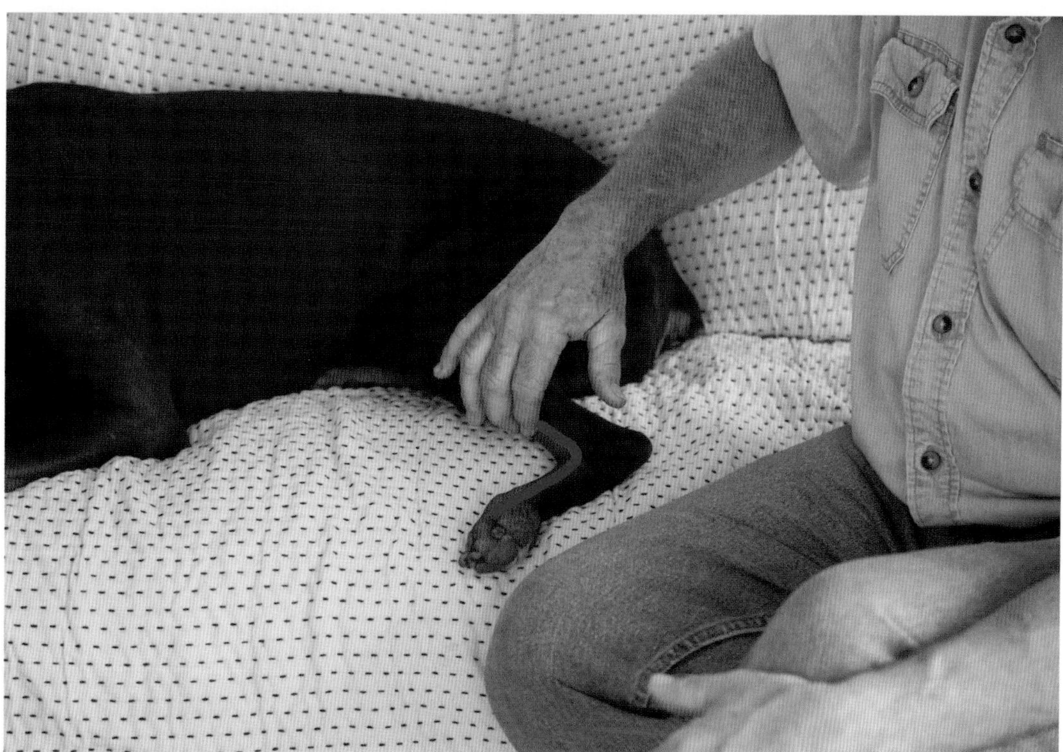

6.16 The Lower Hind Limb Points.

Quick Overview: Step-by-Step

LUMBOSACRAL-PELVIC JUNCTION AND HIND LIMB POINTS

This *SRSR* can be done with your dog standing, sitting, on your lap, or lying down, although it is easier to see what he is telling you when he's sitting or standing. Then choose a place to begin:

- Lumbosacral-Pelvic Junction Points.
- Hind Limb Points.

Step 1. *Search*. Using the tip of either one or two fingers, barely touching the hair, slowly (I said SLOWLY) and gently search with your fingertip(s) in the area of the points (fig. 6.17 A). Your dog will tell you exactly where to stop when you get a…

Step 2. *Response*. Watch closely for a blink or other change of behavior (fig. 6.17 B). In this case, the change in behavior is a blink.

Step 3. *Stay*. Keep your finger over that spot, maintaining Air Gap. Resist the urge to move the finger, push, rub, or stroke. This may take one second or one minute. Be patient. Breathe and relax until you get a…

Step 4. *Release*—in this case, licking, chewing, and a big fidget (fig. 6.17 C).

When you are finished, you can either repeat the process on the opposite side or continue the process in one of the other areas on the same side.

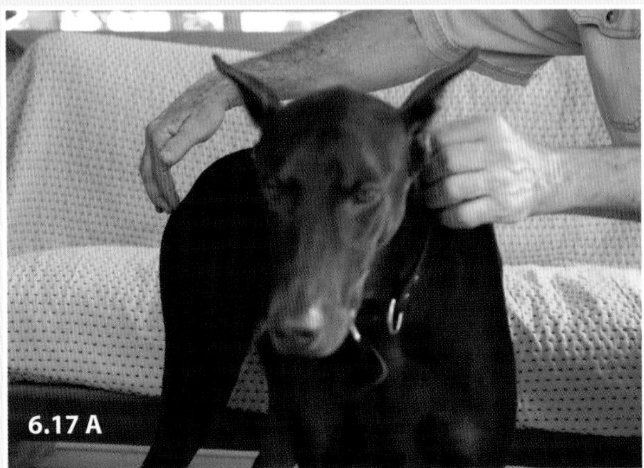
6.17 A

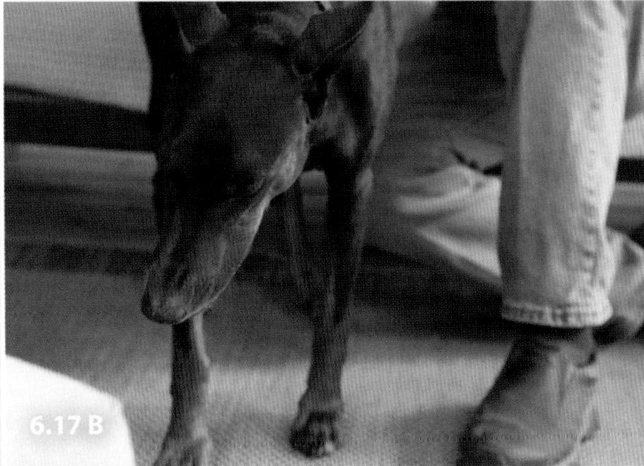
6.17 B

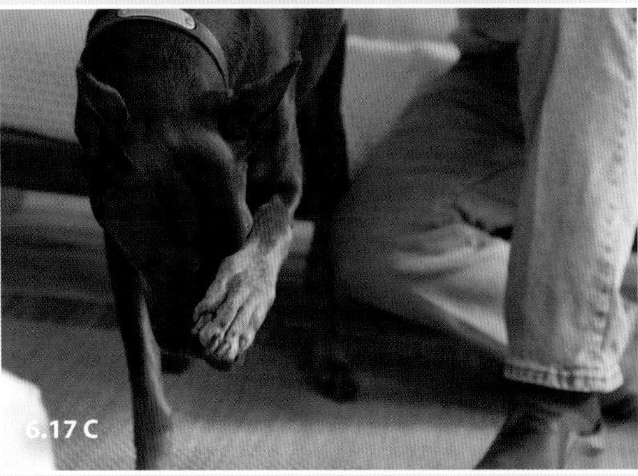
6.17 C

Tips

Remember, barely touch the dog's skin or hair. If you feel you're not getting *Responses*, or if you're waiting and not getting *Releases*, consciously soften your fingers and use even less pressure (figs. 6.18 A & B). Watch the dog's eyes as you do this. Often, you'll get a response where you weren't getting one before. Less is more. Your dog may fuss or fidget or want to get up or walk away as he starts to feel some tension release. Soften your finger even more; ask him to *Stay* with you a little longer.

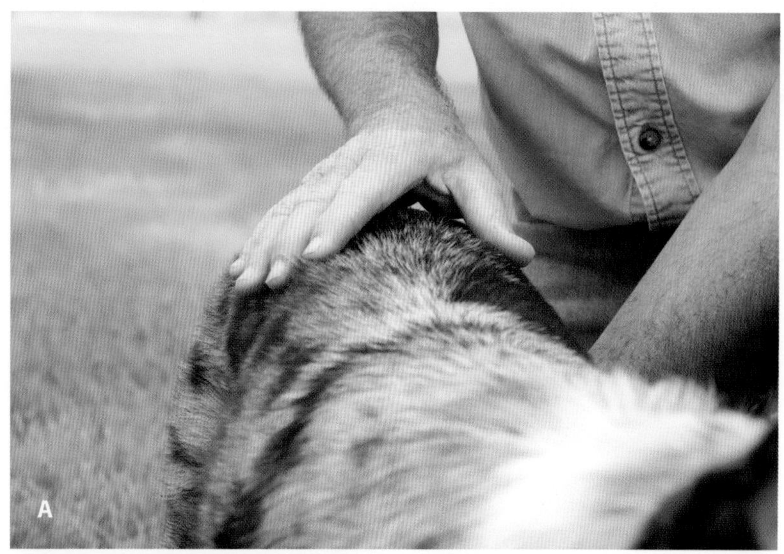

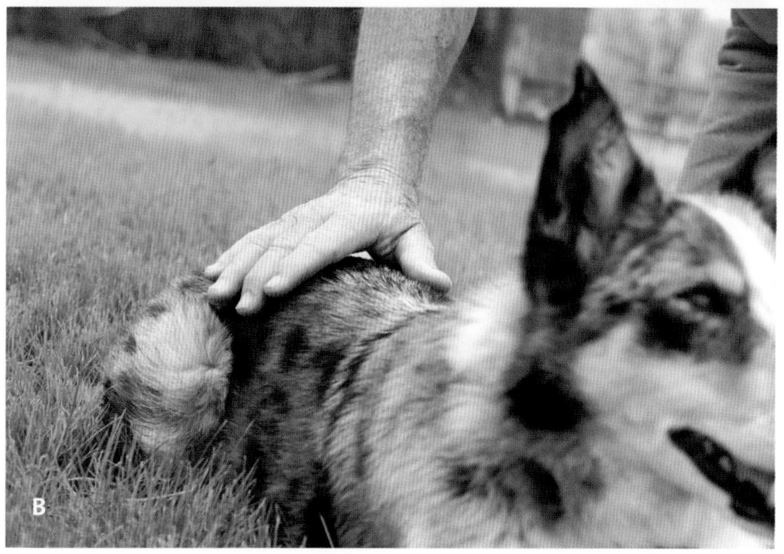

6.18 A & B Using a light touch (A) and even lighter (B).

Movement Techniques

GOAL: With *Movement Techniques*, you *Search* for *Responses* while moving the leg through specific ranges of motion in a relaxed state.

There are three ways you can position yourself and the dog:

- With the dog standing, and you working with the leg that is on the dog's near side.
- With the dog standing, and you working with the leg on the dog's opposite side.
- With the dog lying on his side, and you working with the leg on the upward-facing side.

Quick Overview: Step-by-Step

HIND LIMB MOVEMENT

HIND LIMB MOVEMENT—*NEAR SIDE*

(Shown with the dog standing, working with the leg on the near side.)

You can start with either leg. Let's start with the left hind leg:

Step 1. Sit or kneel at your dog's left side, facing rearward.

Step 2. Place your left hand inside the left hind leg, under the dog's stifle.

Step 3. Place your right hand gently under the lower hind limb below the hock.

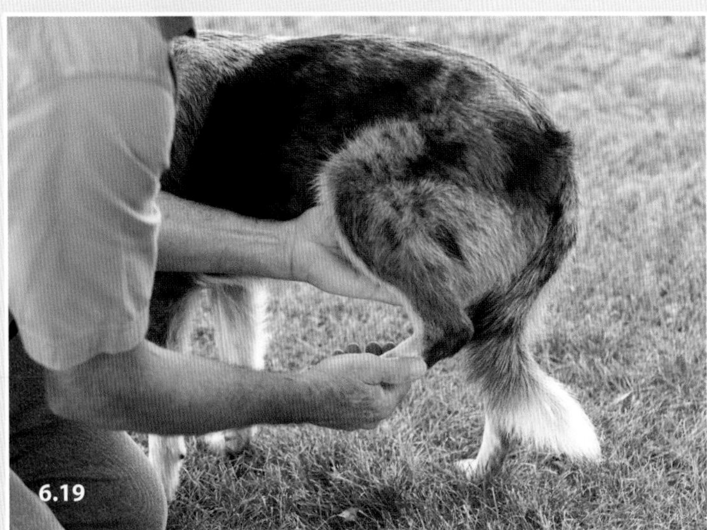
6.19

Step 4. Soften both hands and gently lift upward until you feel weight in the right hand (fig. 6.19). This is the *neutral position*.

Remember, when the dog tenses or starts to pull his leg away, soften and yield.

Lateral and Medial (Hip Joint)—Near Side

Step 1. When you feel the leg is as relaxed as possible (*neutral position*), gently bring the hock and stifle lateral.

Keep the weight of the leg in your hand. If he starts to tense or pull away, soften and yield, then ask again.

Step 2. With your hands in the same position, gently move the hock and stifle medially

Releasing Tension in the Hip Joint

Lateral and medial movement of the hip joint helps to release tension in the ligaments of the joint as well as in important driving muscles such as the *medial gluteal* that attach at the hip joint.

(inward—away from you—toward the opposite hind).

Step 3. Move the hind limb medially and laterally a few times, watching and pausing for the blink (fig. 6.20).

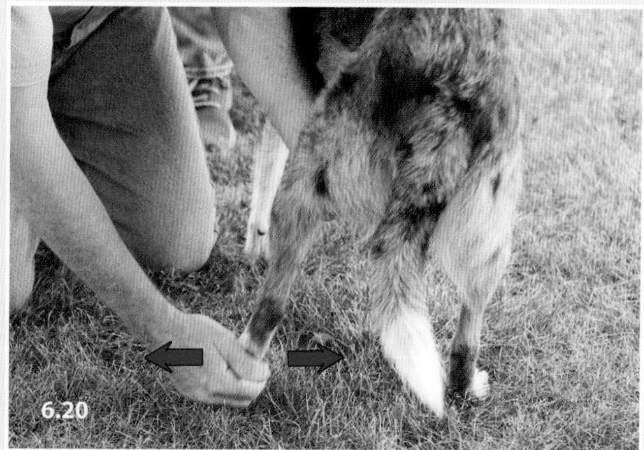
6.20

Flexion and Extension (Hip Joint, Stifle, and Hock)—Near Side

Step 1. With your hands in the same position and the leg relaxed in the *neutral position*, gently bring the foot and hock up toward the belly, flexing or "closing" the hip joint, stifle, and hock (fig. 6.21 A).

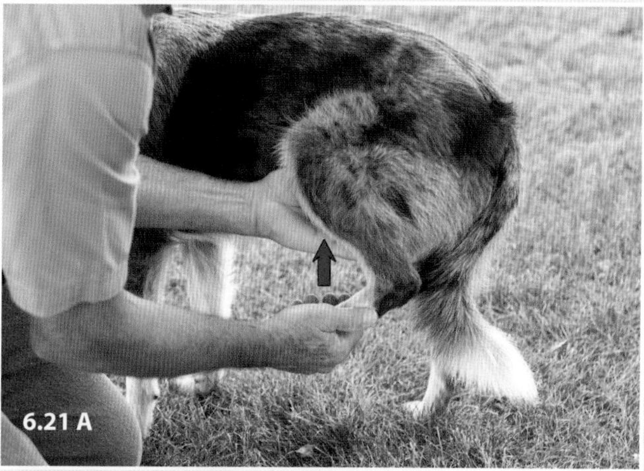
6.21 A

Step 2. With your hands in the same position, gently bring the leg back, extending the leg in a backward direction, "opening" the hip joint, stifle, and hock (fig. 6.21 B).

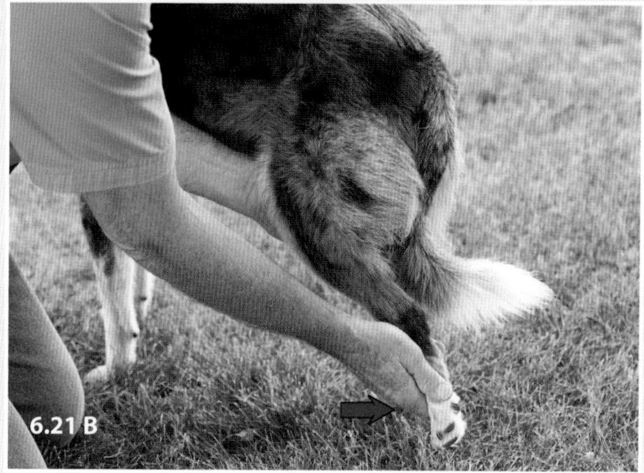
6.21 B

Step 3. You can continue to move the leg up and down, forward, and backward, gently increasing the range of motion as you *Search* for *Responses*.

Set the leg down and see what the dog "has to say." If he needs to move, walk around, yawn, or stretch, let him. When you are finished on this side, you can repeat the process on the opposite side.

HIND LIMB MOVEMENT (continued)

HIND LIMB MOVEMENT—*OPPOSITE SIDE*

(Shown with the dog standing, working with the leg on the opposite side.)

Here, you are basically in the same position as Step 1 on p. 112 but you are reaching around the dog to work with the opposite (right) leg.

Step 1. Sit or kneel next to your dog at the dog's left hind. It's okay to have your body in contact with the dog's.

Step 2. Reach around the dog with your right arm and cup your right hand under the dog's right hock or lower leg.

Step 3. Reach over the dog with your right hand to support the leg and body.

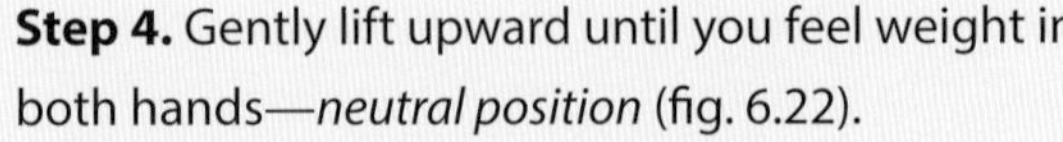

Step 4. Gently lift upward until you feel weight in both hands—*neutral position* (fig. 6.22).

Remember, when the dog tenses or starts to pull his leg away, soften and yield.

Lateral and Medial (Hip Joint)—Opposite Side

Step 1. When you feel the leg is as relaxed as possible, gently bring the hock and stifle lateral.

Step 2. With your hands in the same position, gently move the hock and stifle medially.

Step 3. Move the hind limb medially and laterally slowly a few times, watching and pausing for the blinks (fig. 6.23).

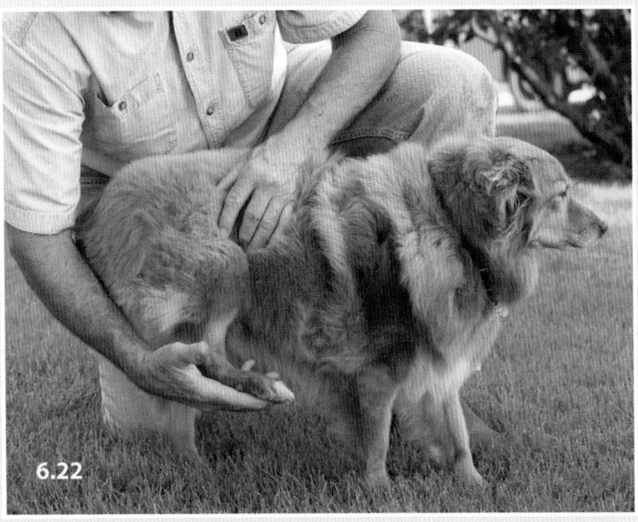

6.22

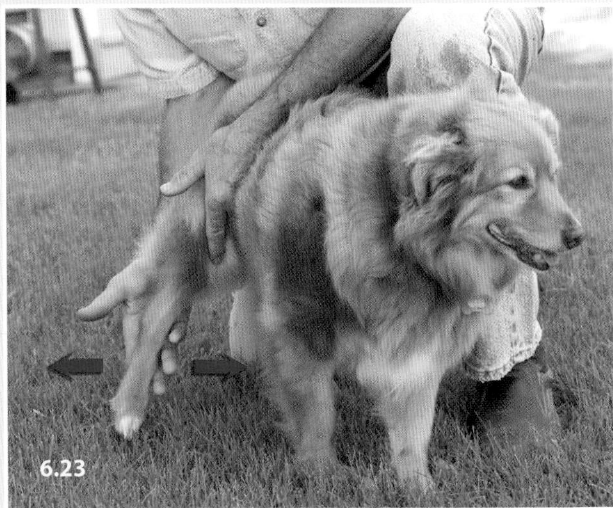

6.23

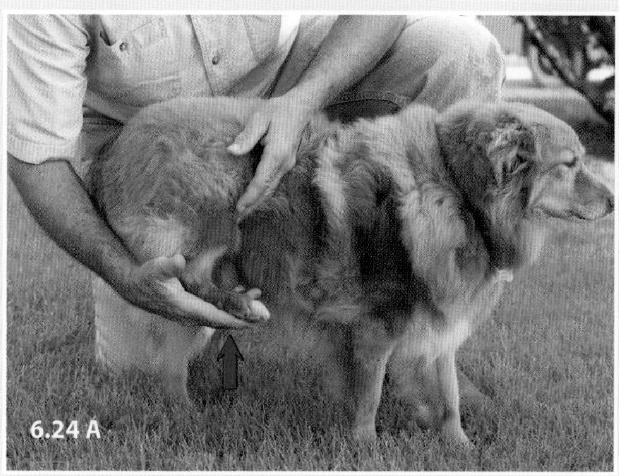

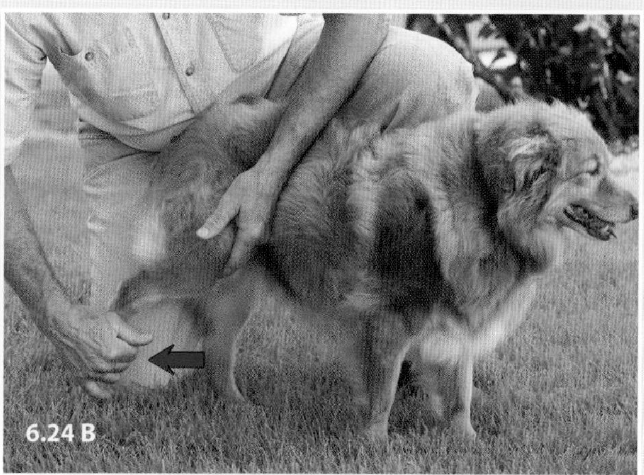

Flexion and Extension (Hip Joint, Stifle, and Hock)—Opposite Side

Step 1. With your hands in the same position and the leg as relaxed as possible, gently bring the foot and hock up toward the belly, flexing or "closing" the hip joint, stifle, and hock (fig. 6.24 A).

Step 2. With your hands in the same position, gently bring the leg back, extending the leg in a backward direction, "opening" the hip joint, stifle, and hock (fig. 6.24 B).

Step 3. You can continue to move the leg up and down, forward and backward, gently increasing the range of motion as you watch and pause for the blinks.

Note: Go slowly and softly as the leg must be completely relaxed.

With larger dogs, you can reach underneath with the stifle hand to do the mobilizations (fig. 6.25).

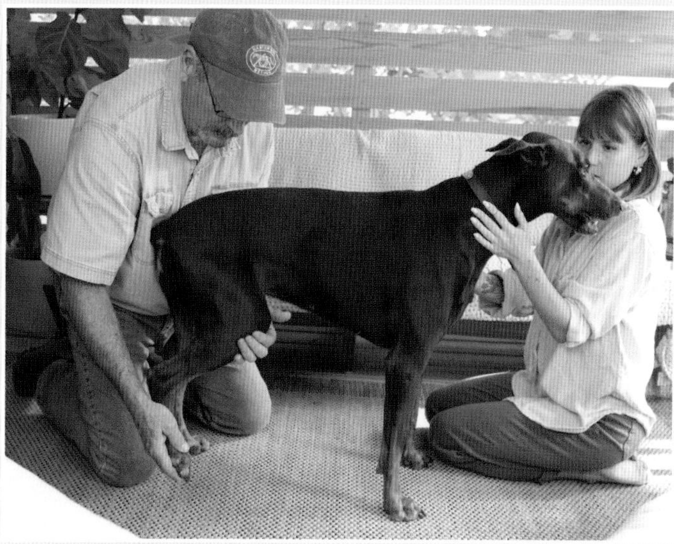

6.25 Reaching underneath to do Movement Techniques on the hind end of a larger dog.

HIND LIMB MOVEMENT (continued)

HIND LIMB MOVEMENT—*DOG LYING DOWN*

(Shown working with the dog lying down.)

To have room for the leg to move, the dog must be lying flat. This is essentially the same as working with the dog on the near side (see p. 112), except that he is lying on his side.

Let's start with the right leg and the dog lying on her left side.

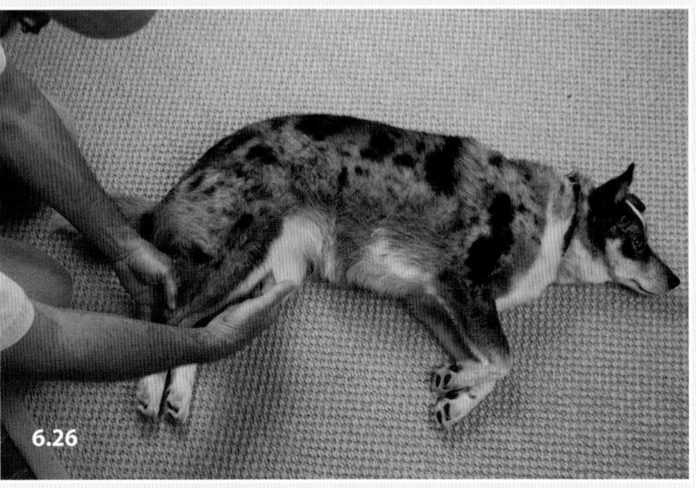

6.26

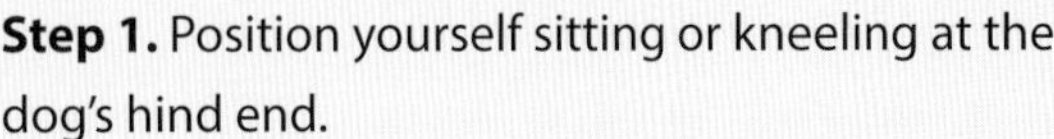

Step 1. Position yourself sitting or kneeling at the dog's hind end.

Step 2. Place your right hand under the dog's stifle.

Step 3. Place your left hand under the hock (fig. 6.26).

Step 4. Gently take the weight of the leg in both hands, lifting it away from the body (yep, you got it, *neutral position*).

Lateral and Medial (Hip Joint)—Dog Lying Down

Step 1. When you feel the leg is as relaxed as possible, gently bring the hock and stifle laterally.

Step 2. With your hands in the same position, gently move the hock and stifle medially (fig. 6.27).

Step 3. Move the hind limb medially and laterally a few times, watching and pausing for the blinks.

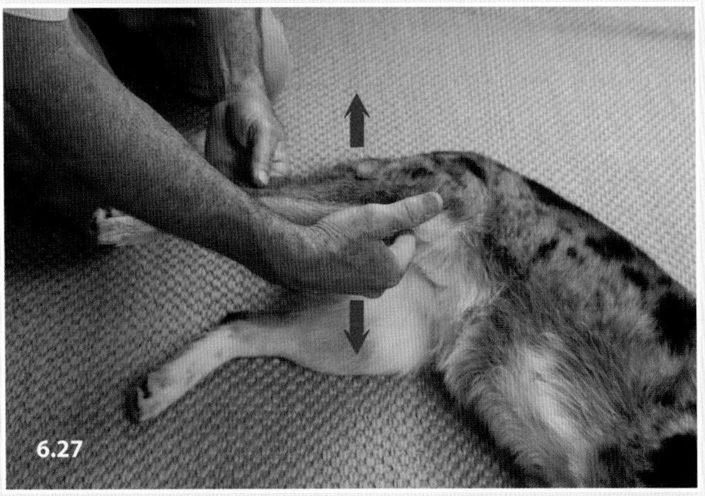

6.27

Flexion and Extension (Hip Joint, Stifle, and Hock)—Dog Lying Down

Step 1. With your hands in the same position, and the leg as relaxed as possible, gently bring the foot and hock up toward the belly, flexing or "closing" the hip joint, stifle, and hock (fig. 6.28 A).

Step 2. With your hands in the same position, gently bring the leg back, extending the leg in a backward direction, "opening" the hip joint, stifle, and hock (fig. 6.28 B).

Step 3. You can continue to move the leg up and down, forward, and backward, gently increasing the range of motion as you *Search* for *Responses*.

Note: Go slowly and softly, as the leg must be completely relaxed.

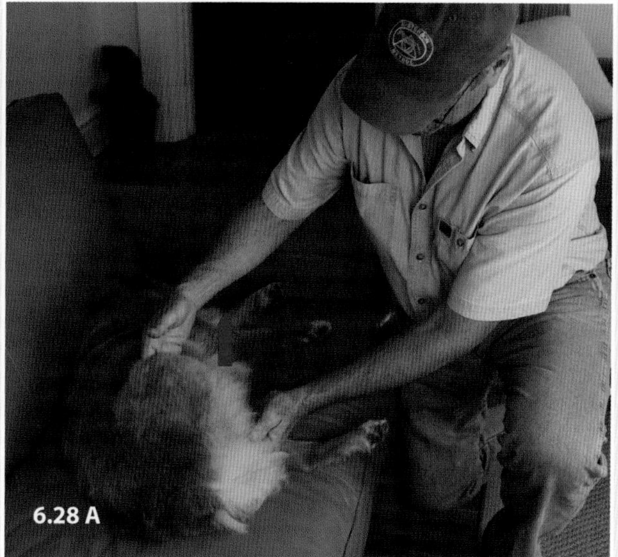

6.28 A

Scan to view Hind Limb Flexion and Extension video

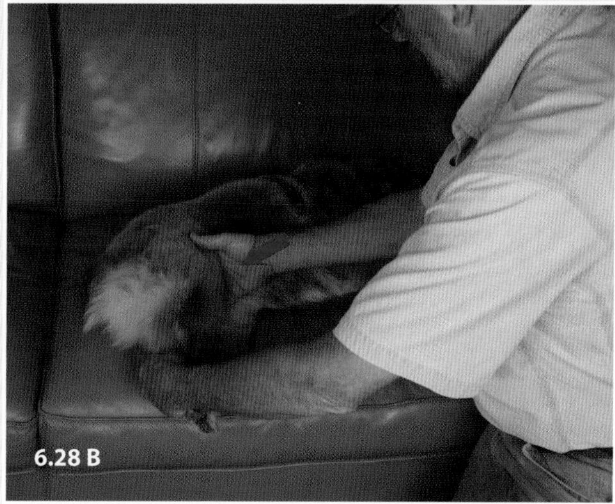

6.28 B

Tips

It doesn't matter which movement you start with. The idea is to gently "loosen" things up while paying attention to your dog's *Responses*.

Start with what is easiest for the dog. If the dog tenses or is having difficulty with one direction or movement, move in another direction. You can then return to the more difficult movement. It's important that this be done with the leg in a relaxed state.

Watch for blinks or other changes in behavior. A blink or fidget means your dog is feeling something in that part of the relaxed movement. Soften or slow down, and gently go back and forth through that part.

Remember this is *not* a stretch, it's a *relaxed movement*. Do not pull on the leg during the extension.

It's the same when doing leg flexions. Do not push against any resistance. Lift softly and slowly so that the movement is in a relaxed state.

Working with Tiny Dogs

As with the forelimbs (see p. 86), tiny dogs can be done on your lap, using the fingers of one hand (fig. 6.29).

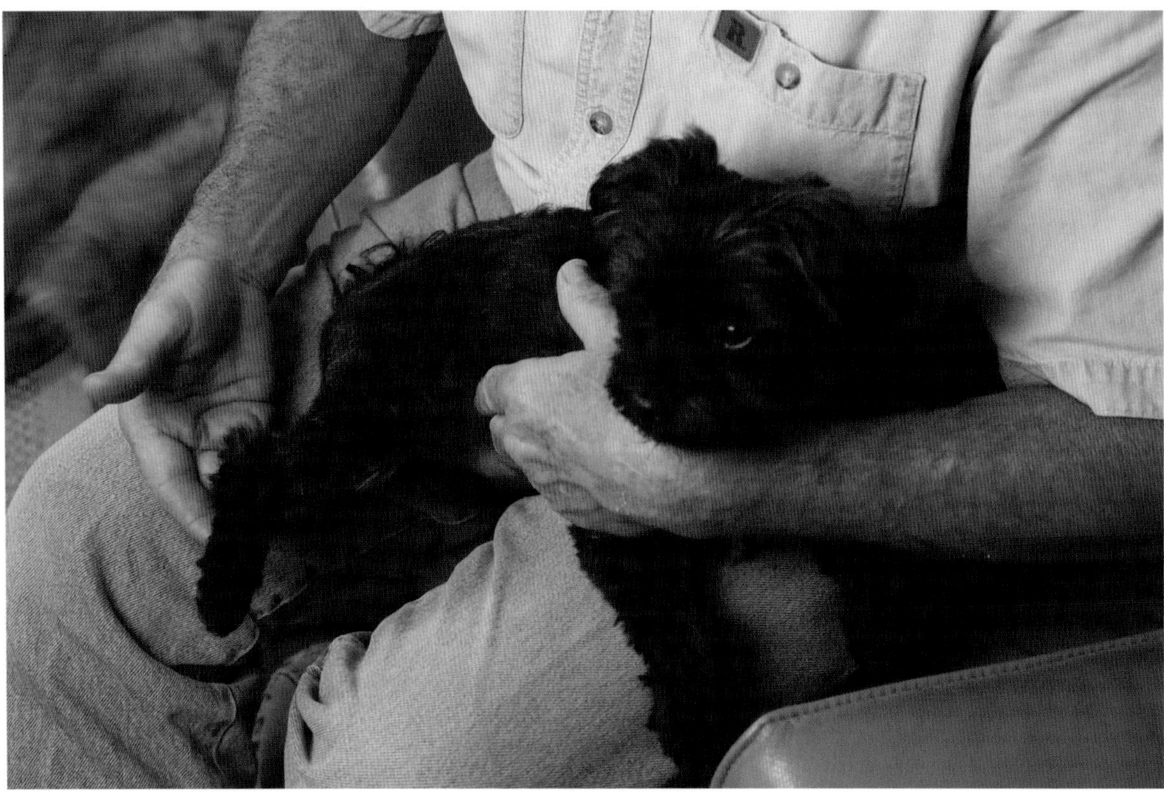

6.29 Tiny dogs can be done on your lap using the fingers of one hand.

Quick Overview: Step-by-Step

LOWER HIND LIMB MOVEMENT

This is easiest when done:

- With the dog standing, and you working with the leg on the opposite side.
- With the dog lying on his side, and you working with the leg on the upward-facing side.

LOWER HIND LIMB MOVEMENT—*OPPOSITE SIDE*

(Shown working with the dog standing, and you working with the leg on the opposite side.)

Let's start with the right hind leg:
Step 1. Position yourself next to your dog's left hind, facing forward.

Step 2. Reach around the dog with your right arm and cup your right hand under the right (opposite) hock.

Step 3. Reach over or under the dog with your left arm and use your left hand to support the dog's foreleg under the paw (fig. 6.30).

Step 4. Soften both hands and allow the dog's leg to relax into your right hand.

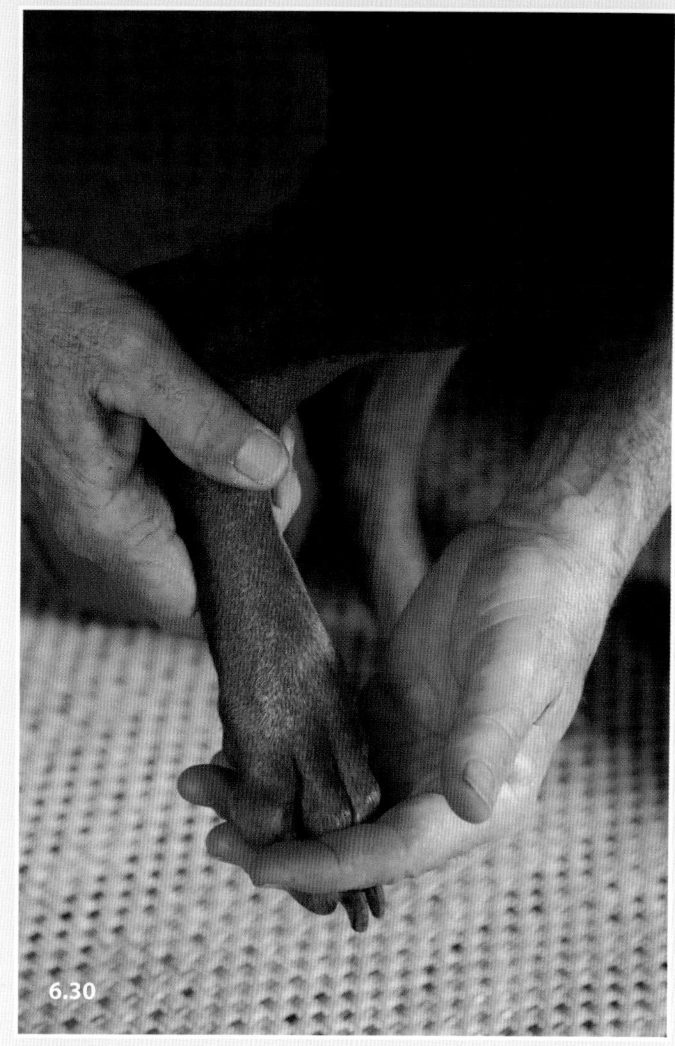

6.30

LOWER HIND LIMB MOVEMENT (continued)

Metatarsal Movement— Opposite Side

Step 1. When the leg is as relaxed as possible, slowly move the paw and metatarsal joints through a gentle range of up-and-down movement with your right hand. Watch for the blink (fig. 6.31).

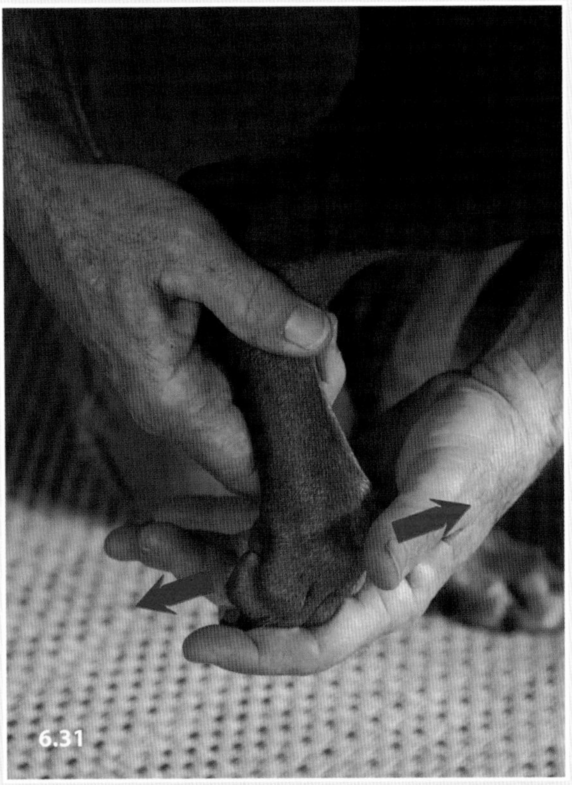

6.31

Toe Micromovement— Opposite Side

Step 1. While continuing to support the leg with the left hand, gently slide the thumb and fingers of the right hand down to the toes (fig. 6.32).

Step 2. Using *very soft fingers*, gently wiggle each of the toes and toenails through a tiny range of motion, continuing to watch for the blinks. Set the leg down and see what the dog "has to say." If he needs to move, walk around, yawn, or stretch, let him.

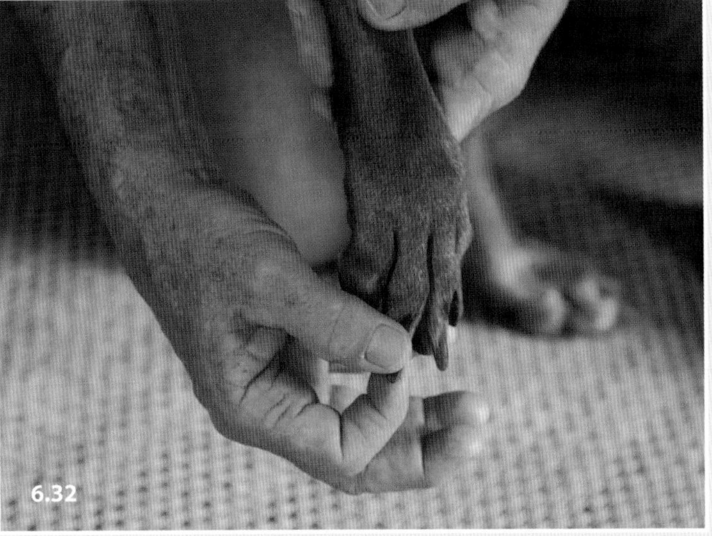

6.32

Tips

As with the front end, you'll find that you can provide a little extra support for your dog while handling the leg when you position yourself next to him to work with the leg on the opposite side.

Make sure, when reaching over the dog, that he's comfortable with this. Some dogs—especially when unfamiliar with the human—feel uncomfortable when being reached over, physically moved, or pushed, or even when held or hugged by a new person.

Also be prepared for the dog to want to sit or lie down as he relaxes. You can let him lean against you while holding the leg up to do the metacarpal and toe movements

Working with Tiny Dogs

As with other techniques, this can be done with smaller dogs on your lap, and with a few fingers.

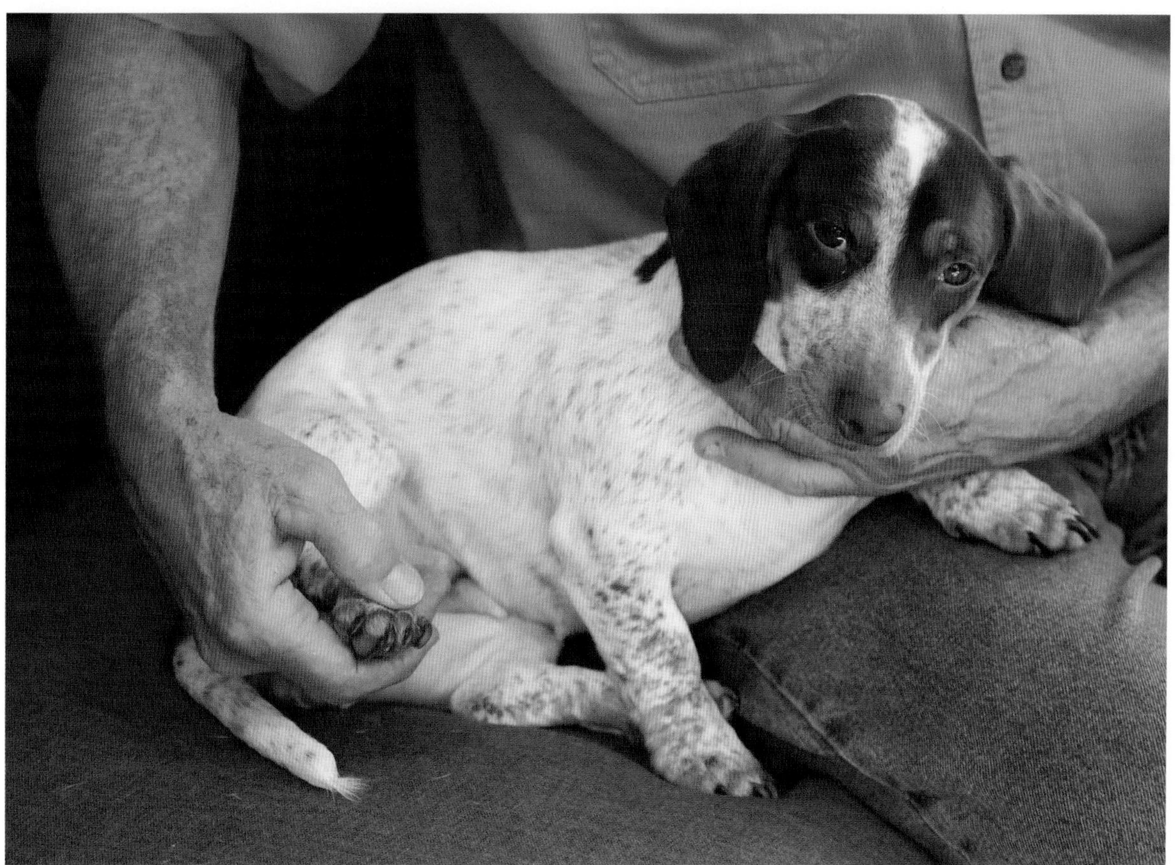

6.33 Toe Micromovement—on my lap!

LOWER HIND LIMB MOVEMENT (continued)

LOWER HIND LIMB MOVEMENT—*DOG LYING DOWN*

(Shown working with the dog lying on his side.)

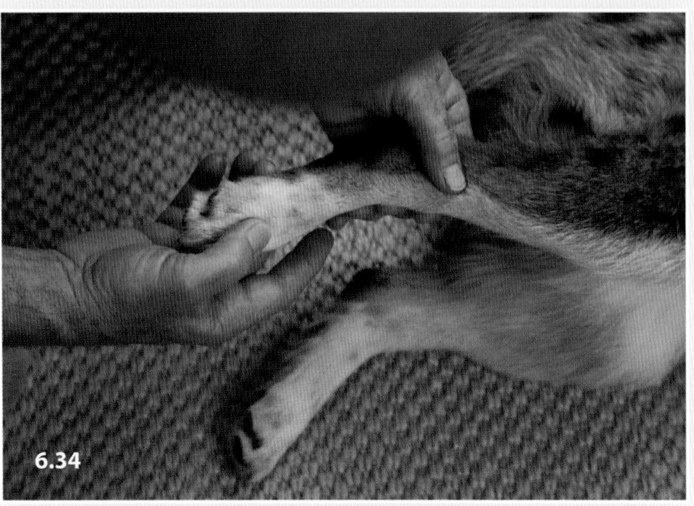
6.34

Let's start with the right leg and the dog lying on his left side.

Step 1. Position yourself sitting or kneeling at his hind end.

Step 2. Place your left hand under his hock.

Step 3. Gently hold the paw with your right hand and place your thumb on the metatarsal joint as shown (fig. 6.34).

Step 4. Soften both hands and allow the dog's leg to relax into your hand.

Remember, if the dog tenses or starts to pull his leg away, soften and yield.

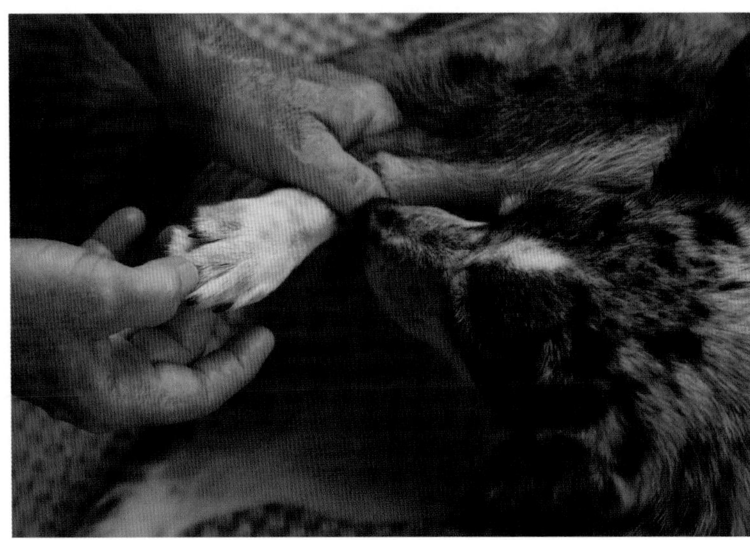

Sensitive Paws and Toes

Be aware that many dogs' lower limbs and paws can be sensitive or sore. Handle them gently (fig. 6.35).

6.35 Soften both hands at the first sign of discomfort.

Metatarsal Movement—Dog Lying Down

Step 1. Slowly move the paw through a gentle forward-and-back movement while watching for the blink (fig. 6.36).

Note: The metatarsal joint doesn't have as much lateral movement as the metacarpals do in the forelimb; however, you can ask for some circular movement behind.

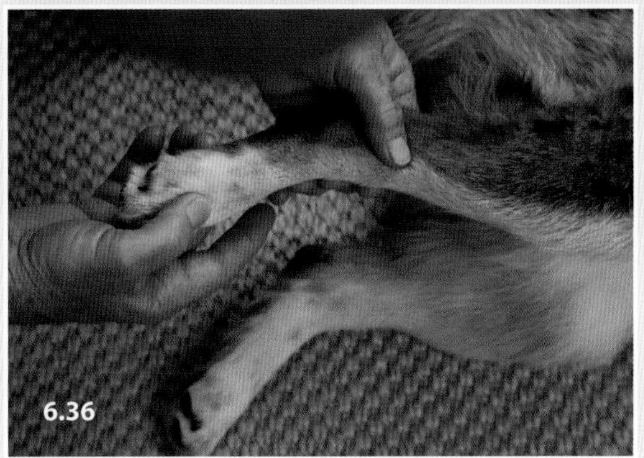

6.36

Toe Micromovement—Dog Lying Down

Step 1. Continuing to support the leg with your left hand, gently slide the thumb and fingers of your right hand down to the toes.

Step 2. Using very soft fingers, gently wiggle each of the toes and toenails through a tiny range of motion, continuing to watch for the *blinks* (fig. 6.37).

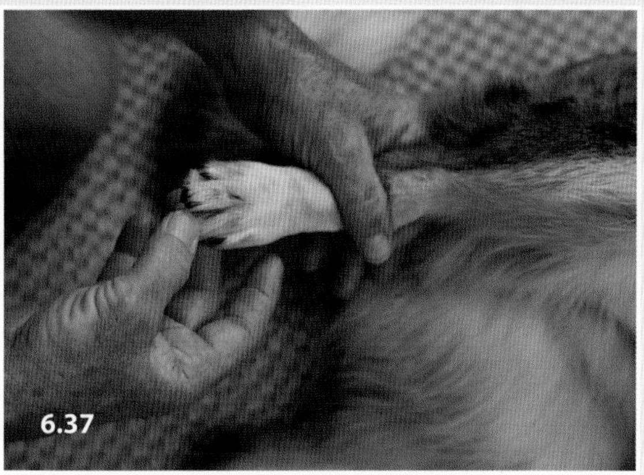

6.37

Hold, Wait, and Melt Techniques

Sacrum Float

GOAL: To apply the process of *Hold, Wait, and Melt* to the sacrum, sacroiliac, and connective tissue associated with the Lumbosacral Junction. You'll get the best results with the dog standing.

WHERE YOU WORK

The first vertebra of the dog's tail is connected to the sacrum. With the *Sacrum Float* you'll be using the tail to bring the dog's awareness to accumulated tension in muscles, tendons, or ligaments that might be putting torque on the dog's sacrum, and consequently, the sacroiliac joints. You do this by gently moving the tail until you see a blink or other subtle *Response* from the dog that indicates he is feeling the tension. When you get that *Response*, hold the tail in that position until the dog's nervous system *Releases* the tension.

Quick Overview: Step-by-Step

SACRUM FLOAT

Step 1. Position yourself sitting or kneeling behind your dog's hind end. When it is a small dog on a table, stand behind him.

Step 2. Gently hold the base of the dog's tail in your right hand (if you are right-handed), as shown.

Step 3. Place the palm of your left hand gently on the sacrum. Wait for the dog to relax the tail into your hand (fig. 6.38 A).

Step 4. Once the tail is relaxed, slowly *(I said, slowly!)* lift it, watching for a blink or other *Response* from the dog (fig. 6.38 B).

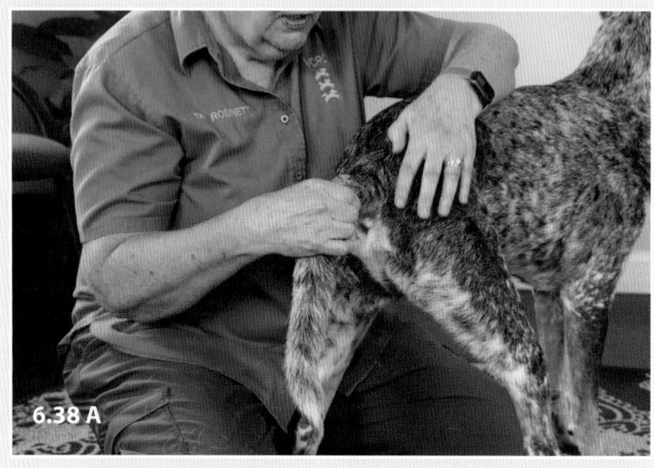
6.38 A

Step 5. When you get a response, *Hold* in this position, and *Wait* for the muscles to relax (fig. 6.38 C).

Step 6. Wait with both hands remaining *as soft as possible* until you get a *Release Response*, fidget, or change in behavior (*Melt*).

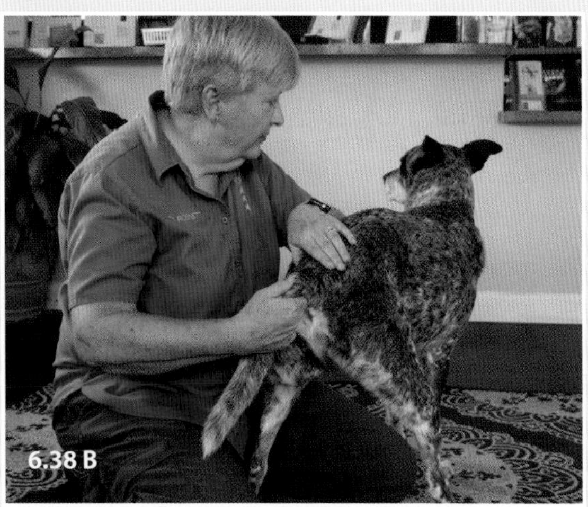
6.38 B

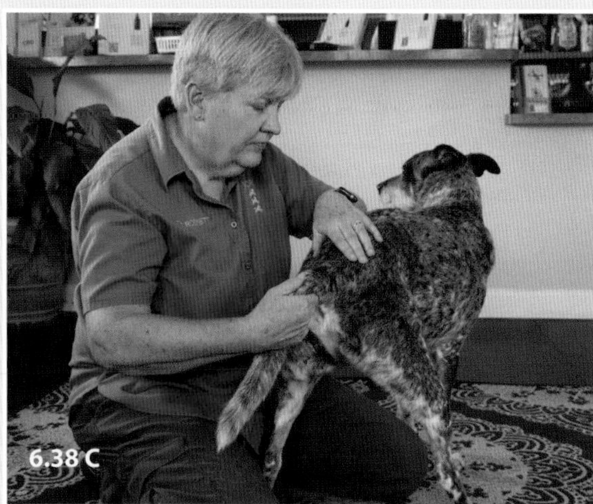
6.38 C

Tips

Take care when first lifting the tail. If your dog has been to the vet and had his temperature taken at this end, he may react uneasily.

When starting, the goal is to get the dog's tail in as relaxed a position as possible before lifting it (fig. 6.39). How you do this depends on your dog's natural tail position. For example, a Shih Tzu or Pomeranian will naturally hold his tail curled up over his back or high in the air, while with a Golden Retriever, not so much. The natural position of dogs' tails can vary anywhere in between.

Keep your hands as soft as possible, use no more than *Egg-Yolk* pressure when lifting, and watch for a blink or subtle change in behavior as you lift.

Some dogs might want to sit down right away as they feel this. If your dog starts to sit down, ask him to stay up a little longer by moving your "sacrum hand" (left hand in this case) under the belly between the hind legs and lifting.

The *Sacrum Float* only needs to be done once but can be done from either side.

Pelvic Release (*Pelvis, Lumbosacral Junction, Pubic Symphysis, Adductor,* and *Groin Muscles*)

GOAL: To apply the process of *Hold, Wait, and Melt* to muscles and ligaments that are putting tension or torque on the pelvis. This Technique is done on both the right and left sides.

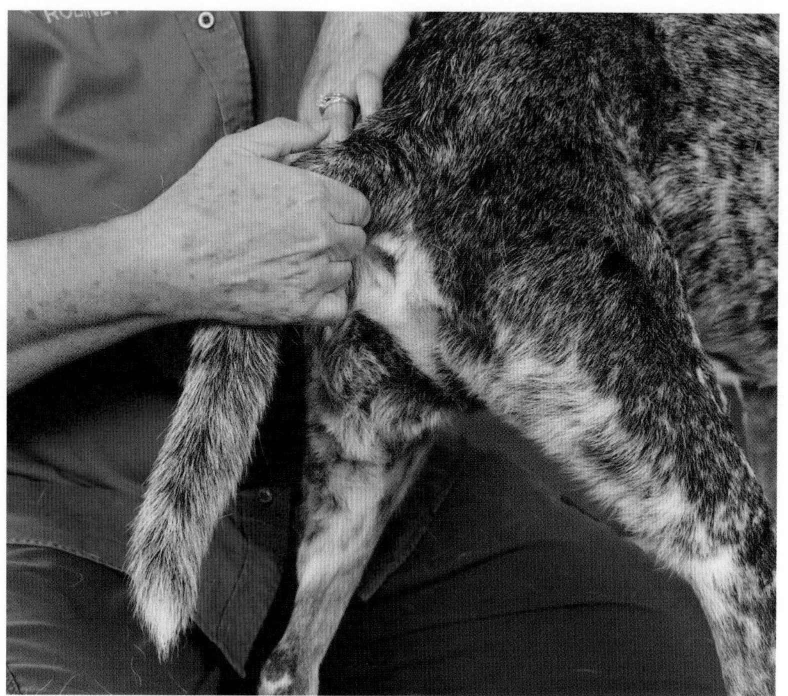

6.39 You can "ask" the dog to relax the tail down by resting the palm of your other hand on top of the tail.

WHERE YOU WORK

Adductor and deeper groin muscles (such as the *gracilis* and *pectineus*) attach inside the hind limb in the area of the pubic symphysis (see fig. 6.4 p. 101). Releasing tension here is done by resting the thumb of the hand on the Pubic Symphysis Point and the palm and fingers inside of the hind leg. The technique should be done on each side.

Quick Overview: Step-by-Step

PELVIC RELEASE

Scan to view Pelvic Release video

You'll get the best results with the dog standing.

Step 1. If working on the left side first, position yourself sitting or kneeling at your dog's left hind end. With a small dog on a table, stand behind the dog.

Step 2. Gently place the thumb of your right hand against the bony, hard area about 1 to 2 inches below the base of the tail on the left side. This is the *Pubic Symphysis Point* at the lower and back part of the pelvis. Rest your thumb softly against this spot (fig. 6.40 A).

Step 3. Place the palm and fingers of this hand on the muscles inside the left hind leg, high up into the groin area. Just rest your hand gently and relaxed against the muscles and *Hold* (fig. 6.40 B).

Step 4. Place your left arm and hand in front of the hind legs under his body to support him and keep him from leaving.

Step 5. Continue to hold with your hand in this position and *Wait*, watching for a blink or *Response* (fig. 6.40 C).

Step 6. Wait with your hand remaining as soft as possible until you get a *Release Response*, fidget, or change in behavior (*Melt*).

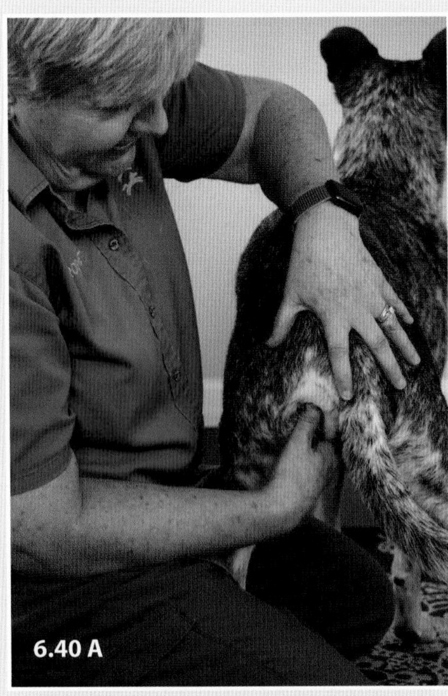

6.40 A

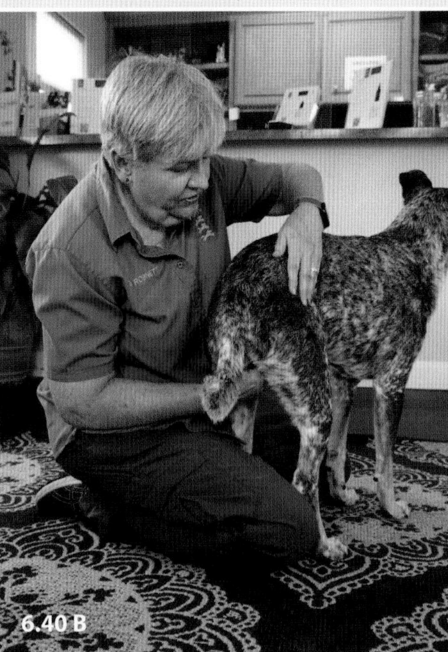

6.40 B

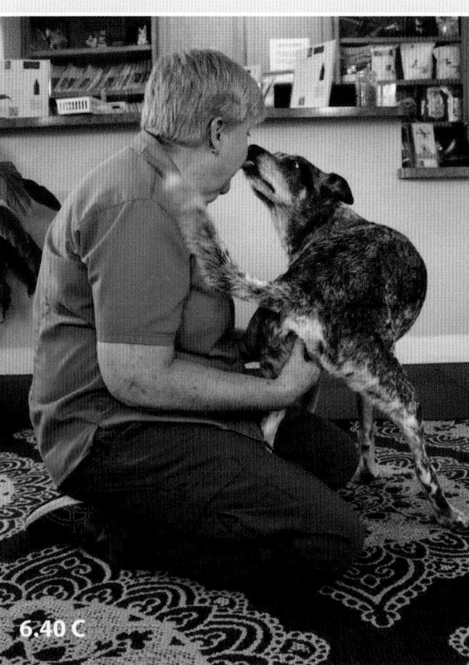

6.40 C

Tips

The left arm underneath the dog is to keep him with you and to keep him standing. He may want to sit.

The *Melt (Release)* will usually only take between 10 to 20 seconds, rarely up to 30 seconds. Often, the dog will rotate the hip outward or might take a step to the side, either toward or away from you (see fig. 6.40 C) when the muscles relax and tension in the pelvis lets go. This is an indication of the *Release*.

Although it is easier to do this with the dog standing, it can be done with the dog lying down using the same steps, and when this is the case, you don't have to worry about using your other hand to help hold him in one place.

If, after 20 seconds, there is no sign of *Release*, exhale and consciously soften the thumb and groin hand. This will often help the muscles soften and let go of the tension.

This work will help to release torque on the pubic symphysis and Lumbosacral-Pelvic Junction.

The *Sacrum Float* and *Pelvic Release* are two of the most effective releases of tension on the *Lumbosacral-Pelvic Junction*.

7

CHAPTER 7

The Midsection

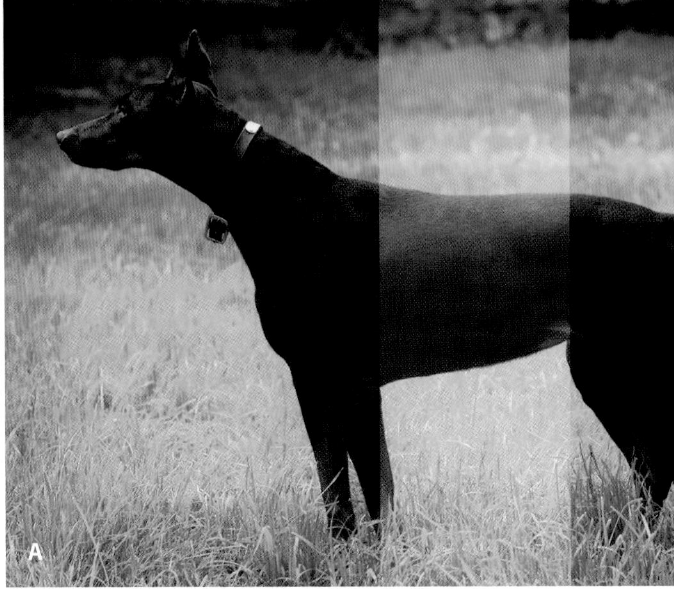

7.1 A–D The midsection.

This chapter discusses the various areas of the dog's midsection that accumulate tension, and offers exercises to release tension in these areas using the three categories of techniques that I outlined in Part One: *Search, Response, Stay, Release (SRSR)*, page 4; *Movement Techniques*, page 5; *Hold, Wait, and Melt Techniques (HWM)*, page 6.

Search, Response, Stay, Release

Shoulder Points, Top of Spine and Back Points, Sublumbar Points, Flank Points

GOAL: To apply the process of *Search, Response, Stay, Release* to muscles on the top of the back along each side of the spine, the lumbar area, and the loin area. (To begin these techniques, see p. 134.)

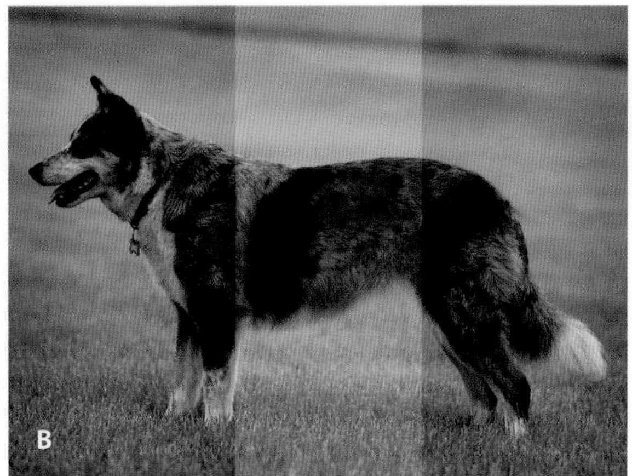

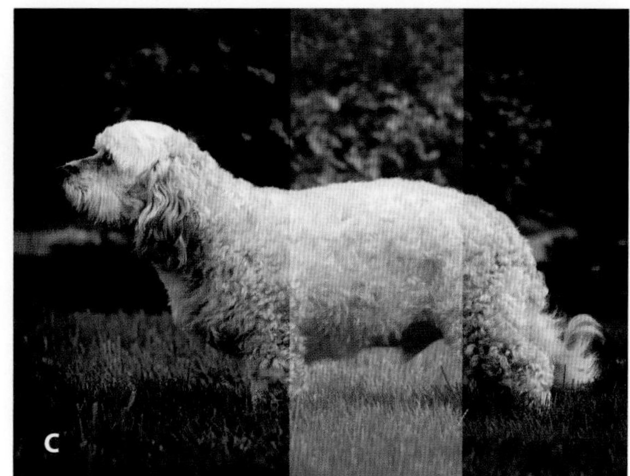

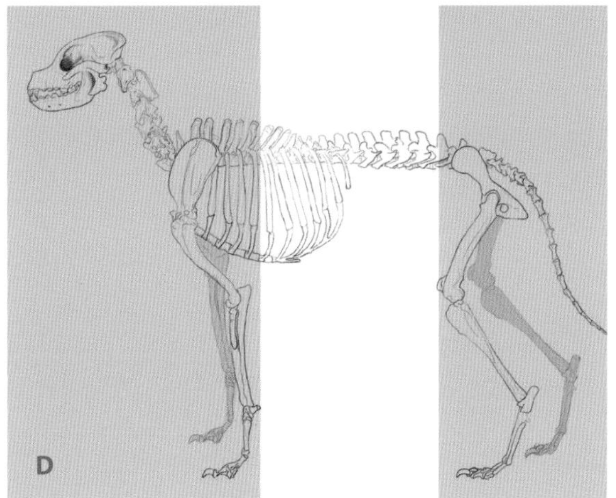

RESULT: *SRSR* on the back releases tension in the muscles and connective tissues of the vertebrae of the spine, the muscles on top of the back, the deeper muscles underneath the spine, and the rib cage. *SRSR* on the flanks and loins releases tension in the muscles of the rib cage and in deeper core muscles in the loin area. This results in improved suppleness of the spine and rib cage and prepares the spine and ribs for the *Movement Techniques* that follow.

Movement Techniques

Lateral (Side-to-Side) Body Rocking and Dorsal-Ventral (Up-and-Down) Body Rocking

GOAL: To get a relaxed and rhythmic rocking of the entire rib cage and spine. (To begin these techniques, see p. 140.)

RESULT: Body Rocking releases tension in all the muscles of the midsection, the Lumbosacral-Pelvic Junction, and the C7-T1 Junction together, and restores natural movement to the trunk in general.

Note: If you've ever had this done to you, you'll know this is really relaxing!

Hold, Wait, and Melt Techniques

Shoulder Release and Lumbar Release

GOAL: To apply the process of *Hold, Wait, and Melt* to the muscles of the shoulders and lumbar spine. (To begin these techniques, see p. 146.)

RESULT: Restores movement and range of motion to the shoulders and lumbar spine.

Note: Some dogs respond better to releasing tension at points on individual muscles associated with a structure or junction, while others respond better to releasing tension on the structure or junction itself. Some dogs respond to both.

More Anatomy and the Effects of Releasing Tension

The back and trunk tie the whole dog together. Almost all major muscles converge and attach to the back and midsection. Don't let this scare you, though. The flip side of this coin is that you've already been releasing tension in many of these areas while working on the front and hind ends. This is one reason you put your attention on the midsection last. It's easier to get the trunk moving once you've released both ends.

The Skeleton

The main parts of the spine you're concerned with here are the:

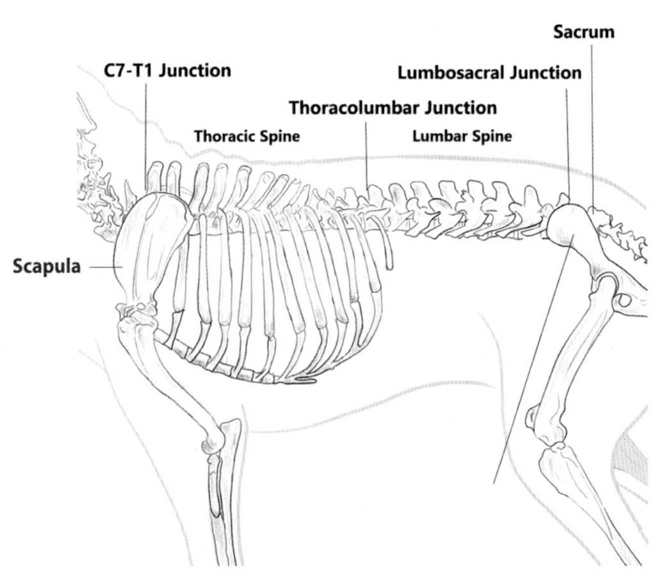

7.2 Midsection spine and junctions.

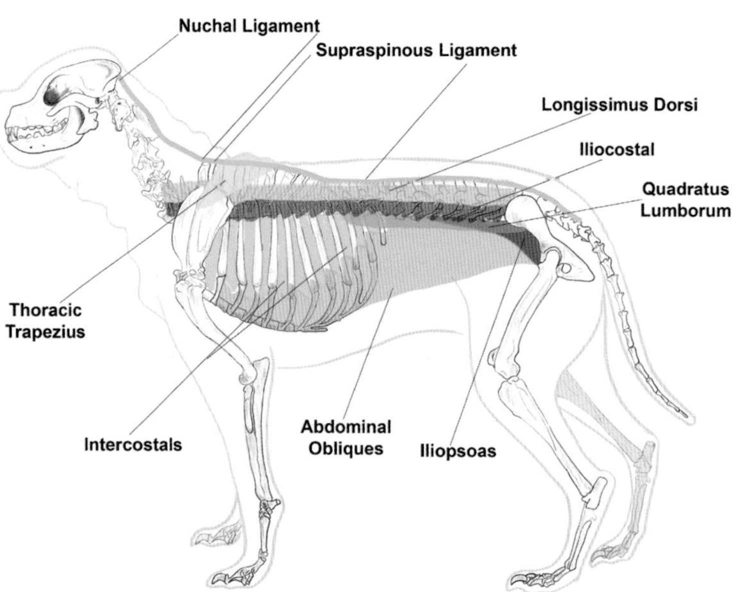

7.3 The muscles of the dog's midsection.

- *C7-T1*
- *Thoracic spine*
- *Thoracolumbar Junction*
- *Lumbar spine*
- *Lumbosacral Junction*

The other parts of the skeleton we're concerned with here are the:

- *Rib cage*
- *Scapula-forelimbs*
- *Hind limbs*

FROM THE VET

Intervertebral Disc Disorder (IVDD)

The *thoracic* part of the spine is relatively stable because of the attachment of ribs and the support of the rib cage.

The *lumbar spine* is more flexible and involved in movement in the hind end.

The *Thoracolumbar Junction* (*T-L Junction*) is a transition point between the two. Because of the increased mobility of the spine at the T-L Junction, it is the most common area for intervertebral disc problems (IVDD) in dogs. Spondylosis or arthritic changes are commonly seen at the T-L Junction area in older dogs as well, for the same reason.

—*Dr. Robinett*

Muscles of the Midsection

Muscles on Top of the Spine and Back

If you remember from chapter 5 (see fig. 5.3—p. 71), there is a *cervical* part of the *trapezius* (cervical traps) that attaches at the top of the neck and a *thoracic* part (thoracic traps) that attaches to the top of the trunk between the shoulder blades. They both attach to the scapula on each side (fig. 7.3).

One of the jobs of the *cervical traps* is to pull the top of the scapula forward, which pulls the forelimb back. When the leg is planted, this propels the dog forward. One of the main jobs of the *thoracic traps* is to raise the scapula back, which assists in raising and bringing the forelimb forward. They are also part of the muscular system that supports the trunk between the forelimbs. This is a busy muscle when it comes to support and movement of the dog.

The *longissimus dorsi* muscles run the full length of the back on top of the rib cage on each side of the spine.

One end of these muscles attaches on top of the lower cervical (neck) vertebrae. They run between the two scapulae and attach at the lower back in front of the pelvis on the other end.

When both *long dorsi* muscles contract at the same time, they cause the back to extend or flatten out as the dog extends forward with the forelimbs and extends behind with the hind limbs. When a *long dorsi* muscle on one side only contracts, it flexes that side of the body, causing a bend in the spine and trunk in that direction.

The *iliocostal* muscles run next to and below the *long dorsi* muscles. These muscles attach on top of the *cervical* (neck) vertebrae on the front end and in front of the *pelvis* at the back end. They have a close relationship with the ribs alongside the trunk, and work individually to assist in lateral (side-to-side) bending.

The *supraspinous* ligament is a band that runs along the top of the spine from the first thoracic vertebra to the top of the sacrum. It attaches to the tops of the thoracic vertebrae along the way. It is a continuation of the *nuchal ligament* (see fig. 7.3—p. 130), which runs from the second cervical vertebra behind the skull to the first thoracic vertebra. This band of heavy-duty ligament stabilizes the spine and helps hold everything together.

The *multifidus* muscles weave in between the vertebrae and support the spine.

FROM THE VET

The Benefit of Core Muscle Exercises

The *multifidus* muscles are major "core" muscles that support the spine. Research in people and animals shows that with a back injury, these muscles start to atrophy or decrease in size and weaken within 72 hours. These muscles have to be activated by doing some type of exercise specifically targeting them to wake them up, strengthen them, and get them working again. This is why core exercises are so important for people and animals, especially after an injury.

—*Dr. Robinett*

Sublumbar Muscles

These are muscles that attach underneath the spine and stabilize and support the Lumbosacral Junction, flex (arch) the lumbar spine, and bring the hind end and legs underneath the body to drive the dog forward, for example, when the dog runs (see sidebar—facing page).

The *quadratus lumborum* muscles ("QLs" in muscle-speak) attach underneath the thoracic and lumbar vertebra on one end, and on the front of each wing of the pelvis on the other. They support the lumbar spine and Thoracolumbar Junction, and flex the spine and Lumbosacral Junction, bringing the hind end underneath the body during the run.

The *iliopsoas* (also called *psoas*) muscles are the major core as well as "gymnastic" muscles in the dog. In addition to supporting and flexing the lumbar spine, these important muscles also attach to the inside of the femur to bring the hind limbs forward when the dog is running.. Tension or weakness in the *psoas* muscles can be a factor in back pain in both people and animals.

Muscles of the Flank, Abdomen, and Rib Cage

The *abdominal oblique* muscles attach in three important areas:

- The area of the *tuber coxa* or *pelvic point.*
- The *pubic symphysis* in the groin area.
- Throughout the ribs and the fascia of the abdominal area.

The *abdominal obliques* assist in flexing and bending the body. They also compress and support

Muscles Working Together

When the muscles on top of the spine contract, they cause the back to extend or flatten out as the dog brings the forelimbs forward and extends the hindlimbs behind.

Muscles on top of the spine contract to extend the thoracic and lumbar spine, helping Nellie to catch the frisbee (fig. 7.4 A). When the opposing *sublumbar* muscles underneath the spine contract, the opposite happens. The back flexes upward as both the forelimbs and hind limbs come under the body as the dog runs. The *sublumbar* muscles contract to flex the lumbar spine and bring the hind end and legs underneath the body, helping Nellie run away with the frisbee (fig. 7.4 B). The *long dorsi* and *iliocostal* muscles on one side contract to bend the body in that direction (fig. 7.4 C).

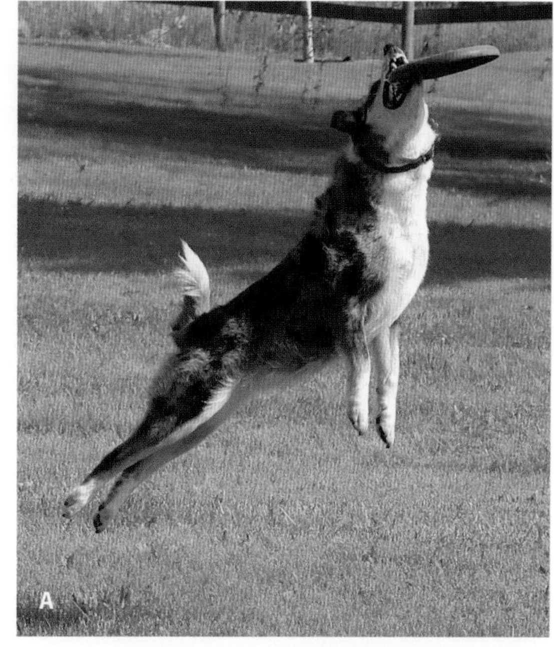

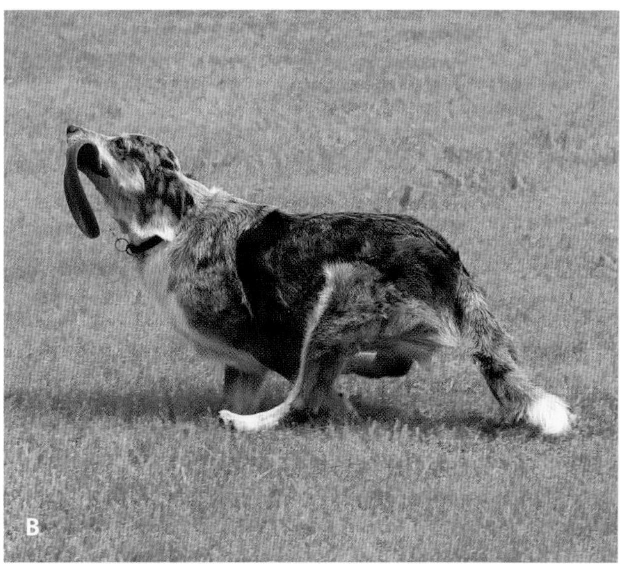

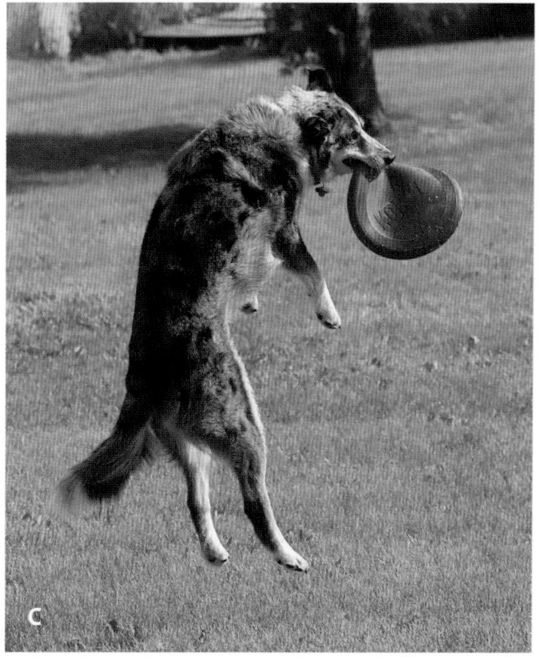

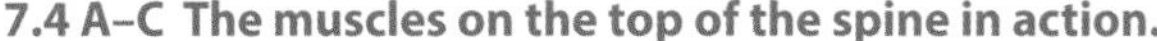

7.4 A–C The muscles on the top of the spine in action.

7.5 A & B The Shoulder Points, Top of Spine and Back Points, Sublumbar Points, and Flank Points, from the top and side view.

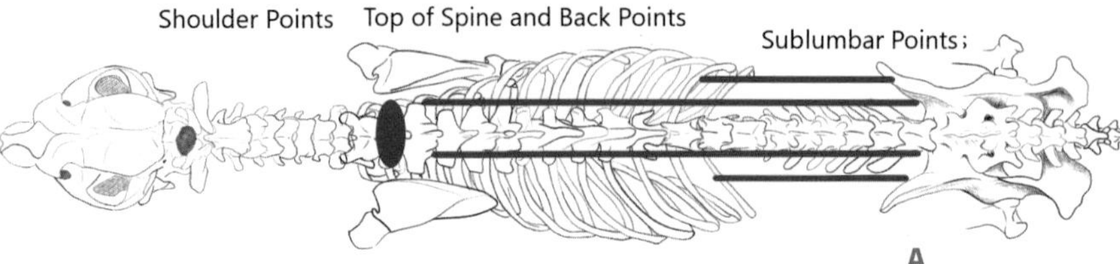

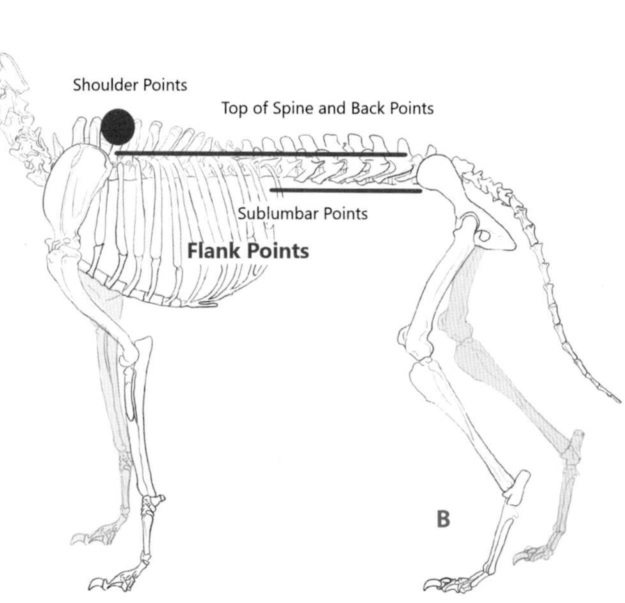

the internal organs of the abdomen during movement.

The *intercostals* are muscles of the thoracic wall or trunk that connect the ribs. Think of them as "rib cage muscles." In addition to holding things together, one of their jobs is to assist the diaphragm with breathing (respiration).

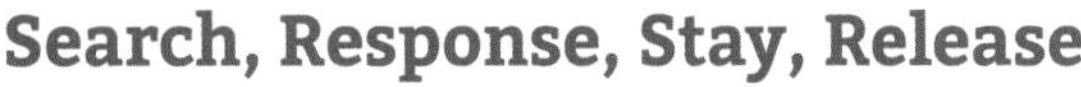

Search, Response, Stay, Release

GOAL: To apply the process of *Search, Response, Stay, Release* to the following areas (figs. 7.5 A & B):

- Top of the shoulders.
- Top of the spine and back.
- Sublumbar muscles.
- Trunk and flanks.

WHERE YOU WORK

Shoulder Points (Thoracic Traps)

These points lie on top of the back just behind the scapula or shoulders on each side of the spine (fig. 7.6).

Top of Spine and Back Points (Long Dorsi, Iliocostal, Supraspinous Ligament)

These points run on and along each side of the

Muscular Balance in the Body

The muscles on the top of the spine and the sublumbar muscles underneath the spine work together to keep the muscles and joints of the body balanced and healthy. This applies to all groups of muscles that work together.

Balanced conditioning (not overworking one muscle or group of muscles), and bodywork to release accumulated tension also work together to keep the body balanced and healthy.

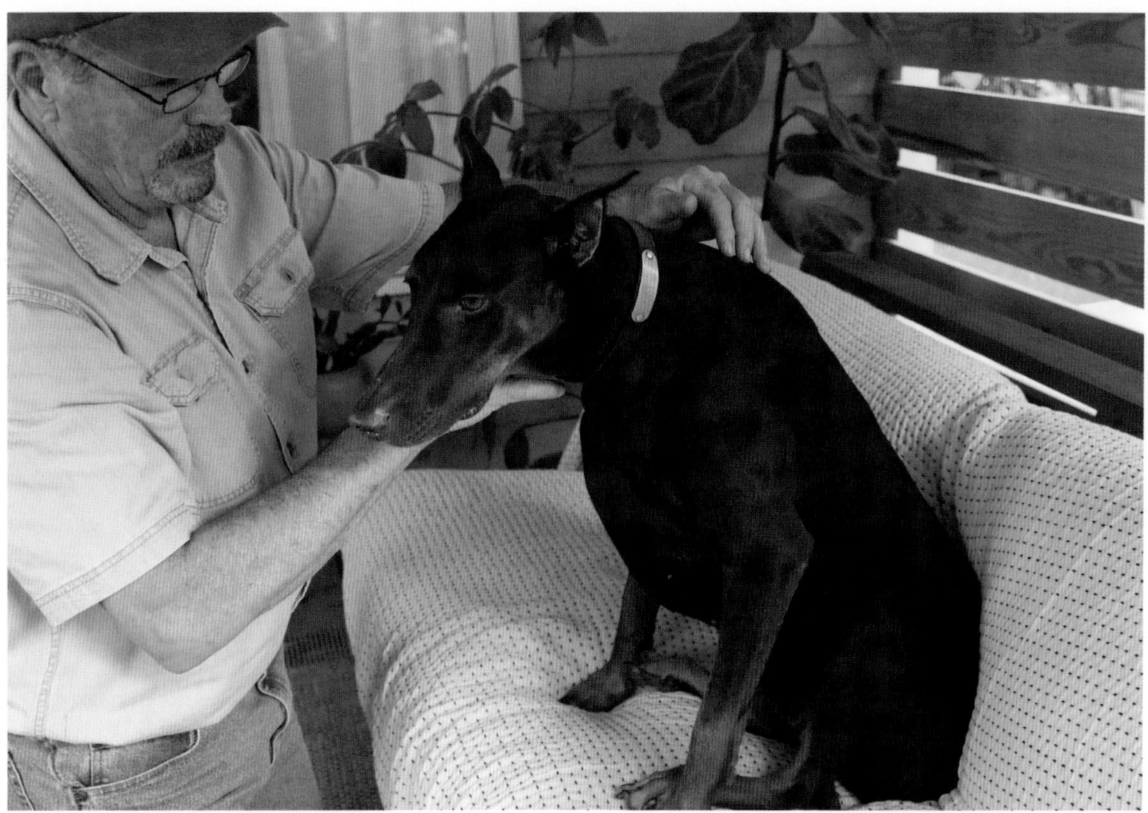

7.6 The Shoulder Points.

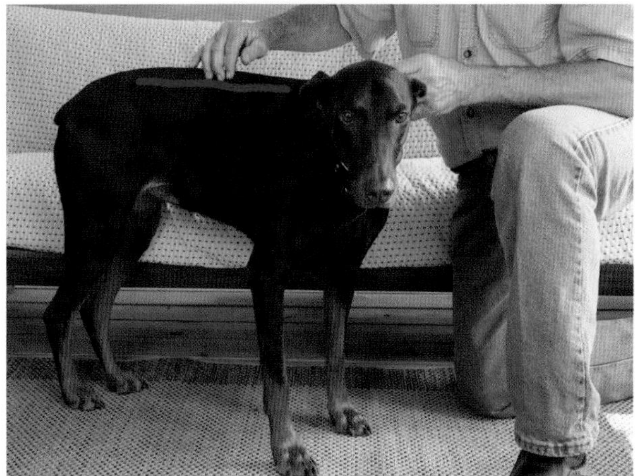

7.7 The Topline and Back Points.

FROM THE VET

Arthritis

The Bladder Meridian runs parallel along either side of the spine. In Traditional Chinese Medicine, the acupuncture point *BL 11* is the back association point for bone. Dogs with arthritis or bony problems in general are often sensitive at this point between the scapulae, just behind the C7–T1 Junction.

—*Dr. Robinett*

Scan to view Top of the Spine, Back, and Sublumbar Points video

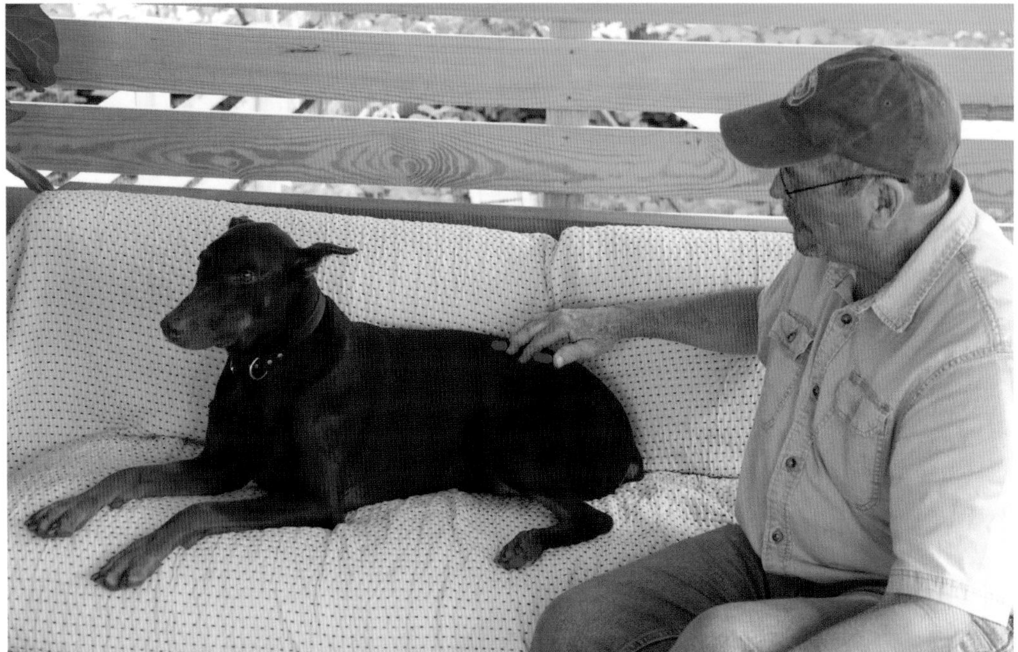

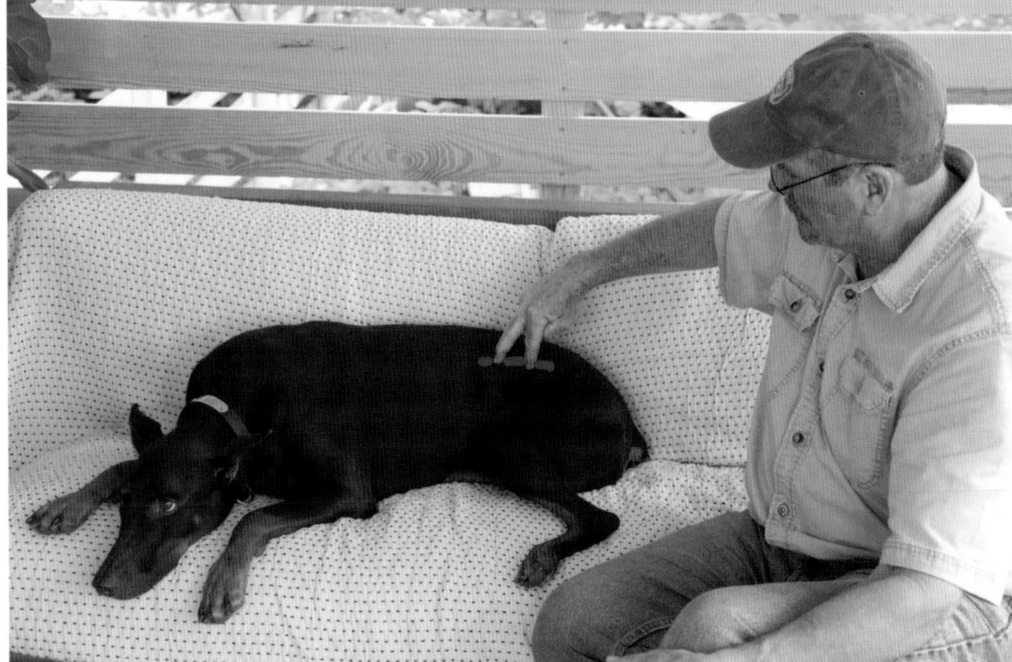

7.8 A & B The Sublumbar Points on top of the lumbar area (A) and on each side of the lumbar area (B).

FROM THE VET

Interconnections

The *abdominal oblique muscles* are also affected by the *Pubic Symphysis Point* on the hind end.

—*Dr. Robinett*

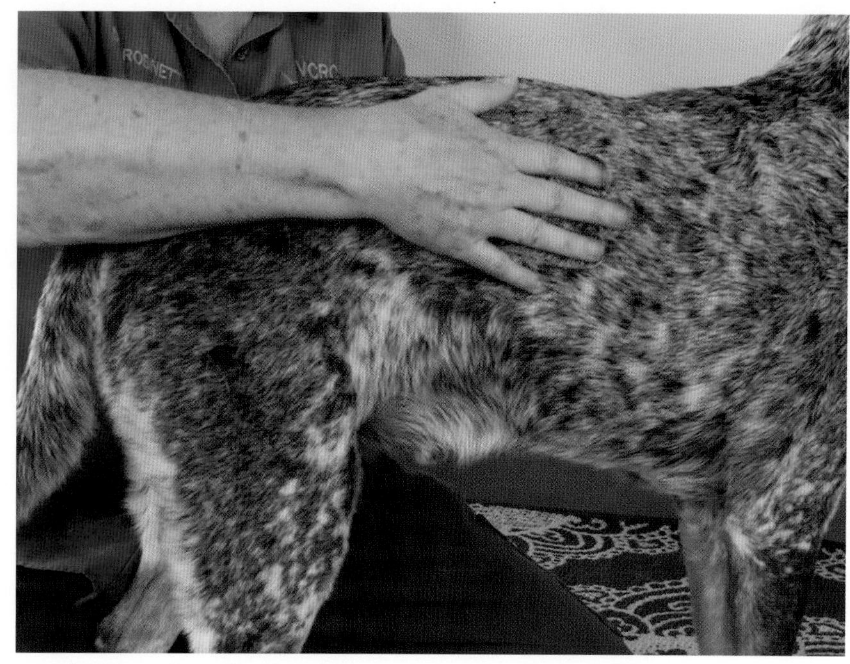

7.9 The area of the Flank Points.

spine, starting behind the scapula and ending at the front of the pelvis (fig. 7.7). The *long dorsi* points lie parallel and directly next to the spine, while the *iliocostals* lie parallel to them and just a little lower. Your dog will tell you which needs attention.

The Sublumbar Points (Psoas, Quadratus Lumborum)

There are two places to access these sublumbar muscles:

1 There are points for sublumbar muscles on top of the lumbar area (fig. 7.8 A).

2 There are points for sublumbar muscles along each side of the lumbar area (fig. 7.8 B).

Search both areas, as they are both effective. The dog will tell you which ones are best for him.

To find the front of the lumbar area, feel along the sides of the spine for the last rib of the thoracic part of the spine (see fig. 7.2—p. 130). This is where the lumbar spine begins.

To find the back of the lumbar area, feel for the *pelvic point* that is on what is commonly called the "point of the hip" (hip bone).

Everything in between is the *lumbar area.*

Flank Points (Abdominal Obliques, Intercostals)

These points start at the *Pelvic Point* and can be found anywhere in front of or below the pelvis, throughout the abdomen, rib cage, and trunk (fig. 7.9).

Note that what I have shown you on these pages are the *general areas* of the points. Your dog's responses will tell you exactly which points need attention and where they are.

Quick Overview: Step-by-Step

SHOULDER POINTS, TOP OF SPINE AND BACK POINTS, SUBLUMBAR POINTS, AND FLANK POINTS

You can do these with your dog standing, sitting, on your lap, or lying down, although it is easier to see what he's telling you when he is sitting or standing. Choose a place to begin.

Step 1. *Search.* Using the tip of either one or two fingers, barely touching the hair, slowly (I said SLOWLY) and gently search with your fingertip(s) in the area of the points (fig. 7.10 A). Your dog will tell you exactly where to stop when you get a...

Step 2. *Response.* Watch closely for a blink or other change of behavior (fig. 7.10 B).

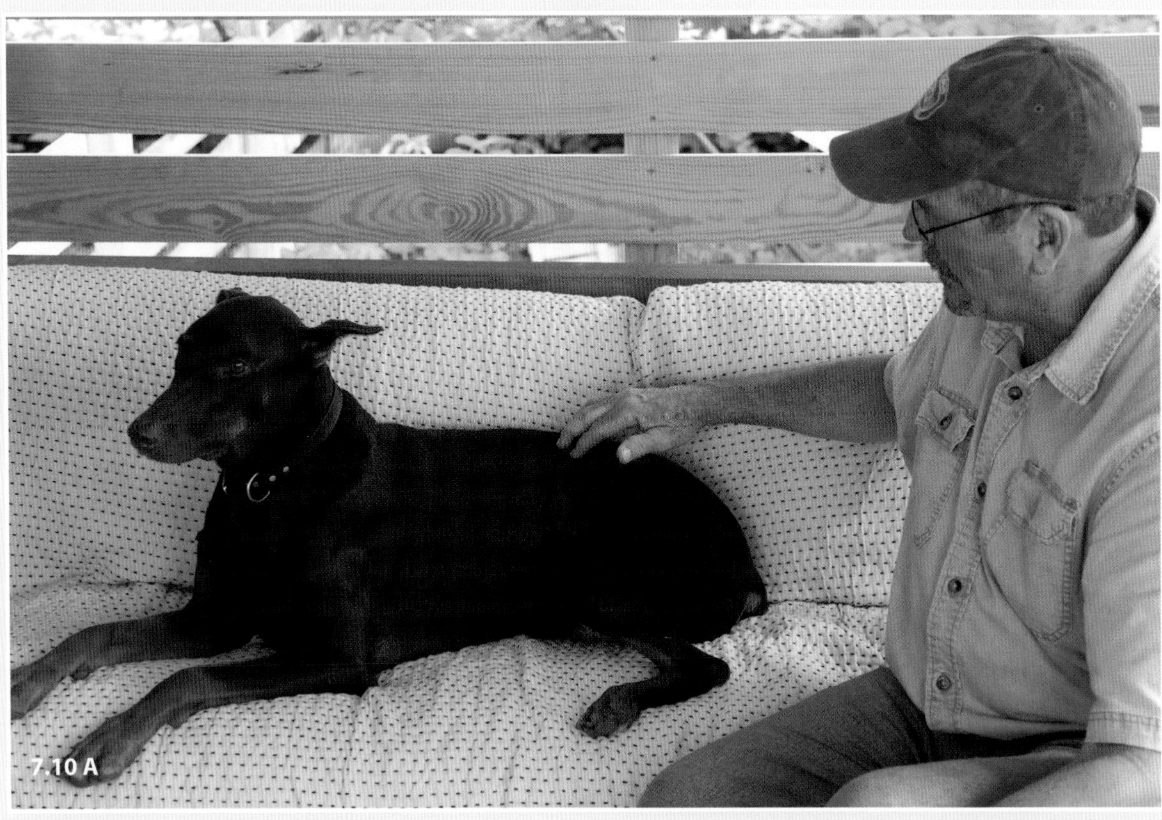
7.10 A

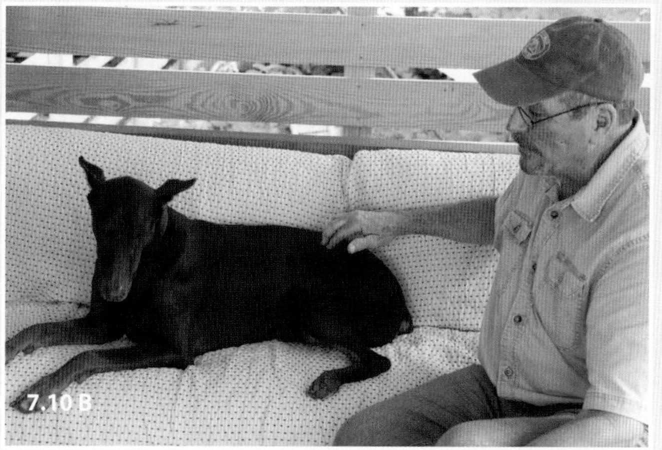
7.10 B

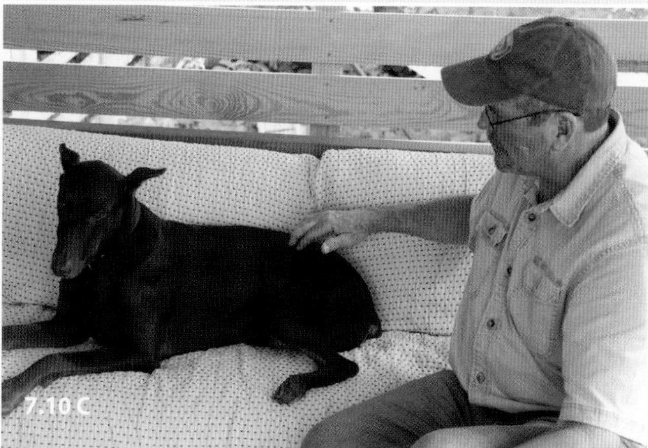
7.10 C

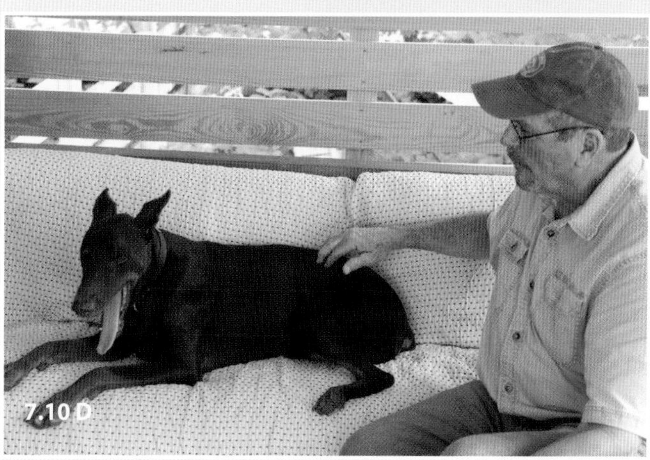
7.10 D

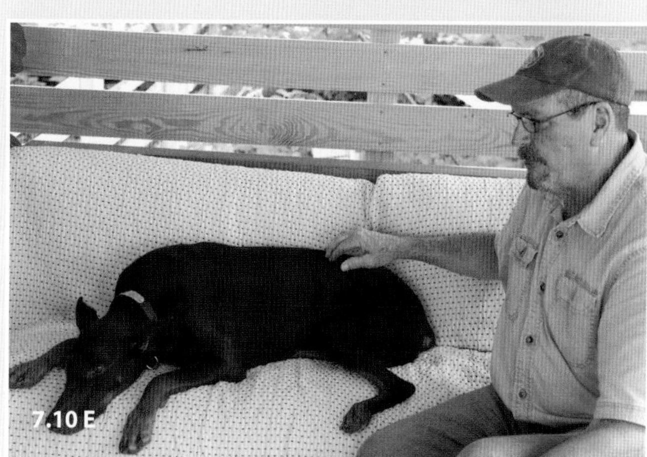
7.10 E

Step 3. *Stay*. Keep your finger over that spot, maintaining Air Gap. Resist the urge to move the finger, push, rub, or stroke (fig. 7.10 C). This may take one second or one minute. Be patient. Breathe and relax, until you get a…

Step 4. *Release*, such as licking and chewing or yawning (fig. 7.10 D).When you are finished, you can either repeat the process on the opposite side or continue the process in one of the other areas on the same side (fig. 7.10 E).

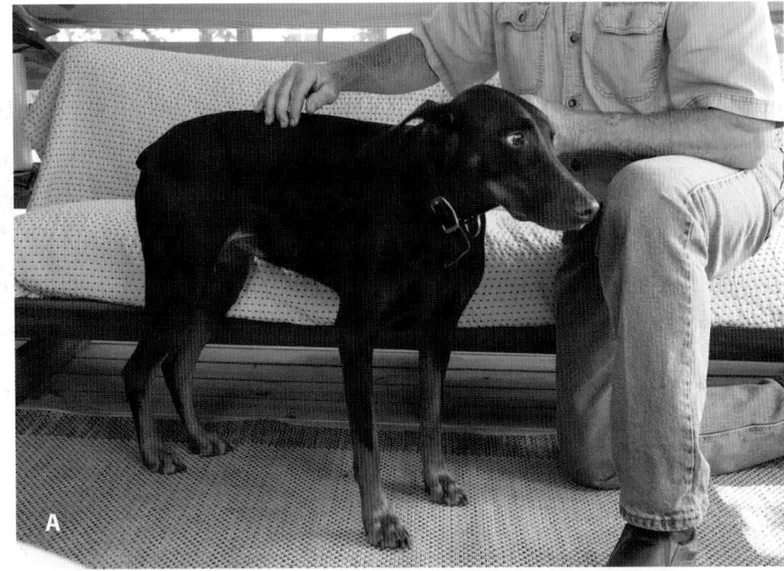

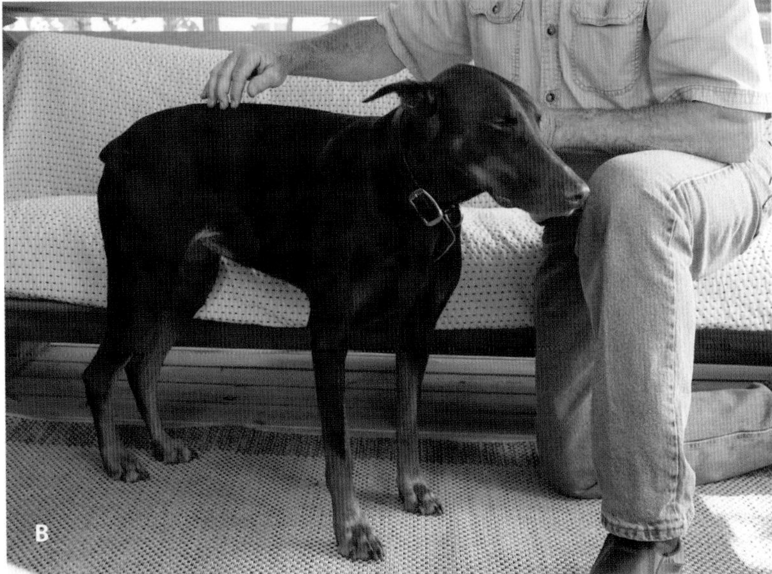

7.11 A & B Search (A) and Response (B). Your dog will let you know. Easy peasy.

Tips

There is no particular order of points or areas that you need to begin on. It's an experiment to see what your dog tells you—that is, *where*. When you find something, you give your dog the opportunity to release it.

Don't worry that you're on the exact point. Your dog will tell you where he's feeling something (figs. 7.11 A & B). *That's* the point!

Start where it's easier for the dog. If you know or suspect your dog is extremely sore in an area, it might be better to start somewhere else first. If your dog fidgets immediately or excessively in an area, move on and come back to the area after you've done the opposite side.

Your dog may fuss, fidget, or want to get up or walk away while you're doing *SRSR* in an area as he starts to feel the tension that has accumulated in that area. This is especially the case in the lumbar area. If this happens, soften, and open the Air Gap even more, and ask him to stay with you a little longer. If he won't stay, don't make him. Let him go and see if he shows you any *Release Responses* after he's moved around.

Movement Techniques

GOAL: *Body Rocking* consists of a relaxed and rhythmic rocking of the entire rib cage and spine. The key to effective rocking is the amount of relaxation in the movement rather than the amount or range of movement. The tiniest relaxed movement is more powerful than a larger range of movement.

Case Study

TRY THE OTHER SIDE

Your dog may fuss and fidget if he feels excessive tension in an area (figs. 7.12 A–C).

The first thing to do is soften your hand and open the *Air Gap* (fig. 7.12 D).

If he's still uncomfortable, then try the other side (fig 7.12 E)…where you might find: "Aah! Release!" (fig 7.12 F).

If you start on his more "accepting" side first, it is often easier for him to release on the tighter side.

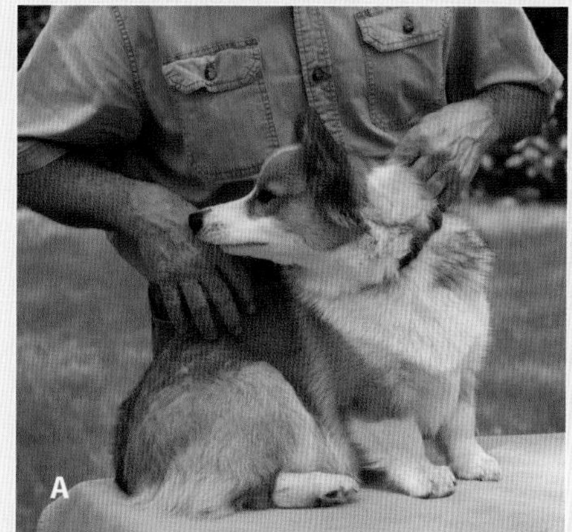

A

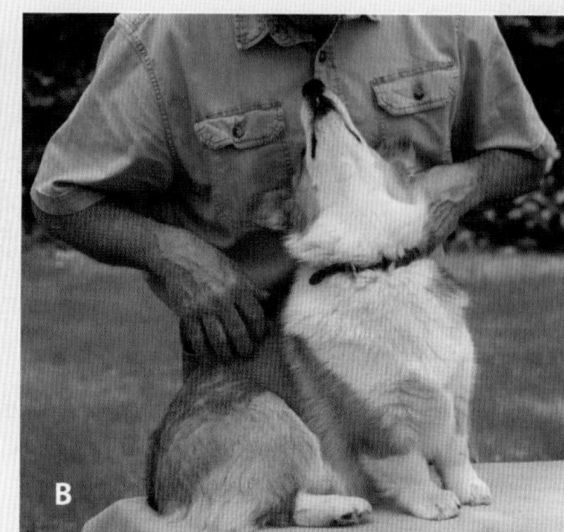

B

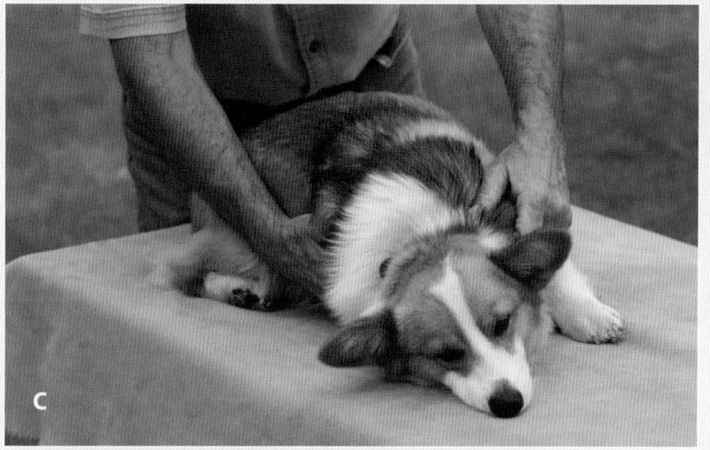

C

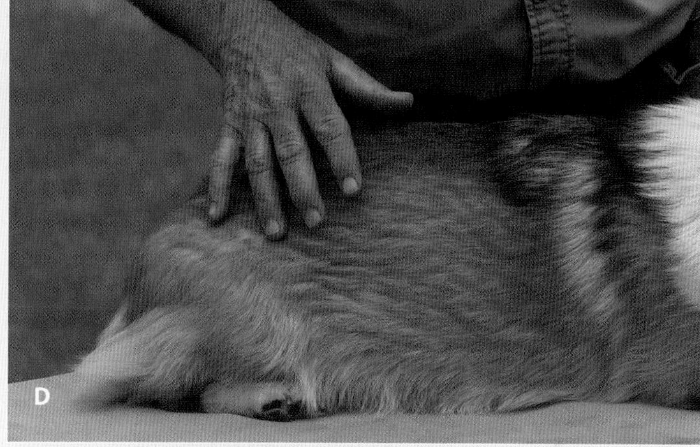

D

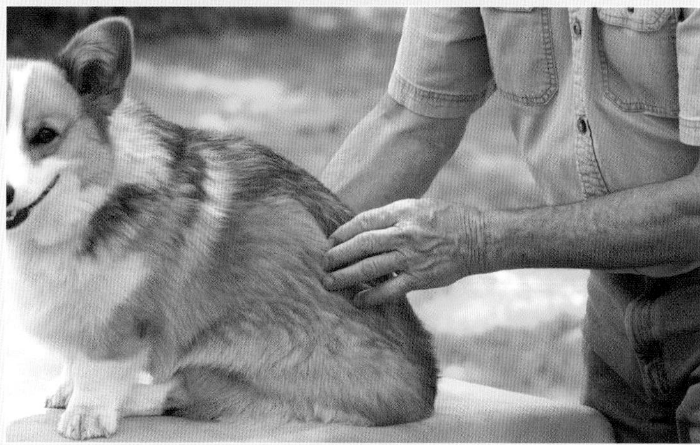

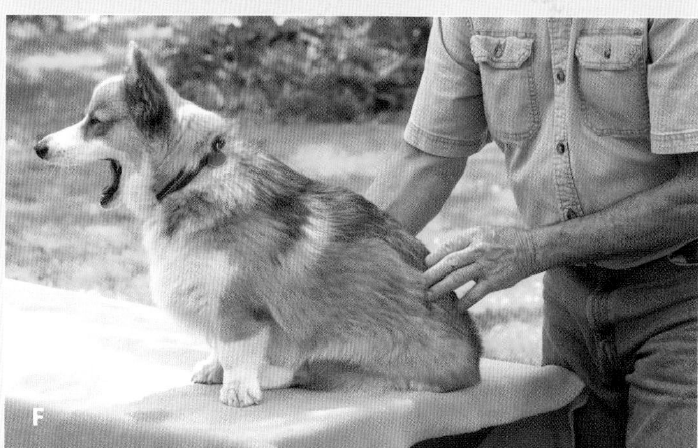

F

Quick Overview: Step-by-Step

LATERAL (SIDE-TO-SIDE) BODY ROCKING

This is more easily achieved with the dog standing but can be done with an extremely lazy dog while he's sitting, and an even lazier dog while he's lying on his back.

The principle here is relaxed, rhythmic movement side to side that creates a tiny bit of movement in the vertebrae of the dog's spine in a completely relaxed state. From this point of view, a dog lying on his back is the best candidate because the spine is as relaxed as it can be. You're going to be using both the front end, and the hind end of the dog to get the body rocking around a fulcrum in the middle.

Step 1. Position yourself next to or behind the dog.

Step 2. Place one hand on the trunk behind the dog's shoulder. This is the "body hand."

Step 3. Place the other hand on the opposite side in the area of the pelvis or rump. This is the "rump hand."

Step 4. Create a gentle side-to-side rocking motion by bringing the body hand toward you while at the same time pushing the rump hand away from you (figs. 7.13 A & B), then releasing both hands to let the body swing back (figs. 7.13 C & D), allowing the dog's body to gently swing back and forth with each "input" and "release."

Step 5. Once you get a gentle, relaxed, side-to-side rhythm going through the body, you can focus where you want the rocking by shifting the placement of your hands up and down the rib cage and flank with each rhythm.

Step 6. If you're gentle enough, you'll be able to watch for blinks as you move the body hand to see where along the body the dog is sensing tension. You can focus on these areas, going back and forth over them with the body hand.

Step 7. Keep rocking until your arms get tired, the dog lies down or goes to sleep, or it's time for dinner.

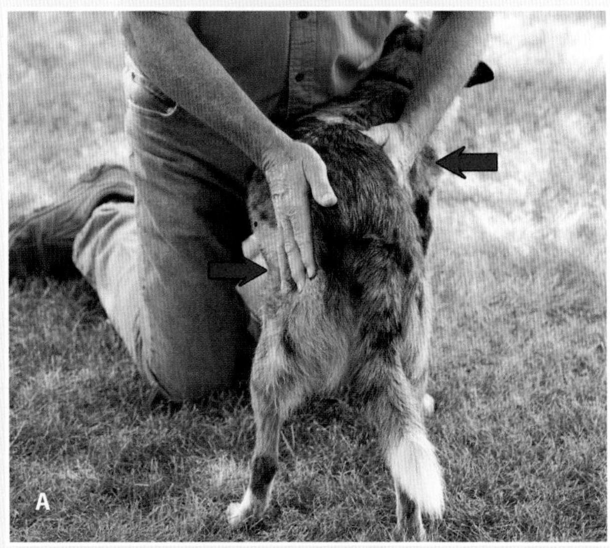
A

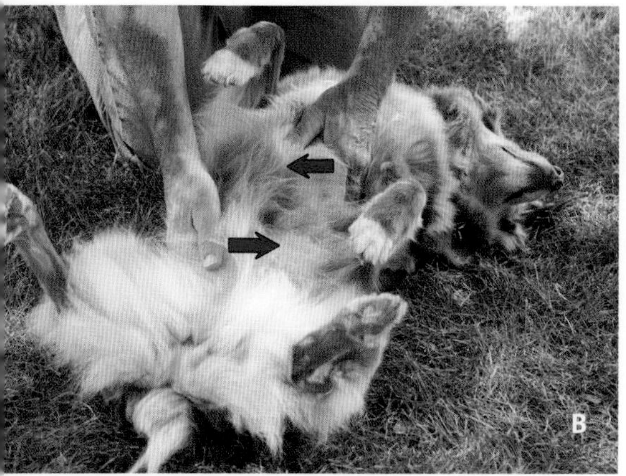

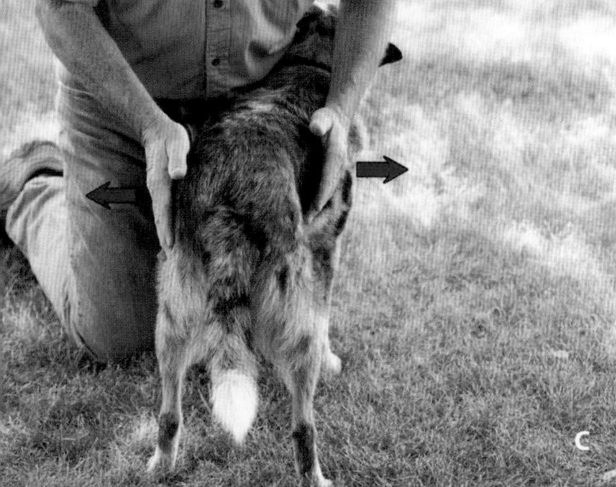

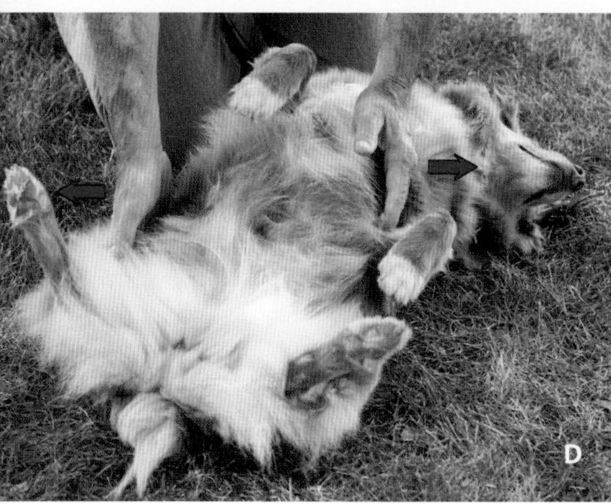

Face Either Direction, As Long As You're "Rocking"

You can do the same thing facing in the opposite direction, with one hand in the area of the lumbar spine, and the opposite hand in the area of the shoulder (fig. 7.14). This puts the focus of the movement farther forward.

Scan to view Lateral Body Rocking video

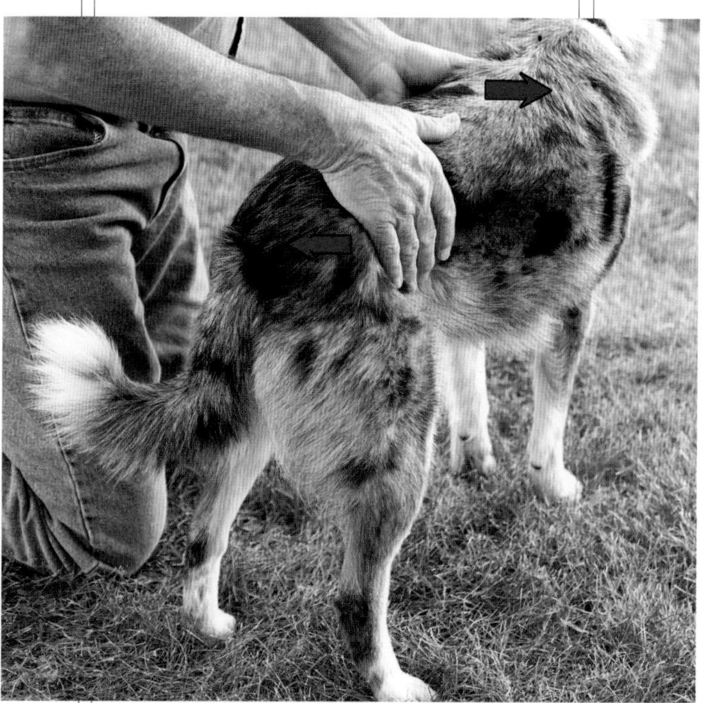

7.14 Switch hands if you change directions, and keep rocking!

Quick Overview: Step-by-Step

DORSAL-VENTRAL (UP-AND-DOWN) BODY ROCKING

Scan to view Dorsal-Ventral Body Rocking video

This should be done with the dog lying relaxed on his side.

Step 1. With the dog lying on his side, position yourself behind or at the feet of the dog.

Step 2. Place one hand on the dog's rump or sacrum. This is the "rump hand."

Step 3. Place the other hand on the dog's chest. This is the "chest hand."

Step 4. Begin by pushing parallel to the floor toward you ("up" on the chest) with the chest hand, while at the same time pushing parallel to the floor in the opposite direction ("down" on the rump) with the rump hand (fig. 7.15 A), then releasing both hands to let the body swing back (fig. 7.15 B), creating a relaxed dorsal-ventral movement with each pressure and release. This will have the effect of bending the dog's rump underneath the hind end, creating a relaxed bending and un-bending of the lumbar spine and Lumbosacral Junction with each movement.

Step 7. Do this until your arms get tired or it's time for dinner. It's possible that after rocking for a while your dog could be completely asleep.

Step. 8. Step back, and if the dog is still awake, see what he has to say. If not, then (sorry, I have to say it) let sleeping dogs lie!

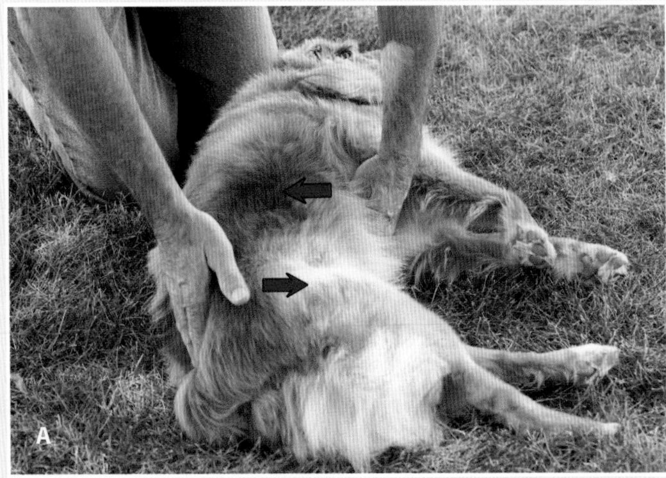

A

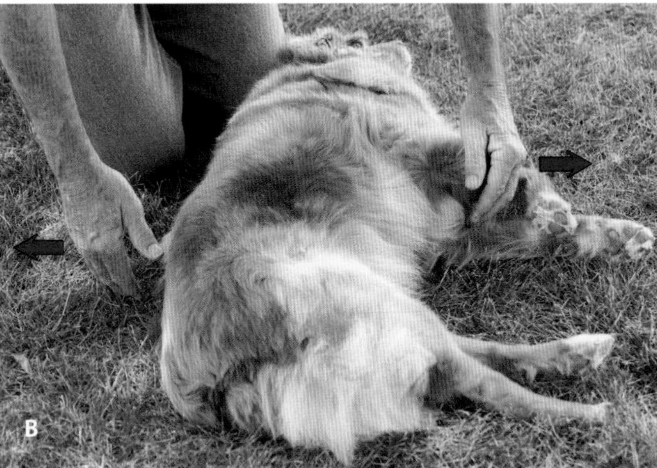

B

Tips

You can start rocking at the front end or the hind end, or in the middle. When the dog is uncomfortable, start again but softer. If he's still uncomfortable, start at the other end. If he's still uncomfortable, go back to *SRSR* (see p. 138) or proceed to *HWM* (see p. 146) on those areas.

With *Dorsal-Ventral Rocking,* the dog will need to be lying relaxed on his side. It's better if he's already lying relaxed, but if you can get him on his side and start with a very gentle rocking, he may relax into it. You'll need to use a little more force to create the movement when the dog is lying on his side, as there is some "drag" caused by the side of his body on the floor.

If your dog has been lying down during any of the other exercises, you can take advantage of this to do either *Lateral* or *Dorsal-Ventral Rocking*. The movement must be as relaxed as possible for this to be effective.

The key words here are "relaxed" and "rhythmic." If you start with too large of a movement, or without relaxation in the rhythm, the dog may be internally bracing against the movement. Start with a very tiny "micro-wiggle." Gently increase the movement from there. Smaller relaxed movement is much more effective than "large" movement.

Keep in mind that the goal of the rocking movement isn't so much to mechanically loosen the connective tissue of the skeleton, but to "wake up" the dog's nervous system in a way that allows him to feel where he's holding accumulated tension that he can begin to *Release*. This is why it's more effective to do tiny rocking movements while the dog is in a relaxed state, than larger movements.

Rocking Tiny Dogs

Small dogs can be rocked even more easily using one hand or a few fingers (fig. 7.16).

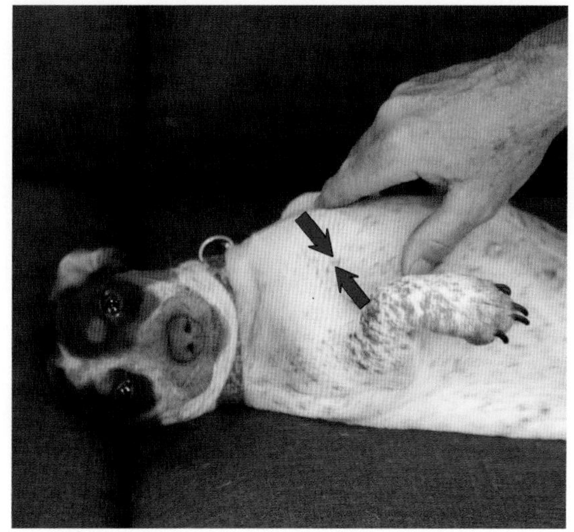

7.16 Doing lateral rocking on a tiny dog.

Keep On Rocking!

You almost *can't* overdo the rocking. The more relaxed movement you get in the spine, the better. Spend extra time on the lumbar spine and the Lumbosacral Junction, as this area tightens up easily in dogs, especially older dogs. But be gentle!

Even if the dog appears relaxed with a large rocking, he could be guarding or tensing internally. If you're not observing any blinks or visual responses when you start, it may be that the dog is "blocking out" any sensation, and you could just be "mechanically" rocking. In this case, soften the rocking and watch the eyes closely for any sign of the dog feeling a sensation along the way.

Hold, Wait, and Melt Techniques

GOAL: To apply the process of *Hold, Wait, and Melt* to the shoulders and lumbar spine.

Hold, Wait, and Melt brings the dog's awareness to tension in a larger area or junction of the body. Allow the dog's *Responses* to tell you where

Quick Overview: Step-by-Step

SHOULDER RELEASE

You'll get the best results with the dog sitting or standing.

Step 1. Position yourself sitting next to the shoulder area or behind the dog.

Step 2. Hold the palm of one hand softly on top of the shoulder area of the dog.

Step 3. Place the palm of the other hand softly on the dog's chest or sternum (fig. 7.17 A).

Step 4. Gently adjust your shoulder hand so that you get a blink or response (*Hold*)...

Step 5. Relax your hands, arms, and shoulders, and wait with your hands as soft as possible (*Wait*)...

Step 6. When you get a larger *Response* such a yawn, fidget, or change in behavior (fig. 7.17 B), that will be the *Release* (*Melt*).

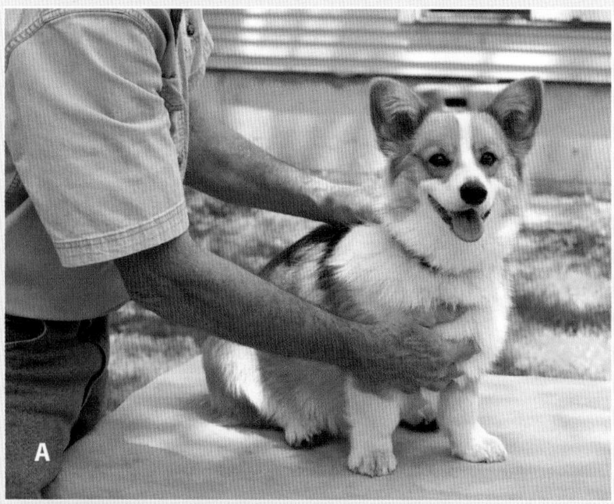
A

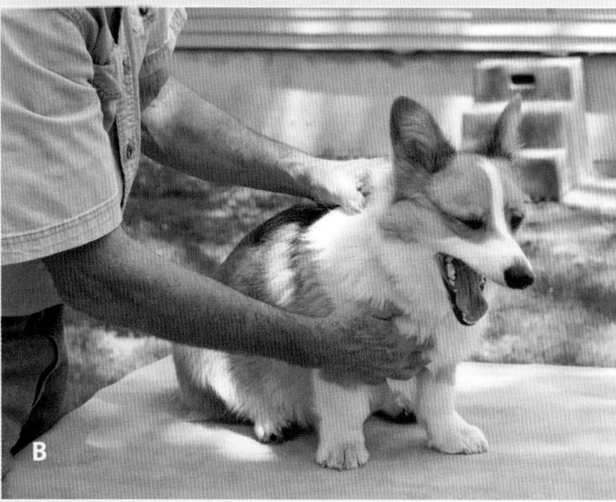
B

Quick Overview: Step-by-Step

LUMBAR RELEASE

Step 1. Position yourself sitting beside or behind your dog.

Step 2. Hold the palm of one hand softly on top of the lumbar area.

Step 3. Gently place the palm of your other hand underneath the dog's hind end (fig. 7.18).

Step 4. If you can softly adjust your hands so that you get a blink or *Response*, even better. If not, just relax both hands (*Hold*).

Step 5. *Wait*, with your hands remaining as soft as possible…

Step 6. …until you get a *Release Response*, fidget, or change in behavior (*Melt*).

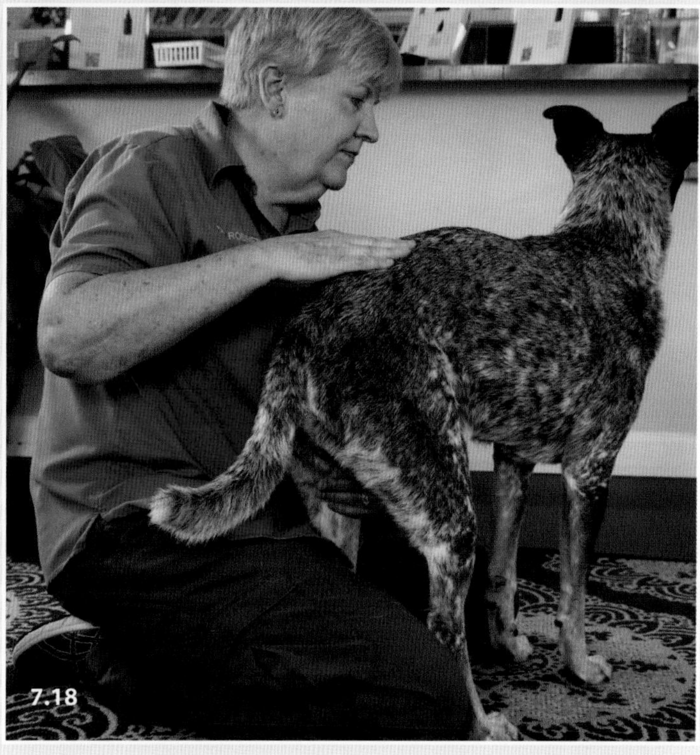
7.18

to position your hands, how much pressure (or non-pressure) to use, and when he has a *Release*.

Tips

Go as lightly as you can but use the level of pressure (or non-pressure) that the dog tells you to use. How much, and where, is determined by the dog's *Responses* (figs. 7.19 A & B).

What Ifs?

- ***What if I would like to work on more than one point at a time?***

Well, the answer is, "Ask your dog" if this is okay. This is also an experiment. Every dog is different, has different things going on, has different levels of trust, and handles discomfort differently. And humans have different levels of feel. So, try it, and see what your dog has to say.

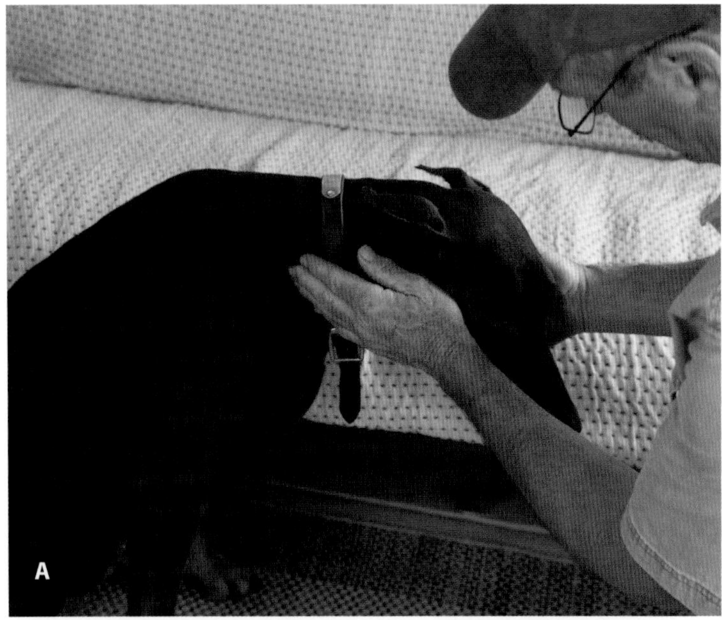

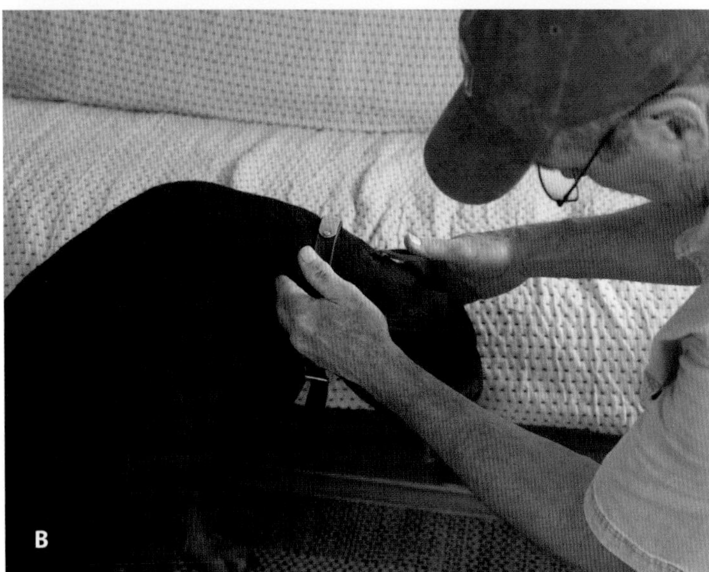

7.19 A & B Use the lightest level of pressure you can (A) and be guided by the dog's *Response* (B).

On these final pages of Part Two are pictures of some examples of combinations of *points* and *Hold, Wait, Melt Techniques* your dog might respond to that will help release some tension he might have been holding on to (figs. 7.20 A–D). Remember, stick with what your dog "says" is working. Have your attention on what's between your hands. But keep your mind and hands soft, don't put anything into it, and don't forget the dog. This method is about results, and the best one to tell you what the dog is feeling about his body is the dog. Your dog will trust you more for it.

Sometimes more than one point or area might be too much for your dog. Other times, not. Go by your dog's *Responses*. Your dog may be able to handle more after he's become used to it. If you don't get *Responses* or it's too much for your dog, go back to where your dog is comfortable or return to what works.

A Fidget Often Accompanies a Release

You can gently use one hand to ask the dog to stay a little longer if he starts to fidget or walk away. Keep in mind that this change in behavior might be the dog telling you he's about to *Release*.

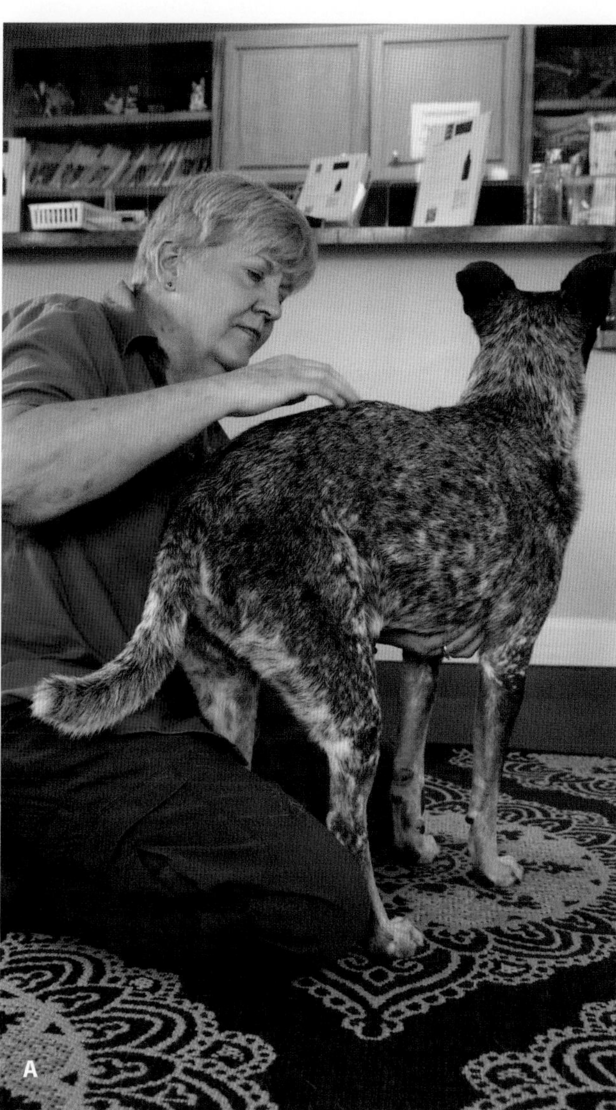

FROM THE VET

Hips

As the back muscles tie to the hip joint, dogs with hip dysplasia or arthritis also often have a sore back.

Counterpoint: if the back is sore, then the posterior limbs can also be weak, sore, or stiff.

—*Dr. Robinett*

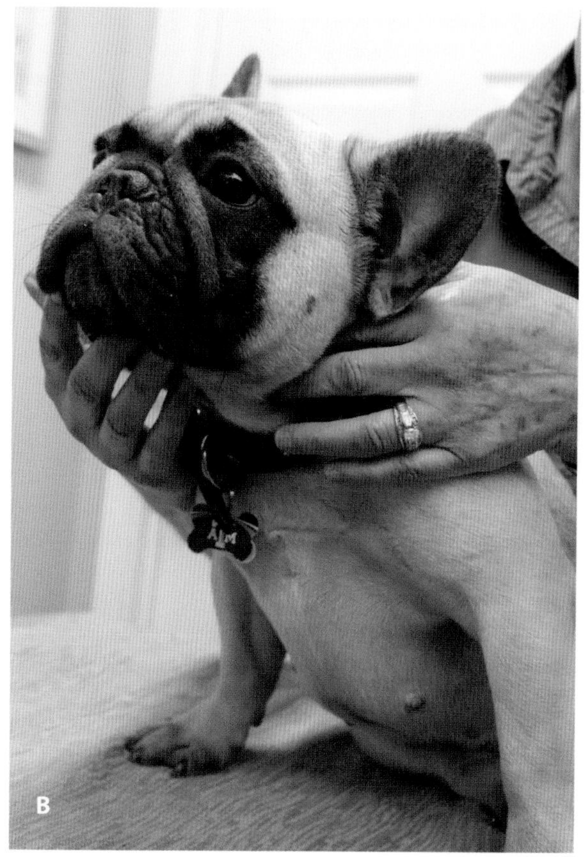

7.20 A & B Top of Spine Points and pectorals/sternum (A), and the Hyoid Release and Hyoid Movement (B).

Scan here to view the Accordions bonus video

FROM THE VET

Stifles

Dogs with chronic *cranial cruciate ligament* (CCL) injuries or stifle problems commonly develop spondylosis or arthritic changes in the lumbar spine—especially at the *Lumbosacral Junction* area. This is due to compensation and stress in the lumbar back.

—*Dr. Robinett*

Now that you have a better idea of what your dog has to say about all of this, relax, and have some fun with it.

Combinations

Now that you've finished this section, absorbed EVERYTHING in it, and practiced ALL the bodywork tirelessly, you have permission to experiment with all you have learned. As I said at the beginning of this book, everything you do is an experiment. You're trying something to see what the result is and whether it is something that can help your dog to feel better.

PART THREE

Problem Solving with the Masterson Method

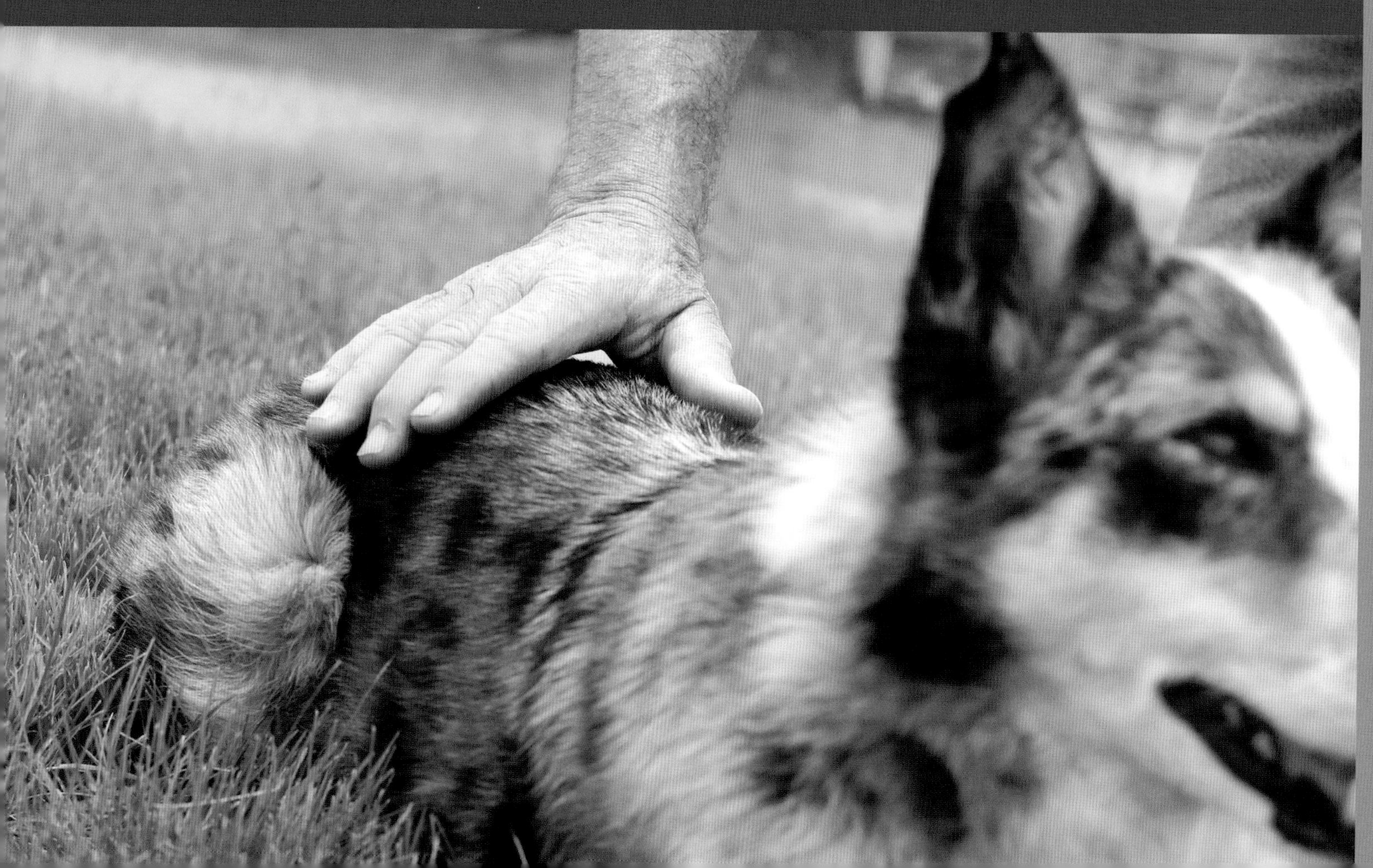

8

CHAPTER 8

From the Vet

Solving Mobility and Performance Issues with Dr. Robin Robinett

Primary Issues vs. Secondary Issues

Much of what you will work on are going to be secondary issues caused by a primary issue or issues. This most commonly is due to compensation from physical issues such as hip or back pain, or caused by a direct issue such as poorly fitted harness.

When dogs compensate for discomfort or pain caused by a primary issue, secondary issues are created—for example, pain, tension, and restrictions that affect mobility. Releasing this pain, tension, and restriction improves your dog's mobility and performance, but to prevent these secondary issues from returning, you need to determine where the primary issue is and address that problem. In some cases, you might be able to prevent the primary issue from becoming a serious physical problem or one for your veterinarian to address.

On the following pages are some examples of primary issues (this is by no means a complete list of issues).

Common Primary Issues

Hip and Hind Leg Pain

- Pain from the hips due to hip dysplasia or arthritis.
- Pain from the stifle, or knee problems due to *cranial cruciate ligament* injury (CCL) or a luxating patella.
- Pain from the lower lumbar back or sacrum due to *spondylosis* or *arthritic changes* in the spine, or from *sacral instability.*

Front Leg Pain

- Pain in the upper leg due to neck problems, shoulder, or elbow arthritis, or elbow dysplasia.
- Pain in the lower leg from carpal or wrist arthritis, or sprains due to toe (digit) injury or inflammation.

Dental Issues

- Pain from teeth due to a fracture or chip.
- Pain from periodontal disease.

- Pain from *temporomandibular joint inflammation* (TMI) or arthritis.
- Pain from muscles around the jaw, due to *myositis* of the *masseter muscles*.

Harness or Collar Issues

- Improperly fitting harnesses can impede shoulder movement and change the gait.
- Collars can be too tight or too wide and put pressure on the neck. Collars can cause pain for dogs with cervical (neck) arthritis or cervical intervertebral disc problems (IVDD).
- Dogs that pull when walking should use a properly fitted harness instead of a collar in order to prevent neck problems.

Overwork or Overtraining

- With sporting and competition dogs, unbalanced training, for example, going too much in one direction or doing too many repetitions of a certain obstacle, may cause an imbalance in the muscles or repetitive motion injury.
- Overtraining can cause muscle fatigue and possibly change the dog's gait—both leading to injury.

Conformational Issues

- Crooked front legs turned out at the carpal joints (wrists). This is often seen in hound breeds and Dachshunds.
- Long back, short legs (common in Basset Hounds, Dachshunds, and Corgis).
- Straight back legs, bow-legged in front or back.

Congenital or Inherited Issues

- Hip problems: Hip dysplasia (common in large breed dogs).
- Elbow problems: Elbow dysplasia (common in Labrador retrievers and other large breeds).
- Spine or back problems: vertebral malformations, extra or missing vertebrae, curvatures of the spine such as *scoliosis* or *kyphosis* (common in Pugs, French Bulldogs, and other *brachycephalic* breeds with short, rounded heads, short muzzles, and more protruding round eyes).

Muscle-Tension Patterns

Tension in the body can develop from the effects of the dog's daily activity. Muscle-tension patterns arise from repeated contractions and when some muscles end up working more than others, imbalances occur. Dogs, like people and horses, tend to be right-handed or right-sided so they have a natural asymmetry and a stronger or predominant side. This imbalance can become emphasized through daily activity and training for sports competition, so over time larger imbalances get created. These contribute to physical issues or lameness.

Finding the Culprit

When trying to detect the location of possible primary issues, remember that dogs instinctively do not want to show outward signs of pain or weakness. Because of their nature, the majority of dogs are stoic and don't show pain, but because of domestication and breeding for small toy breeds, there are some that may be overly sensitive and seem to be in pain everywhere you touch them. Consequently, primary issues may go undetected for some time, and the longer this goes on, the more tension accumulates.

Sometimes, determining if there is a primary issue and what or where it might be is like putting together a puzzle or solving a mystery. The more clues or information you gather, the better the chances of finding the underlying cause of the pain and tension as well as being able to do something about it. Here are some things to consider when looking for the culprit:

> ### It Is Almost Never One Thing!
>
> As all parts of the body are interconnected, one area of tension or pain is connected to another. When a dog has a hind leg issue, he will shift weight and compensate with his front end. Same if there is a front leg problem: he will compensate with the rear legs and accumulate tension there. When doing bodywork, be sure to remember this, and while focusing on the primary area, spend time on the areas of compensation.

Diagonal or Pacing Gaits

Observe your dog's movement to gain an insight into how he moves. Does he move in a diagonal gait pattern, or does he have a natural pacing gait, moving from side to side? Most dogs move in a diagonal gait pattern with one front leg paired with the opposite hind leg in motion, but some move with the front leg paired in motion with the rear leg on the same side. Also, watch to see which side your dog turns toward more often when moving freely. This will help you determine which side is his predominant side and help you find out where tension accumulates, where primary issues may be, and where to watch for future problems.

Pain vs. Restriction

Some mobility and performance problems are related more to *pain* or *discomfort,* while others are due to *restriction* and *stiffness.* In general, stiffness is due to an older issue, or one that developed over time, while pain is related to a newer or current issue. Determining the difference between pain and restriction can help you find the primary issue (fig. 8.1).

Other Considerations

While using Masterson Method Techniques on your dog, note where he has the most trouble *Releasing*. If he *Releases* easily behind but has difficulty doing so in the neck, atlas/occiput, or shoulder, you should focus on his front end. When the front end

Releases easily, but the hind end is difficult, he is sensitive over the hips or stifles, the hamstring and inner thigh muscles are tight, or he is sensitive over the pelvis or sacral area, focus on the hind end. The primary issue is commonly located wherever the dog has the most difficulty with *Releases*. This helps you narrow down where the culprit may be hiding.

Look at the whole dog and pay attention to the connections pointed out in this book, including the relationship between the front-to-hind-end diagonals, or the side-to-side connections.

- Tension in the *atlas* is connected to tension in the *sacrum*. (When the atlas or sacrum is not moving well from tension or restriction, the flow of cerebrospinal fluid from the brain down the spinal cord is disrupted, so the entire nervous system can be affected).
- Often tension at atlas/occiput or neck on one side is connected to spasm in the muscles over the hip/pelvis on the opposite side.
- Shoulder, elbow, or carpal joint issues often go along with increased soreness or tension over the lumbar back (the spine, including muscles and associated soft tissues), pelvis, and hip on the opposite side.
- Tension in the Neck-Shoulder-Upper Thoracic Junction is connected to tension at the Thoracolumbar Junction of the spine, lumbar spine, pelvis, and sacrum.
- Dogs with hip or stifle issues will frequently have tension in the lumbar back and excessive tightness and tension in the hamstring muscles.
- Stifle issues often go along with excessive soreness or tension in the inner thigh muscles, lumbar back and hamstring muscles. (There is ongoing research on the role of the *Iliopsoas* muscle in stifle injuries in people and dogs. The *Iliopsoas* is one of the core muscles of the back that attaches to each lumbar vertebrae then attaches to the medial or inner part of the femur or hip.)

Masterson Method Solutions for 16 Mobility and Performance Problems

The one thing that should always be done during the course of addressing any mobility problem, no matter which part of the body you are focusing on—the head/neck, back, front or hind end—is to release tension at the Atlas/Occiput (skull) Junction (or poll). Releasing tension at the atlas helps to release tension in the entire body, thus making releases in other parts of the body easier, and allowing the releases to last longer. Everything connects to the occiput/atlas.

Note: When addressing any of the problems listed next, remember you may be dealing with the dog's way of compensating for an underlying problem, so the dog could seem to "get worse." However, once you remove how the dog may have been "hiding" his underlying problem, it may finally be able to be diagnosed and treated by your veterinarian.

Is My Dog's Mobility or Performance Problem Caused By...?

Pain or Restriction?			Primary or Secondary Issue	
Problem	**Restriction**	**Pain**	**Primary**	**Secondary**
1. Stiffness	**X**	x	x	**X**
2. Not jumping	**X**	x		**X**
3. Hunched or sore back		**X**	**X**	
4. Shifting weight to front end	**X**			**X**
5. Short-striding behind	**X**	x		**X**
6. Holding head down		**X**	**X**	
7. Intermittent lameness	**X**	x	**X**	
8. Short-striding in front	**X**	x		**X**
9. Short choppy gait all four legs	**X**			**X**
10. Lameness, holding leg up		**X**	**X**	
11. Decreased activity, slower times on runs		**X**		**X**
12. Not sitting square	**X**			**X**
13. Needs assistance to stand		**X**	**X**	
14. Dragging toes		**X**	**X**	
15. "Bunny-hopping" or skipping with back leg(s)	**X**		**X**	
16. Back legs turn out with hocks turning in (cow-hocked)	**X**		**X**	

Note: A bold capital "X" indicates that the issue is more likely. A small, light "x" indicates less likely.

This chart is by all means not complete and not to be used to diagnose actual physical problems. That is the job of your veterinarian. Please call your veterinarian when your dog is experiencing any physical problems.

1 Stiffness

The dog is moving slowly, slow to sit, and slow to get up from sitting or lying down. He is not be as active or agile as usual.

Possible Primary Issue

This is one of the most common complaints I hear from clients. There are many things that can cause this. I consider the age of the dog: with younger dogs, stiffness is most likely caused by his being overly active and more of a temporary problem or more recent injury; with an older dog, it is more likely due to a chronic ongoing problem or problems that have become aggravated.

When a primary issue is not severe enough to create an obvious lameness, it can still bother a dog enough that he compensates for it and creates muscle problems that show up as overall stiffness and reluctance to move. Tension patterns develop in the compensatory muscles, creating a muscle imbalance and changing the way the dog moves.

Stiffness is usually a whole-body concern that may have developed from one or more primary issues and has created tension in the muscles causing restrictions. The primary issue may be in the neck and front end, the back, or the hind end. A careful and thorough exam is needed in order to indicate where to start looking.

Neck and Front End

Some examples of primary issues with the neck are pain from cervical *intervertebral disc disease (IVDD)*; inflammation from *spondylosis*; an arthritic change in the ligaments holding the vertebrae together; or inflammation from arthritic changes in the cervical vertebrae. Muscle tension can also be a primary issue causing stiffness and neck pain, especially with a younger dog, or could be a secondary issue from compensation because of the primary problem. Compensation causes increased tension in the muscles that connect the foreleg to the neck, atlas, and poll. Prolonged contraction and increased tension in the *brachiocephalicus, omotransversarius*, and *trapezius* muscles will cause soreness and restrictions in the neck, atlas, and poll, which can be unilateral or bilateral, resulting in stiffness.

Primary issues with the front end may also include forelimb problems involving the shoulder, elbow, carpal joint, or wrist, as well as problems with toes (digits) or nails. Problems with the foreleg can be due to recent injury, such as soft tissue bruising, tendon or ligament sprains, or muscle strains. Chronic or long-term problems because of arthritic changes in a joint can be aggravated, creating compensations and causing stiffness.

When unilateral tension on the atlas or poll causes a dog to become tight or more restricted on one side—or misaligned—it affects not only the function of the front end but also the hind end. For example, when the atlas is misaligned or restricted by muscle contractions on one side, it often causes muscle spasms and tension in the *gluteal* muscles and *biceps femoris* muscle around the hip joint on the diagonal or opposite hind leg. When the tension or misalignment of the poll and atlas is cleared up, the spasm or muscle tension in the muscles around the hip often clears up as well.

When a dog compensates for foreleg discomfort, a restriction in movement will show up in the C7-T1 (neck–trunk) Junction. This restriction will create increased tension in the muscles connecting the front end to the hind end, such as the *longissimus dorsi* and the *Iliocostal* muscles (see fig. 7.2—p. 130), leading to more discomfort and creating overall stiffness.

HOW TO ADDRESS

Techniques to use to release tension in the neck and front end:

- Head Up (Occiput-Atlas) Release (p. 58)
- Jawline Groove and Lateral Cervical Microflexion (p. 61)
- Scapula and Forelimb Movements (p. 80)

Back

Back problems in dogs are one of the most common problems seen in my practice. Dogs have a high instance of intervertebral disc disease (IVDD) and spondylosis, which are arthritic changes in the back. The most common location for these problems is at the Thoracolumbar Junction of the back (at back of rib cage) and in the lumbar spine (see Appendix I for more information—p. 179). After the acute or immediate phase with IVDD, it becomes a chronic, or "old" problem, and most of the time the dog does not show any signs of discomfort or restrictions from it, but he will always have some compensation patterns due to the problem. If the dog overdoes it and plays too hard, too much jumping or certain movements can aggravate the issue, and he can become very sore and need veterinary care, but it could just show up as stiffness. An analogy is a man with an old or chronic disc problem in his back who bends over to tie his shoe and his back "gives out."

HOW TO ADDRESS

Releasing tension in the front end and hind end (see p. 130) helps to release tension in the back, along with specific techniques for the back, such as:

- Bladder Meridian (p. 36)
- Head Up (Occiput-Atlas) Release (p. 58)
- Pubic Symphysis (p. 106)
- Pelvic Release (p. 126)
- Top of Spine and Back Points and Sublumbar Points (p. 138)
- Lateral and Dorsal-Ventral Body Rocking (p. 142)

Hind End

Common primary issues in the hind end of the dog are most often due to hip or stifle issues. Some of the muscles the dog uses to compensate for discomfort or pain in the hips or stifles include the groin or inner thigh muscles, such as the *iliopsoas*

(*psoas*), *pectineus*, *adductor*, or *gracilis* muscles. Other muscles that hold tension for hip or stifle problems include the hamstrings (*semitendinosus, semimembranosus*), lumbar back muscles (*longissimus dorsi*), *gluteal* muscles, cranial or front thigh muscles (*sartorius, quadriceps*), and outer or lateral thigh muscles (*biceps femoris*).

When these muscles put enough tension on the sacrum, especially unilaterally, it creates torque on the sacrum, pelvis, and Lumbosacral Junction. When this area becomes "torqued," it can affect all the muscles of the hind end and back and cause stiffness. As a chiropractic veterinarian, I see this very commonly. This "torque" or chiropractic subluxation of the sacrum and pelvis can happen first or be the primary issue, causing the secondary muscle tension. In other cases, the muscle tension and imbalances can be the primary cause of the pelvic and sacral subluxations or "torque" (see Primary or Secondary Issues—p. 156).

When you release tension on the sacrum or pelvis, you release tension in the muscles of the back and hind end. You will also get release of tension in muscles in other areas of the body leading to the stiffness by moving the hind legs through a range of motion in a relaxed state.

HOW TO ADDRESS

Techniques to use to release tension in the hind end:

- Hind End (p. 97)
- Head Up (Occiput-Atlas) Release (p. 58)
- Lumbosacral-Pelvic Junction Points and Hind Limb Points (p. 110)
- Hind Limb Movement (p. 112)
- Sacrum Float (p. 124)
- Pelvic Release (p. 126)
- Lateral and Dorsal-Ventral Body Rocking (p. 142)

2 Not Jumping

This is probably the second most common complaint I hear—agility and other competition or sporting dogs not wanting to jump obstacles in training or events; dogs pulling poles on jumps; dogs not wanting to jump up on the bed or couch—or trying to jump on the furniture but not making it up all the way.

Possible Primary Issues

There may be several primary causes for a dog not wanting to jump, but most commonly I look for hind-end problems. Back problems can also be the primary problem. (Or the back issue can be a *secondary* problem from compensation for the *primary* hind-end problem. Neck or front-end problems can be a possible cause, but usually not as likely as hind-end or back problems. Dogs with front-end issues are usually more reluctant to jump off the furniture.)

The primary problem can be muscle tension or imbalance because of the way a dog moves, or compensation from an old injury or fall causing "torque" in the pelvis, sacrum, or hips as discussed in the previous section (see p. 159). Hip, stifle, hock, or paw issues can also be the primary cause of a dog not wanting to jump. However, the most common primary issues are:

- Pelvic and sacral "torque."
- Hip problems: hip dysplasia or hip arthritis.
- Stifle problems: chronic or old cranial cruciate ligament (CCL) injury; stifle arthritis; medial luxating patellas (MPL) with small dogs.
- Back problems: IVDD, spondylosis.
- Lower hind leg problems: hock or paw problems.
- Possible front-end or front-leg problems.

HOW TO ADDRESS

- Head Up (Occiput-Atlas) Release (p. 58)
- Lumbosacral-Pelvic Junction Points and Hind Limb Points (p. 110)
- Hind Limb Movement (p. 112)
- Sacrum Float (p. 124)
- Pelvic Release (p. 126)
- Lateral and Dorsal-Ventral Body Rocking (p. 142)
- Top of Spine and Back Points and Sublumbar Points (p. 138)

CCL Injuries

With an acute or recent CCL injury or tear, a dog will be in pain and very lame—even not bearing weight or using the rear leg. He should be seen by a veterinarian as soon as possible.

3 Hunched or Sore Back

A hunched or sore back is one of those whole-body issues. When the dog's back is painful, the front end and hind end are also affected. His gait changes, compensating for the pain and restrictions in the muscles.

Possible Primary Issues

A dog with a hunched-looking back most likely has a primary back problem. When the dog is in pain but without a hunched appearance to the back, he can have a primary back problem, or the back issue can be *secondary* to a hind-end or front-end problem.

It is important to determine the location of the primary problem and have your dog examined by his veterinarian for a diagnosis. Otherwise, the soreness will return no matter how much bodywork you do on the dog's back, and the condition can progress and worsen. These are the primary issues commonly seen:

- Old injury: arthritis, chronic IVDD, spondylosis, muscle injury (see Stiffness—p. 157).

- New or acute back injury: acute IVDD, muscle injury.
- Compensation for feet or leg injuries: front or hind leg.
- Possible neck problems.
- Muscle tension in back, caused by overwork, overtraining, or rough play.
- Dental problems: fractured or infected tooth, TMJ or jaw pain.

Core Exercises: Not Just for People

Studies on back injuries in people and other animals show that the deep core muscles of the back, the *multifidus* muscles, start to atrophy within 72 hours following a back injury. The muscles have to be activated in order to start to function again. Core-strengthening exercises are important for animals (just like people), especially after a back injury, to reactivate those deep core muscles and strengthen them. When core muscles are not reactivated, other muscles have to take over to support the back, and they become overworked, leading to muscle contraction, tension, and pain (see fig. 7.3—p. 130).

Note: The back is an essential part of proper movement—any back tension or restriction prevents it.

The more longstanding the soreness in the back, the more stiff or rigid the back becomes, and over time this can lead to muscle atrophy or muscle loss. With muscle loss over the back, it looks like the spine sticks up because of the loss of muscle around the back. Often, there may not be as much pain at this point because the muscles of the back might be "shut down" and the nerves damaged.

In some cases, the primary cause might have been already treated or removed and is no longer an issue, yet the back is still tight and rigid in compensation because of the prior issue. Once you have done the work described in this book to free up the back, it can remain loose and begin to function more naturally again.

HOW TO ADDRESS

- Bladder Meridian (p. 36)
- Head Up (Occiput-Atlas) Release (p. 58)
- Scapula and Forelimb Movements (p. 80)
- C7-T1 Release (p. 94)
- Lumbosacral-Pelvic Junction Points and Hind Limb Points (p. 110)
- Hind Limb Movement (p. 112)
- Sacrum Float (p. 124)
- Pelvic Release (p. 126)
- Top of Spine and Back Points and Sublumbar Points (p. 138)
- Lateral and Dorsal-Ventral Body Rocking (p. 142)

Often, simply by doing some *Bladder Meridian* work (p. 36) and *Lateral Body Rocking* (p. 142) to loosen up the back, you will see improvement. For deeper or more longstanding back problems, it helps to loosen up the front and hind ends, then work toward the middle with the *Releases* you learned in chapter 7 for the back (p. 128). Once both ends are loosened up, the back will let go.

Remember: when the dog's back is sore, there can still be a primary issue that needs to be dealt with. Find the primary issue and keep the back released and loose on a regular basis.

(Note: With a dog that has recurring back pain or issues, I highly recommend having a veterinarian do radiographs of the back to determine if there are any bony changes. If there are, doing these techniques regularly may prevent the dog from having episodes of severe back pain and help the back from getting worse, or at least slow the progression. Even when there are no bony changes or abnormalities seen on radiographs, these exercises can help prevent or delay the development of changes in the back.

4 Shifting Weight to Front Legs

Dogs will often shift their weight forward, putting more weight onto the front legs when there is pain or discomfort somewhere in the hind limbs or in the muscles of the hind end, trying to keep the weight off their hind end.

Possible Primary Issues

Dogs normally carry 60 percent of their weight on the front end and 40 percent of the weight on the rear. If they have pain anywhere in the hind legs or in the muscles of the hind end, they shift their weight forward, putting more weight on one or both front legs.

Older dogs with hip arthritis or dogs with hip dysplasia commonly shift their weight more to the front end. These dogs also use the front legs to pull themselves up when sitting or lying down, rather than pushing up from the rear end to stand.

Releasing tension in the hind end allows it to work more efficiently and relieves the need for dogs to shift weight to the front end. When there is a serious primary issue with the hind end, they will continue shifting weight to the front end and need to be seen by their veterinarian to determine the problem.

HOW TO ADDRESS

Techniques to use:

- Lumbosacral-Pelvic Junction Points (p. 110)
- Hind Limb Movement (p. 112)
- Sacrum Float (p. 124)
- Head Up (Occiput-Atlas) Release (p. 58)
- Scapula and Forelimb Movements (p. 80)

5 Short-Striding with Hind Legs

For a dog to be able to use his hind legs efficiently, his whole body must work together. He must be able to round the back, engaging the deep core muscles in the back and abdomen to step under his body with his hind legs to use the hind end effectively. An inability to do this can be the result of overwork with the hind legs and a lack of core strength.

Possible Primary Issues

When a dog is short-striding with both hind legs but moving them both forward evenly with no evidence of lameness or limping on either leg, it is most likely due to a sacral-pelvic hind-end issue or a lower lumbar issue. The dog is not able to round or lift his back in order to step under himself because of muscle tension, pain, or restriction in the hind end or lower back.

Other primary issues causing this are recent or chronic back injuries, muscle injuries or tension, other soft-tissue injuries or joint issues. Hind-end issues involving the sacrum, pelvis, or hips are the first place to look for tension or restrictions causing short-striding with both hind legs. Lower-back problems, especially in the lumbar area and Lumbosacral Junction area, also cause short-striding with the hind legs. Front-end issues can cause short-striding with the hind end, but not as commonly as with hind-end or low-back problems. Whatever the cause, tension or "torque" on the sacrum and pelvis will be a key part of the dog not being able to step under himself and move well with the hind legs.

HOW TO ADDRESS

Techniques to use:

- Bladder Meridian (p. 36)
- Head Up (Occiput-Atlas) Release (p. 58)
- Lumbosacral-Pelvic Junction Points (p. 110)
- Hind Limb Movement (p. 112)
- Sacrum Float (p. 124)
- Top of Spine and Back Points and Sublumbar Points (p. 138)
- Lateral and Dorsal-Ventral Body Rocking (p. 142)

Your strategy is to release tension in the back and at both ends. The best way to start to release tension in the sacrum and pelvis is to release tension at the occiput/atlas. The back will release more easily once the tension at the occiput/atlas releases. Once the back is released, it can do its job so the body can work together, allowing the dog to use his hind end more effectively.

Starting at the atlas/poll area begins the process of releasing in the sacrum, pelvis, and hind end. Then when you go to work on the hind end, start with the *Release Points* of the hind end (p. 106).

Pay close attention to the *iliopsoas* (*psoas*) and medial thigh muscles, such as the *gracilis* and *pectineus* creating "torque" and tension on the pelvis (see fig. 6.4—p. 101). Also, check tension in the hamstring muscles (*semitendinosus*, *semimembranosus*) that can create "torque" on the sacrum (see fig. 6.5—p. 102).

Once you have loosened things up by using the *Release Points*, go on to the *Hind Limb Movements* (p. 112), paying close attention to where your dog has the most restriction, discomfort or gives the best

Releases. This is the area you should focus on to help him let go of tension.

Also pay close attention to the lumbar back. Often, the lumbar back may not show any signs of soreness or sensitivity, but it may be stiff or immobile. Restriction in the lumbosacral area blocks motion from the hind end through the back, affecting the dog's ability to use the whole body.

After the *Hind Limb Movements*, spend a lot of time on *Lateral Body Rocking* (p. 142) to help relax all the muscles of the back. It may take a while for the dog to stop guarding his low back, but once he does, the releases can be large.

6 Holding Head Down

This includes the dog holding the head to either side, crookedly, or tilted. He might also not want to turn or bend the neck to one direction and will move his front legs to look to one side, rather than turning his head and neck.

Dogs, like people, carry a lot of tension in their head and neck with stress and with pain or resistance anywhere in the head or neck region, or anywhere else in their body.

Treat for Mobility

I often check the mobility in a dog's neck by having him reach and follow for a treat to see how well he can turn his head and neck.

Possible Primary Issues

Excessive unilateral tension in muscles and ligaments in the Occiput-Atlas Junction and neck can lead to bending and unilateral resistance issues. A muscle that is tight and contracted on one side—for example, the *brachiocephalicus*—will cause crookedness in the neck.

As discussed earlier, this contracted muscle can be due to the dog compensating for foot or leg pain, or discomfort elsewhere in the body, but if it is in the neck, it is usually from a problem located on the same side the dog can't bend toward.

We've already discussed how dogs are like people in that they have a stronger, more predominant side, so they can develop unilateral tension patterns over time that may manifest as a mobility issue or abnormal posture, such as holding the head down or crookedly. Regular releases of these tension patterns help to keep the dog moving more evenly and in balance.

During the *Lateral Cervical Microflexion* (p. 63), look for locations with restrictions in movement or less flexibility, and especially pay attention to the differences from one side to the other. Remember to start releasing tension on the easier side that is opposite from the side with the issue and then go on to work on both sides of the neck.

HOW TO ADDRESS

Techniques to use:

- Head Up (Occiput-Atlas) Release (p. 58)
- Jawline Groove and Lateral Cervical Microflexion (p. 61)
- Scapula and Forelimb Movements (p. 80)
- C7-T1 Release (p. 94)
- Hyoid Release (p. 65)

By focusing on the Occiput-Atlas Junction and the scapula at the C7-T1 Junction, you are working the attachments at both ends of the major muscles in the area, the *brachiocephalicus* and the *trapezius*. Releasing the muscles at both ends where they attach to bone will make your *Releases* easier and more effective. Releasing the muscles with these exercises will begin to release the area of restricted motion at the upper neck. Use a very light touch when releasing tension over the upper neck O-A Junction and it should release easily.

Note: Remember, any time you are having trouble working on an area, or the dog seems uncomfortable, try going to the opposite side to release tension there first. After having worked on the easier side first, the dog will have released much of the tension on the difficult side. Don't attack the problem area first; save it for last! Go to where it is easier first to make this a more enjoyable experience for your dog.

7 Intermittent Lameness (Front End or Hind End)

Intermittent lameness usually happens after the dog has had some sort of lameness in the front or hind end for a fairly extended period of time. After the injury or issue causing the lameness has been treated and healed, the dog will sometimes limp on that leg for quite a while afterward—sometimes for months. The longer the lameness has gone on, the longer the subsequent intermittent lameness may last.

Possible Primary Issues

Compensation for lameness over a long period of time creates a muscle-tension pattern that puts unilateral tension or "torque" on the Occiput-Atlas

Vestibular Syndrome

If a dog has a sudden, severe head tilt, with eyes that may or not be twitching, and is having problems with walking and with balance, seeming to fall over, then he needs to be seen by a veterinarian as soon as possible. Older dogs may have a condition called *idiopathic vestibular syndrome*, where inflammation in the inner ear or in the brain causes a loss of balance, usually with a head tilt and twitching movement of the eyes (*nystagmus*). I find these cases respond well to acupuncture. Conventional medical treatment may include medication for nausea and an anti-inflammatory.

and C7-T1 Junctions if in the front end and on the Lumbosacral Junction and pelvis if in the hind end. Once the primary lameness is gone, this tension pattern or torque remains until it releases. It may relax and release on its own, but most of the time it requires some type of intervention or therapy to release these restrictions.

HOW TO ADDRESS

Techniques to use for intermittent front-leg lameness:

- Head Up (Occiput-Atlas) Release (p. 58)
- Scapula and Forelimb Movements (p. 80)
- C7-T1 Release (p. 94)
- TMJ Point (p. 55)
- Scapula Trunk Points, and Sternum and Pectoral Points (p. 74)

Releasing the tension at the C7-T1 Junction, the area where the last cervical vertebrae joins the first thoracic vertebrae of the body, often helps with this and may even be the key to clearing up this problem. After releasing tension in the Occiput-Atlas Junction and the vertebrae of the neck, it is important to release as much tension as possible at the C7-T1 Junction by doing the *Scapula Raise and Lower* (p. 80).

When doing the *Scapula Raise and Lower/Forelimb Movement* (p. 80), ask the dog to relax the leg in front and just across the midline of the chest. If there is "torque" at the C7-T1 Junction, the dog might be uncomfortable doing this, so lighten up some and move the leg slightly to a more comfortable position where the dog is able to relax. Wait and hold for the signs of a *Release.*

After this *Release*, go to the *C7-T1 Release* (p. 94). Proceed slowly with light contact and allow the dog to relax into it. Start on the side with less tension before doing the *Release* on the side with the lameness. When you feel you have achieved some

Neuroplasticity

Injuries that cause long-term lameness can change the posture and gait of a dog (or person) long term, or even permanently, due to the compensation patterns created by the injury. The brain and central nervous system begin to register the new posture as normal, so trying to change these postures back to the "true" normal can take many sessions over a long period of time, and may take more extensive physical rehabilitation. There are studies about these effects and retraining the brain, based on principles of *neuroplasticity* (the ability of neural networks in the brain to change through growth and reorganization—in other words, the brain can be rewired in response to stimuli or trauma in the brain or body, so that compensation postures such as limping may be perceived as normal with long-term injuries).

Release, check to see if there is any improvement in releasing the leg forward and across the midline. If there is, you have probably made an improvement in the intermittent lameness issue, or may have even cleared it up.

HOW TO ADDRESS

Techniques to use for hind-leg intermittent lameness:

- Head Up (Occiput-Atlas) Release (p. 58)
- Lumbosacral-Pelvic Junction Points and Hind Limb Points (p. 110)
- Hind Limb Movement (p. 112)
- Sacrum Float (p. 124)
- Pelvic Release (p. 126)
- Top of Spine and Back Points and Sublumbar Points (p. 138)
- Lateral and Dorsal-Ventral Body Rocking (p. 142)

I find that releasing tension in the hind end using the *Pelvic Release* (p. 126) often improve—or may clear up—intermittent hind-leg lameness. It is important to let go of as much tension as possible in the large muscles of the rear end first, so start with *Hind End Points*, using SRSR Technique (p. 00), then *Hold, Wait, and Melt* until the dog shows signs of *Releasing* (p. 11). Then use the *Pelvic Rlease* (p. 126) on each side and *Release* over the medial thigh or groin muscles. Next, do the *Sacrum Float* (p. 124), which releases tension at the sacrum, including the pelvis and Lumbosacral Junction areas as well.

Once the tension is released around the hips, medial thigh, gluteal, and other muscles of the rear end, do the *Hind Limb Points, Hind Limb Movements,* and *Lower Hind Limb Movements* (pp. 110, 112, and 119). By moving the leg in a relaxed state, it further releases the tension over the hips, pelvis, and sacrum. When doing the *Hind Limb Movements*, try moving the hind leg down and back, then slightly across the midline. If the dog is uncomfortable doing this movement, there may still be tension due to some remaining torque in the pelvis, so slightly shift the position of the leg until the dog is more comfortable, then wait and hold, watching for the *Release*.

After releasing tension in the hind end and mobilizing the hind leg, relax the dog's back by performing *Lateral Body Rocking* to further release tension in the hind end and hind leg (p. 142). By using these exercises, you will improve—or clear up—the compensations and restrictions causing the intermittent lameness. Maybe it will go away altogether over time with more sessions.

8 Short-Striding in Front

Also: Not extending with the front legs; restricted in the shoulders.

Possible Primary Issues

Restrictions in the front end can cause a dog to short-stride, or not extend out with the shoulders, and can:

- Develop over time, especially after having a previous injury and developing a change in gait from a compensation pattern.
- Be the result of front-leg pain involving the shoulder, elbow, carpus (wrist), or paw/digits (toes, including nails).
- Be sometimes caused by neck pain.
- Result from the dog shifting weight to the front end, trying to compensate for hind-end pain.

In my experience, the first two points above are more common.

Compare the effect that front-end restriction has on a dog's mobility and performance to asking a swimmer to swim a mile with a stiff neck or knot between the shoulder blades. The swimmer's time will not be very good and his strokes not as effective. All parts of the front end—the head, neck, shoulders, and legs—need to work together to keep the front end moving well and efficiently.

Dachshunds and Short-Striding

In my experience, Dachshunds are notorious for not wanting to stretch out their shoulders, and they tend to move with a short stride in front with restrictions in both shoulders. Trying to resolve this issue can take time and a lot of patience. Maybe, since they have such short legs, this is their natural tendency.

The dog's head and neck are important for movement of the front legs and to help balance the whole movement of the dog. The soft tissue connection of the scapula to the dog's body needs to be loose and flexible for proper locomotion. The C7-T1 Junction and the dog's trunk are the anchors for this support of the scapula, and are also a key to moving the dog forward.

All the front-end techniques help keep these essential components moving freely. Working on the *Occiput-Atlas Release* lets go of tension in the large muscles that insert at the other end at the foreleg and at the C7-T1 Junction. *Scapula Raise and Lower* helps with extension and suspension, or shock absorption with the front end. *C7-T1 Releases* are key to keeping the Neck-Shoulder-Cervicothoracic Junction moving freely. As all these areas loosen up, the muscles and tendons in the front legs will also begin to release tension. This will allow for better extension

HOW TO ADDRESS

Techniques to use:

- Head Up (Occiput-Atlas) Release (p. 58)
- Jawline Groove and Lateral Cervical Microflexion (p. 61)
- Scapula and Forelimb Movements (p. 80)
- C7-T1 Release (p. 94)
- Hyoid Release (p. 65)

with the front legs and enable all the components of this junction to work together more effectively.

9 Short Choppy Gait

In other words, short-striding with all four legs.

Possible Primary Issues

This is considered a whole-body problem and is seen more commonly in older dogs. It is due to long-term or chronic issues causing compensation. The primary issue could be in the front end, hind end, or back—or (more likely) be due to problems in multiple areas of the dog's body. I commonly see this type of movement in older dogs with arthritis in multiple joints or in the back.

HOW TO ADDRESS

Releasing tension in the dog's neck and shoulders will improve motion in his front legs. Releasing tension over the sacrum, pelvis, and hips will improve motion in the hind legs. As with all the other techniques, relaxing and releasing the occiput, atlas, and sacrum will always make a difference in movement, so start with these.

Techniques to use:

- Scapula and Forelimb Movements (p. 80)
- C7-T1 Release (p. 94)
- Hind Limb Movement (p. 112)
- Pelvic Release (p. 126)
- Lateral Body Rocking (p. 142)

10 Lameness and Holding a Leg Up

This can be the result of acute or recent injury, or due to aggravation of an old injury or problem. No matter the cause, it needs to be seen by a veterinarian first to diagnose the cause and receive medications for inflammation and pain. After seeing the veterinarian, releasing tension in the dog's body will help with overall motion and decrease pain.

Possible Primary Issues

Concentrate on either the front end or hind end, depending on which leg the dog is not using. Be careful and use very light touch over the affected area, and watch him closely for his reaction to your work. When asking for motion in the affected joint, only do as much as he can and will do at the time; don't ask for too much too soon.

Maintaining mobility in the muscles, tendons, and ligaments around the injured joint is important for healing and returning to full function, but take your time and be patient. Most injuries take six to eight weeks, if not longer, to heal.

Techniques to use depend on whether a front or rear leg was injured, but as usual, start by releasing the occiput, the atlas, and then the sacrum. Releasing tension in the back also helps with an injury to either a front or hind leg.

HOW TO ADDRESS

Techniques to use for front-leg lameness:

- Head Up (Occiput-Atlas) Release (p. 58)
- Scapula and Forelimb Movements (p. 80)

- C7-T1 Release (p. 94)
- Scapula Trunk Points (p. 74)
- Sternum and Pectoral Points (p. 77)

Techniques to use for hind-leg lameness:

- Head Up (Occiput-Atlas) Release (p. 58)
- Lumbosacral-Pelvic Junction Points and Hind Limb Points (p. 110)
- Hind Limb Movement (112)
- Sacrum Float (p. 124)
- Pelvic Release (p. 126)
- Dorsal-Ventral Body Rocking (p. 144)

11 Decreased Activity; Slower Times for Competitive Dogs

There can be many causes for this, but it is most likely another whole body-type problem.

Possible Primary Issues

Overall body stiffness, soreness from overwork, and short- or long-term compensation for an issue can all be reasons for decreased activity and slower times for competitive dogs. Older dogs show decreased activity from age-related issues and tend to sleep more than when they were younger. Consequently they become stiffer from inactivity as well as arthritis.

A trip to your regular veterinarian is in order to confirm there is nothing other than stiffness causing this issue.

Case Study

SLOWER AGILITY TIMES

I had an agility dog patient whose times on agility runs had become slower, but she was not showing any signs of disease or injury. On further examination, she was found to have developed a heart murmur. She was referred to a veterinary cardiologist and diagnosed with mitral valve disease and put on medication. The dog returned to competition with a more limited show schedule and did well.

This demonstrates how, in some of these cases, there may be more going on than just musculoskeletal issues causing slower run times and decreased activity, so a visit to your veterinarian is in order.

12 Not Sitting Square

This is also called "puppy sitting," because growing puppies tend to sit this way, especially when they are in a growth spurt. Most puppies do outgrow this and as they mature, they start to sit squarely with both hind legs up underneath their body.

Possible Primary Issues

This is usually due to a hind-end, hind-leg problem. Dogs with a previous stifle injury or CCL tear tend to sit with the injured leg cocked out because they don't want to flex the painful stifle joint. They often tend to do this even after the injury has healed. Relaxing the muscles of the hind end and mobilizing the hind leg releases the tension around the stifle and improves the range of motion of the joint. Once the tension is released around the stifle, the dog will usually start to sit squarely again.

HOW TO ADDRESS

Any of the techniques for releasing tension in the hind end and lower lumbar back will help with this problem. Be sure to try:

- Head Up (Occiput-Atlas) Release (p. 58)
- Lumbosacral-Pelvic Junction Points and Hind Limb Points (p. 110)
- Hind Limb Movement (p. 112)
- Sacrum Float (p. 124)
- Pelvic Release (p. 126)
- Lateral and Dorsal-Ventral Body Rocking (p. 142)

13 Needs Assistance to Stand

Usually, this is an older dog's problem with arthritis in the lower back or hind end.

Possible Primary Issues

I think of this as mostly a hind-end issue with pain, muscle tension, and weakness in the hind end. As a dog gets older, he is less active and sleeps more and loses muscle. He gets stiff after sleeping so it can become difficult to get up after lying down for so long. He will sometimes need assistance to stand. Once up, he can walk on his own without assistance and the more he walks, the more he warms up and walks better.

Older dogs should be encouraged to get up, then walked for five to ten minutes several times a day to prevent them from getting so stiff. Several shorter walks a day are much better for them than going for one long walk a day.

These older dogs also tend to walk with short, choppy strides once they do get up to walk, so refer back to that problem (see p. 169).

Arthritic older dogs have a lot of areas of muscle tension and compensations, depending on which joints are affected, but hind-end weakness is a common problem.

HOW TO ADDRESS

Try any and all Masterson Method techniques!

You can improve flexibility and comfort in older, arthritic dogs by asking for small increases in range of motion without forcing anything. You are just looking for an improvement. Go slow, be patient, and do a full treatment from head to toe, remembering to stop and soften when you find resistance. It is so rewarding working on older arthritic dogs and seeing how much better they feel and their improvement in mobility. They are so grateful for your help!

Look to the Front End for Standing Up

I get dogs referred to me when they are having problems standing up and need assistance because their hind legs have finally given out. After examining them, I often find they have been compensating for hind-end problems for so long, their front end is a *secondary* problem because it has given out too and can no longer compensate for the weak hind end that is the *primary* problem.

After having tension released in the neck and front limbs, these dogs can again pull themselves up with the front legs. Make sure to release tension over the hind end and back for these dogs as well, but at this point, it is the front end giving out that is causing the standing-up problem. So make sure to release the front end when you have a dog with issues standing.

14 Dragging Back Toes When Walking

This problem is where the dog is scraping or dragging his nails or toes on one or both back paws when walking. Note that this is different from a dog that is "knuckling," or flexing his toes and paws, and walking with the top of the paw contacting the ground. ("Knuckling" is a more severe problem.)

Possible Primary Issues

Dogs wear their nails down more on one of the hind paws as compared to the other because of increased muscle tension in the hind end causing a structural imbalance or "misalignment." This results in more restricted motion on one side, effectively making one leg functionally shorter than the other leg. As a chiropractic veterinarian I see this commonly with sacral and pelvis misalignments. Releasing tension in the Lumbosacral Junction, pelvis, and sacrum improves the gait.

Older arthritic dogs can drag their toes due to inflammation or pain in the back or hind end, such as the hips. They may have spondylosis or arthritic changes in their back. And when they are too active or jump off the couch or out of the car, they can get to a point where muscle tightness and tension causes them to start dragging their toes. At times, arthritis in the back or hips causes muscle weakness, so this also results in dogs dragging their hind toes. Releasing muscle tension in the back and hind end will help these older dogs, improve their mobility, and decrease their pain.

Sometimes dragging toes can be due to an old injury where the muscles have had to compensate long term and have become contracted and tight.

Regular bodywork will help improve the function of these muscles and correct the imbalance. How much of an improvement depends on the severity of the injury and how long the dog has been unbalanced. Multiple treatments will be needed, and the dog's movement pattern will take time to improve. It might not resolve completely, but releasing this muscle tension always makes the dog more comfortable and improves mobility.

HOW TO ADDRESS

All front-end, back, and hind-end Masterson Method techniques can help in this scenario.

It always helps to release the occiput and atlas before working on the hind end. In some cases, there is so much tension around the atlas, it has created muscle spasms in the *gluteal* muscles that may be the reason a dog is dragging his back toes while walking.

Lateral Body Body helps to release imbalances or restrictions in the lumbar region and Lumbosacral Junction area that may be a part of the problem.

Working on *Hind-End Release Points* helps with longstanding hind-end issues. It seems that older, more chronic issues respond better to more subtle input. The dog's body has been guarding and protecting an area for so long that signals to the nervous system to "let go" (using *Release Points*) may work better for getting a *Release* than using movement or mobilization techniques that are difficult for the dog to do.

Possible Spinal Cord Injury

When a dog is "knuckling" with one hind paw or both hind paws and acting as if he doesn't know how to correctly place the paw, he could have a back or neck problem involving the spinal cord. In these cases, he should be seen by his veterinarian as soon as possible.

15 "Bunny-Hopping" or "Skipping" with Hind Legs

This is where a dog trots or runs with the hind legs moving together. The dog may also "skip" with one or both hind legs when moving at a gait faster than a walk.

Possible Primary Issues

"Bunny-hopping" or "skipping" is much more common in the toy breeds and other smaller breeds of dogs and is due to a hind-end problem. This is the result of a condition called *medially luxating patella (MPL).* We are taught during our veterinary education that this is a developmental problem with small breeds of dogs because their bone structure is so diminutive that the groove the patella sits in is not deep enough. This means the patella does not stay in place and "pops" out of the groove, going toward the inside of the leg because of the stronger pull of the medial thigh muscles.

Over years of working on many of these dogs

Chiropractic Recommended for Patella Problems

Dogs with medial patellar luxations (MPL) greatly benefit from regular chiropractic treatments, so all dogs with this problem should be referred to a certified animal chiropractor. Rehabilitation and exercises to help improve the dog's gait and posture are usually needed to help prevent recurrence and resolve this condition. Routine and repeated bodywork makes a big difference with these dogs' mobility, as well. These types of treatments may prevent dogs with MPL from needing surgery and from developing severe arthritis as they get older.

and successfully treating them without surgery, I find that this condition develops over time due to muscle and postural imbalances, resulting in muscle tension and compensations pulling the patella out of place. Using techniques to release muscle tension in the hind end helps to improve—or may correct—this condition, depending on how long it has been going on.

Regular bodywork to relax the hind end, along with exercises to strengthen the outer thigh or hip and stifle flexor muscles, help these dogs immensely and may prevent them from needing surgery to correct the condition.

Case Study

CLARK

When I was taking the certification course for veterinary chiropractic, I had a retired racing Greyhound named Clark that I'd adopted from the Houston SPCA when I'd worked there. Clark was 14 years old when I first started learning chiropractic for animals. He was my willing patient and teacher, and I practiced my new techniques on him as I was learning. Sometimes he would come and ask me when he needed his adjustment by backing up to me and standing there looking at me over his shoulder, waiting for me get to work on his rear end! Other times I knew it was time for his adjustment because when I let him in from the back yard, I would hear him dragging the nails on his right hind paw along the concrete patio. When his pelvis was out of alignment, he would drag on his right hind paw. This was always his signal to me to do my job!

I know that Clark would definitely have benefited from Masterson Method techniques to keep him moving better.

HOW TO ADDRESS

Any of the techniques for releasing tension in the hind end and lower lumbar back will help with this problem. Also, do not forget to release the occiput and atlas, because these dogs are often very tight and carry a lot of tension in the neck. Releasing tension in the neck and front end help to release the hind end.

Specific techniques to use:

- Head Up (Occiput-Atlas) Release (p. 58)
- Lumbosacral-Pelvic Junction Points and Hind Limb Points (p. 110)
- Hind Limb Movement (p. 112)
- Sacrum Float (p. 124)
- Pelvic Release (p. 126)
- Lateral and Dorsal-Ventral Body Rocking (p. 142)

16 Hind Legs Turn Outward or Stifles Turn Inward

These dogs may have a "bow-legged" type of appearance or appear to be "cow-hocked."

Possible Primary Issues

This condition is a primary hind-end and low-back issue caused by muscle imbalances and excessive tension in the medial thigh or hip adductor muscles, especially the *psoas* (*illiopsoas*), *pectineus*, *gracilis,* and *hamstring* muscles. Other muscles are involved, such as the *sartorius* at the front of the stifle, but the former tend to be the muscles that are the most problematic (see figs. 6.4 and 6.5—pp. 101 and 102).

Dogs with this condition may tend to tear their CCL or *cranial cruciate ligament* over time because of more stress on the stifle joint from the increased muscle tightness and contractions of the muscles and the abnormal posture. This is the large- and medium-breed equivalent of "bunny-hopping" (see p. 173). As mentioned, larger breeds of dogs don't usually develop the MPL problem with the increased muscle tension, muscle contractions, and muscle and postural imbalances in the hind end like the small breeds do. They can instead have some low-grade lameness issues, problems with jumping, not be as active as usual, and feel pain in the hind end and lumbar area of the back.

Chiropractic Recommended

The hind legs turning outward or stifles turning inward is another problem where I recommend referral to a certified animal chiropractor to correct the misalignments in the pelvis, sacrum, and spine. See also the previous discussion of "bunny-hopping" (p. 173), because this is almost the same type of problem, but here seen in larger dogs.

Releasing tension in the lumbar back and hind end helps and, with repeated bodywork sessions, may even be able to correct the problem. Correcting the muscle imbalances and improving the dog's posture, when the issue is caught early and an appropriate bodywork routine is maintained, also decreases the likelihood of the dog tearing his CCL.

HOW TO ADDRESS

Any of the techniques for releasing tension in the hind end and lumbar back will help with this problem. Also, do not forget to release the occiput and atlas, because dogs with this problem are often very tight and carry a lot of tension in the neck. Releasing tension in the neck and front end helps to release the hind end.

Recommended techniques:

- Head Up (Occiput-Atlas) Release (p. 58)
- Lumbosacral-Pelvic Junction Points and Hind Limb Points (p. 110)
- Hind Limb Movement (p. 112)
- Sacrum Float (p. 124)
- Pelvic Release (p. 126)
- Lateral Body Rocking (p. 142)

APPENDIX I

Bodywork for Individual Breeds, Competition, and Different Sports with Dr. Robin Robinett

The Masterson Method will benefit any of the numerous dog breeds and can be used to improve the performance of dogs competing in any canine sporting event. The variations in dog breeds and the many different kinds of canine activities and sporting events lead to a wide range of considerations when doing this work. What follows are some guidelines of what to look for overall, which areas of the dog tend to accumulate tension, and bodywork I recommend to loosen those areas up before and after competitions.

While it is beyond the scope of this book to discuss all dog breeds, here I will address a number of issues that are often seen in specific breeds. I will also talk about some of the injuries and issues with dogs who participate in certain activities, competitions, dog shows, and sporting events. Like the breeds mentioned, the list of competitions and events is by no means complete, so do not be offended if the sport you are interested in is not discussed.

AKC and UKC

The American Kennel Club (AKC) website (www.akc.org) has information about many of the sporting events for dogs, descriptions of all the breeds, advice on picking out a dog, and lots of other useful information.

An additional source of information and another dog registry group is the UKC—United Kennel Club (www.ukcdogs.com). The UKC registers many of the same breeds that the AKC recognizes, but also recognizes some breeds not included by the AKC. The UKC includes both purebred dogs and those of "unknown ancestry." The UKC is the largest performance dog registry in the world, recognizing 300 different breeds from the United States and 25 other countries. It also puts on many different types of sporting events and competitions.

So Many Dogs...

There are 360 to 400 different breeds of dogs worldwide. Officially, there are 360 breeds recognized by the FCI (*Federation Cynologigue Internationale*), the international association of kennel clubs. The American Kennel Club recognizes 197 different breeds as of December 2021.

The Labrador Retriever has been the most popular dog in the United States for 31 years, according to AKC statistics. Popularity of different breeds may vary according to regions of the country and the world, and depends on whether people live in the city or more rural areas. Larger breeds tend to need more room to run so may not be as popular as smaller breeds in the city where people live in high-rise apartments and live closer together without yards.

Dog breed registries in general do not recognize the many mixed breeds or the so-called "designer breeds," many of which are Poodle crosses, such as the Maltipoo, Labradoodle, and Golden Doodle. People pay a lot of money for these mixed breed puppies that can't be registered with the AKC or other registries. Labrador mixes are very common, as are Shepherd mixes. In addition, more people are adopting mixed breeds from rescue organizations or shelters around the country instead of buying purebred puppies from breeders.

Mixed breed rescue dogs and terrier mixes are some of the most commonly seen dogs in my practice. Probably the number one dog breed seen in my practice—since we do chiropractic, acupuncture, and rehabilitation—are Dachshunds, since they are highly prone to back problems.

Different breeds are more prone to different problems and certain breeds are more commonly used for different sports, which can lead to specific problems. On the pages ahead I discuss the Masterson Method Techniques that can be helpful to keep all kinds of dogs competing at their best.

Different Breeds and Common Health Problems

Individual dog breeds tend to have different health problems, but most dogs will develop arthritis as they age, just like people. In general, any large breed dog can have hip dysplasia problems, and good breeders screen the parents for this and other diseases before breeding them. Their goals are to improve their breed and eliminate diseases and problems.

Because I cannot include a discussion of all dog breeds in these pages, instead I have addressed common issues with the top five AKC breeds at the time of writing, and then included problems typical to a number of other breeds that I often see in my practice.

Labrador Retriever

Labrador retrievers and Lab mixes are generally friendly, fun-loving dogs with good temperaments that make good pets and were bred for hunting and retrieving birds. Lab puppies tend to be energetic and need appropriate toys to play with and chew on or they may chew up shoes and other inappropriate things. They are probably the most common

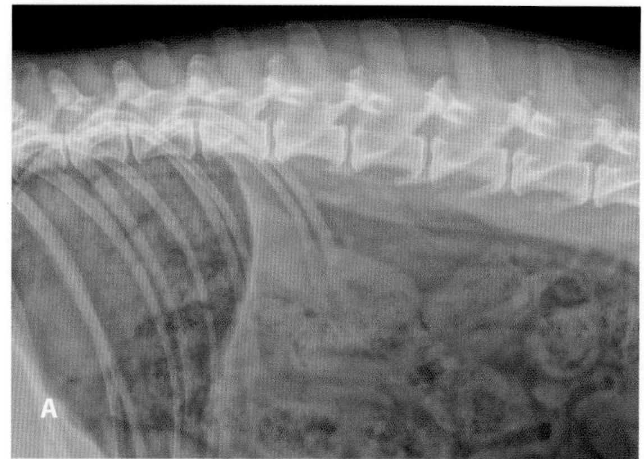

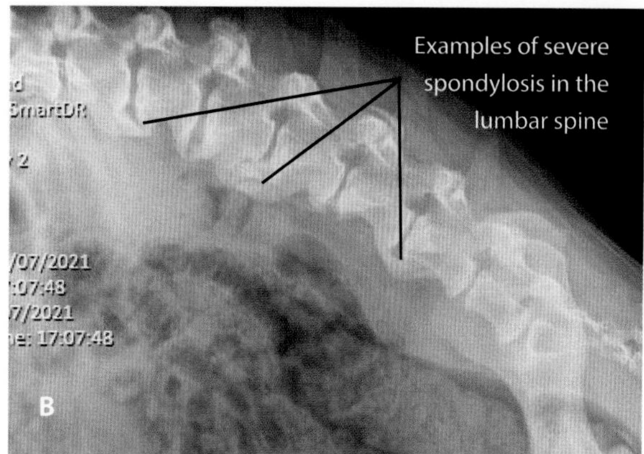

AI.1 A & B A Labrador Retriever's normal lumbar spine (A) and one showing severe spondylosis (B).

breed requiring surgery to remove foreign bodies from their intestinal tract, including toys, towels, underwear, and socks. I have even removed rocks from the stomach of a Lab puppy! They truly will eat anything, so make sure you "puppy-proof" your house, just like you would make your house safe for young children, or you could end up with an expensive vet bill!

Labrador Retrievers, like most large breeds, can have *hip dysplasia*, a congenital hip problem where the hip joint is not formed correctly so it is not as stable as it should be. With age, Labs tend to develop arthritis of the hips, back, or other joints, termed *degenerative joint disease* by veterinarians. They also can develop *spondylosis,* arthritic changes in the spine that look like bone spurs or "bridging" off the vertebrae (figs. AI.1 A & B). *Elbow dysplasia* is a congenital problem that a lot of Labs may need surgery to correct when they are young to prevent a lifetime of limping and pain.

Labs are often used for hunting and retrieving birds. They compete in "field trials," which simulate hunting conditions and test the dog's ability to find and retrieve birds in different conditions. They are also popular choices for other sporting competitions, including obedience trials, rally, agility, flyball, and nose work. Labradors are used in police work as drug-sniffing dogs, for search and rescue, and as cadaver dogs, among other jobs. They are very versatile, easy to train, excel at many sports, and make great companions, which is why they have been one of the most popular breeds for so many years.

When doing Masterson Method bodywork with your Labrador, refer to chapter 8 to address specific problem areas he may have (see p. 152). For front-end or elbow issues, release tension at the occiput/atlas with *Head Up Technique* (p. 58), with *Lateral Cervical Microflexion* (p. 63), and *Scapula and Forelimb Movements* and *Lower Forelimb Movements* (pp. 80 and 88) to keep him more flexible and allow him to move better.

For hip issues, use the *Pelvic Release* (p. 126) and

Hind Limb Movement and *Lower Hind Limb Movement* (pp. 112 and 119), as well as others to relax the hind end. For front-end or hind-end problems, don't forget the middle of the dog, and relax the back as well, since everything is connected. Labs in general enjoy any kind of bodywork and will "train you" to work on them when they need it (or anytime they want attention!).

French Bulldog

French Bulldogs have recently exploded in popularity. They are members of a group termed *brachycephalic* breeds. Brachycephalic breeds have large heads, flat, wrinkled faces with short, wide muzzles or "smushed-in" noses, and tend to have smaller nostrils and shorter airways. They also have fairly large eyes that may bulge out somewhat. Because of their shortened noses, these dogs tend to have breathing problems and can overheat easily in the warm weather or with exercise. They are also prone to eye problems, such as scratches or ulcers on the cornea or surface of the eye.

French Bulldogs and some of these other brachycephalic breeds are prone to congenital problems (problems that they are born with), such as malformed vertebrae, too few vertebrae, or extra vertebrae in the spine that cause back problems and pain. These types of breeds also tend to have a lot of allergy issues, which cause itching and skin problems or digestive or gastrointestinal problems. When breeding for smaller size and specific characteristics over time, humans have bred more problems into some of these breeds. Also, the more popular certain breeds become, the more likely the people who breed them do not know how to breed for good-quality dogs, so be aware of this when searching for a puppy.

"Frenchies" are fun-loving dogs with big personalities that love people, children, and attention. They make wonderful companions and can also compete in agility, scent work, and are good therapy dogs. If competing with your French Bulldog in any sport, or even just playing in the yard or at the dog park, avoid going during the hottest time of day, make sure they have plenty of water, and take multiple breaks so that they do not overheat.

Any of the bodywork exercises described in this book would be appreciated by your Frenchie. With their large heads and heavier front ends, their necks do tend to get tight from holding up their head, so releasing tension in the occiput, atlas, neck, and at the C7-T1 Junction will always make them feel better (pp. 58, 61, and 94). Work over the back to relax it would also be in order, especially if they do have back issues (p. 128).

Golden Retriever

Golden Retrievers, or "Goldens," are a large breed with longer hair than a Lab, and are usually very sweet, happy, friendly dogs that like to play. Like Labs, they were bred to retrieve birds when hunting and are commonly seen in hunting field trials, agility trials, dock diving, rally, obedience trials, nose work, and many other sporting events. They *love* to play fetch. You may commonly see them being walked by their owners with one (or more!) tennis balls in their mouths.

Goldens are prone to hip dysplasia; elbow

Case Study

STELLA

I have a French Bulldog named Stella. She was given to me by a client because at nine months of age, Stella jumped off a couch and suddenly couldn't use her back legs. She was taken to her primary veterinarian where radiographs were taken, and she was given pain and anti-inflammatory medication (figs. AI.2 A–C). The radiographs showed three malformed hemivertebrae, or "butterfly" vertebrae, in her lumbar spine and severe hip dysplasia.

Stella was brought to my clinic and treated with chiropractic, acupuncture, and other rehabilitation therapies, and she gradually regained the use of her back legs. The owner subsequently gave her to me since Stella will always need such treatments to maintain her mobility.

To be honest, a French Bulldog was never on my wish list because of their tendency to have health problems. I must admit, though, that Stella is the funniest and most entertaining dog I have ever had, and she even knows how to get along with my bossy little Corgi!

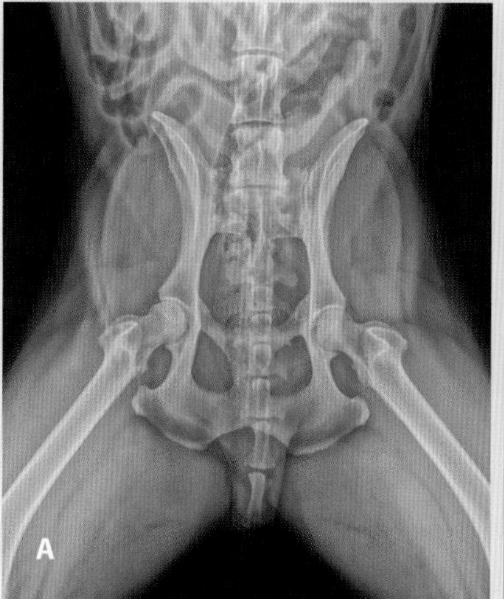

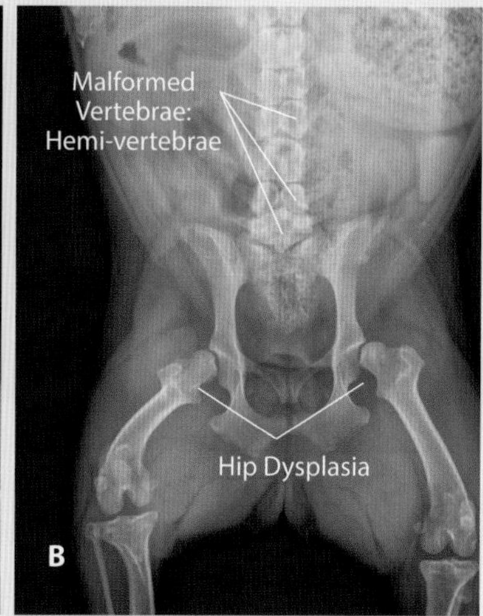

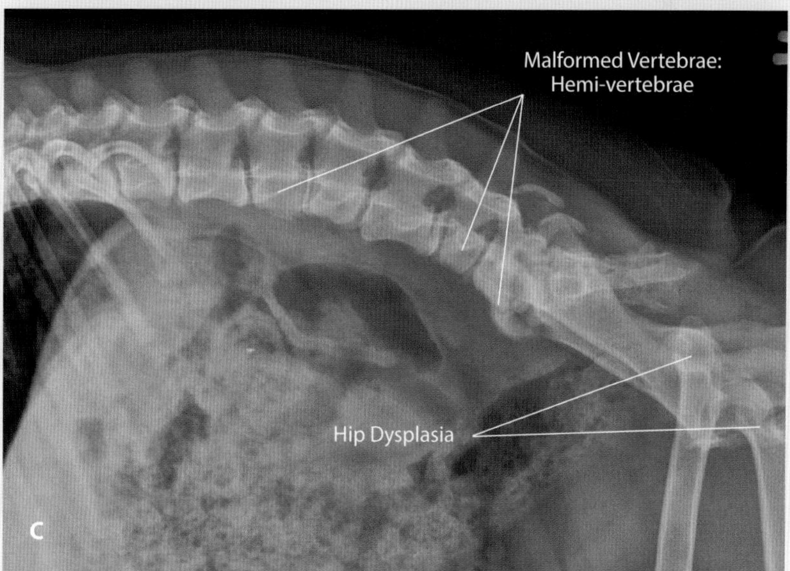

AI.2 A-C A radiograph of a normal French Bulldog spine and hips (A). Stella's spine, showing hemi-vertebrae and malformed vertebrae and severe hip dysplasia from two views (B & C).

dysplasia may also be a possibility, but they are not as prone to elbow problems as Labs. Goldens, unfortunately, tend to be very prone to all types of cancer, especially hemangiosarcoma of the spleen, lymphoma, and osteosarcoma (bone) cancer. The Morris Animal Foundation began a study in August 2012, The Golden Retriever Lifetime Study, which is the first breed-specific, life-to-death research project of its kind and has 3,000 dogs enrolled. Over 2,000 veterinarians in the United States are participating in the study, collecting samples and data from the enrolled dogs and sending it to Colorado State University College of Veterinary Medicine's Flint Animal Cancer Center, whose veterinary oncologist specialists oversee the research. It is hoped that this work will help determine why Goldens in North America are so prone to cancer, what factors contribute to the problem, and ways to help prevent it.

Bodywork for Goldens is always appreciated. They love the attention and are easy to work on. Time spent on the hind end and hips is always a good place to start, using the *Pelvic Release* (p. 126), *Hip Joint Points* (p. 110), and *Hind Limb Movements* (p. 112). Like most dogs (and people!), they really appreciate a nice neck massage, so use the *Head Up Release* (p. 58), *Lateral Cervical Microflexion* (p. 63), and any *Hold, Wait, and Melt Techniques*. Your Golden will let you know when to stop…when he falls asleep!

German Shepherd

The German Shepherd breed dates back to the late 1800s in Germany and are known for their loyalty to their owners. They are intelligent, confident, courageous, and protective of their family. They were bred for herding, but are more commonly used as protection, police, and service dogs. They were the first breed of dog to be used as guide dogs for the blind.

German Shepherds do well in obedience and rally competitions due to their intelligence and being easy to train. *Schutzhund* is a challenging sport that was originally designed as a breed test to measure a German Shepherd's abilities at obedience, tracking, and protection. (It has grown into a popular sport, which includes other breeds now as well.) German Shepherds are seen competing in other sports, such as agility and herding, but are mainly thought of and used as working dogs or simply as family pets.

German Shepherds can be born with hip dysplasia or may develop arthritis of the hips as they get older, along with spondylosis or arthritis in the back. They also are one of the most common breeds to inherit a genetic disease called *degenerative myelopathy (DM),* which causes a progressive hind leg weakness leading to paralysis. DM is very similar to ALS (Lou Gehrig's Disease) in people. There is a DNA test for this disease to be able to differentiate it from lumbosacral disease, hip problems, or intervertebral disc disease (IVDD) that all can be causes of the hind limb weakness commonly seen in Shepherds as they age.

German Shepherds usually enjoy massage and bodywork if they know you. They tend to be vocal and will probably direct you to where they want you to work and for how long. Any Masterson Method Techniques would be helpful, especially those that release muscle tension in the hind end (see p. 97).

Poodle

Poodles, although the national dog of France, were first bred in Germany. There are three types of Poodles recognized by the AKC: Standard, Miniature, and Toy. Standard Poodles were bred as retrievers and for swimming. The Toy and Miniature types were bred down from the larger type to be pets.

One of the most appealing features of Poodles is that they have a single coat of short, curly hair, rather than most dogs, which have a "double coat." This means they do not shed and are hypoallergenic, so they make great pets for people with pet allergies. Since they do not shed, they need to be clipped regularly.

Poodles are very intelligent dogs and are highly trainable, very athletic, and agile. Standard Poodles are still commonly used for retrieving birds and competing in field trials and hunting trials. All sizes of Poodles can be seen competing in obedience, rally, and agility trials. Because Poodles are smart, athletic, and energetic, they need a lot of attention and exercise to keep them from inventing inappropriate activities if left home alone.

Because of Poodles not shedding and their hypoallergenic properties, their good temperaments, high intelligence levels, and trainability they have been bred with many other breeds to develop the "designer breeds" I mentioned earlier.

Common health problems seen in Poodles are cataracts in the eyes as they age (this is more common in the smaller varieties but may be seen in the Standards as well). As with all, they may develop arthritis as they age, especially if they compete in sporting events. The Toy and Miniature Poodles may develop heart valve problems when they are older and require medication to support heart function. The smaller Poodles are also prone to luxating patellas (see p. 173), which regular bodywork will help control or may even prevent.

Poodles, no matter their size, usually enjoy massage and bodywork and are good patients. You may want to be cautious at first when starting work on smaller Poodles, as they may be a little feisty. In general, all Poodles respond well to releasing tension over the head and neck, using the *Head Up (Occiput-Atlas) Release* (p. 58) and relaxing the hind end with the *Pelvic Release* (p. 126). All the Poodles I have ever worked on really love having their head and face massaged and love the light-touch type of bodywork described in this book.

Issues to Consider with Other Common Dog Breeds

Dachschund

Dachshunds are fun-loving, energetic small dogs that think they are the size of a Great Dane. Dachshunds were bred in Germany to go into burrows to hunt badgers and other animals, so they were bred to be tough. Be careful with your Dachshund around unfamiliar dogs, as they can be protective and think they are bigger and tougher than anyone else! Keep these personality traits in mind when starting to do bodywork on a Dachshund, because they can be reactive and some may be nippy, so watch their reactions carefully. Once they are used to the Masterson Method Techniques, they will love them and benefit from them.

Veterinarians commonly see Dachshunds for back problems as they are very prone to herniating or "blowing out" discs in the back, causing intervertebral disc disease (IVDD). A dog with IVDD will show signs of moderate to severe back pain, reluctance to walk, and possibly weakness in the hind legs. Some cases of IVDD can be treated conservatively with medications and restrictions on activity. Acupuncture, chiropractic, and other rehabilitation therapies like Masterson Method Techniques work well in cases of IVDD, along with medications. With a severe disc problem, the spinal cord damage may be more significant, and these dogs can progress to hind-leg paralysis that may require surgery.

Since Dachshunds are so prone to back problems, get yours used to all the bodywork in this book as a puppy, if possible. It may help prevent him from having problems, or lessen the severity of back issues if they do develop later.

Boxer

Boxers are a medium-to-large breed and usually sweet, energetic, active, and fun dogs that I commonly see in my practice. Boxers were initially bred as working dogs and used as guardian dogs. They are very loyal and may be very protective of their owners and have been used as police dogs. They are athletic dogs, so do well in obedience, rally, agility trials, and other sports.

Like any larger breed, Boxers may develop hip problems and arthritis as they age. Like Golden Retrievers, unfortunately, they are also prone to different kinds of cancer at a higher rate than other breeds.

Boxers are always game for any kind of attention, so any form of bodywork will be welcomed and greatly appreciated, but a focus on the hind end can be most helpful (see p. 97).

Border Collie

Border Collies are a member of the herding group and are a very active, energetic, and athletic breed. They are one of the most common breeds used in competitive sporting events for dogs. The Border Collie is generally considered and has been tested to be the smartest breed of dogs. Since Border Collies are so smart and energetic, they need a "job," so if considering one for your family, know that they need a lot of activity, exercise, socialization, and interaction to keep them from getting into trouble.

Border Collies are commonly used in agility, flyball, herding trials, and frisbee or disc. I see a lot of Border Collies at my clinic for maintenance and preventive chiropractic, bodywork, and conditioning work, as well as rehabilitation from injuries from competing. They are great patients in general but may try to distract you to avoid having a problem area worked on. They will also try to convince you that they are fine and try to go back to work before they are ready, so they tend to have relapses when recovering from an injury. With bodywork, most of them like to lie down and roll around on their backs while you work, so I recommend *starting* a Masterson Method session with techniques that are more easily done with the dog standing—because he won't be standing for long!

Terrier

Terriers are a large group of different breeds, and I see a lot of Terriers and Terrier mixes in my practice. Terriers are mostly small-to-medium breeds, although there are a few large breeds also included in this group. In general, they were bred to hunt small animals, and to even go into burrows after animals, so they tend to be feisty, energetic, and tough dogs. They are usually highly intelligent but can be stubborn, so training can be somewhat challenging and may require a lot of patience. They commonly compete in flyball, agility, nose work, barn hunt, and earthdog competitions. Terriers make great pets if you make sure they get plenty of exercise and stimulation to keep them out of trouble.

When doing bodywork on Terriers, go slowly and use very light touch techniques. They like to be asked for permission before being touched and then only after a proper introduction. They tend to be reactive and are very fast, so they may react first and apologize later, if they have a sensitive or painful area. Do not grab a Terrier or startle him, or he may snap. Terriers tend to be the boss, so they will tell you where they want you to work and for how long, but they do appreciate bodywork—on their terms.

Pit Bull Terriers (or American Pit Bull Terriers) are a member of the Terrier group, but I would like to discuss them briefly, since they have become so common and have a bad reputation in some respects. Pit Bulls and Pit mixes are generally sweet-natured and love people, but they were originally bred for hunting wild or feral livestock, including wild boars. They were used in "bull baiting" and "bear baiting," which were outlawed in the 1800s. They were bred to be aggressive toward other animals, so unfortunately, they have been used in many countries for illegal dog fighting. Because they are a very strong muscular breed, today they are commonly used in weight-pulling competitions, and may also participate in agility or nose work, or be used as police or service dogs.

The Pit Bull Terrier is one of the most common breeds or mixes seen in the United States, and unfortunately, in the southern part of the country, it is probably one of the most common breeds seen loose on the streets or in rescue shelters. They can make excellent pets but need to be well socialized and receive appropriate training and attention.

Avoidance Behavior

I have several Border Collie patients that will roll over on their back or turn around to offer their hind end instead of allowing me to work on their neck when it is more tight than usual. They are very good at avoidance behavior and think they are fooling me by looking cute and trying to distract me! After using the Masterson Method to relax their neck, they often give lots of kisses to show their appreciation—and to apologize for their avoidance behavior.

Since they were bred to hunt other animals, some do not do well in homes with other pets, such as cats or smaller dogs. Pit Bulls may be aggressive toward other dogs, so owners need to be responsible and take precautions when having their dogs in public areas.

Most Pits and Pit mixes love attention and bodywork and tend to be big babies. The ones I've worked on love Masterson Method Techniques. They tend to have a high incidence of hip problems, so they do like work over the hind end (see p. 97) and usually enjoy having their heads and necks massaged (see p. 48). I find they prefer to be worked on while sitting—or while lying in your lap!

Competitions and Sporting Events for Dogs

There are a wide range of competitions and organized activities that people can participate in, whether they have a purebred dog or mixed-breed rescue dog. There are sports that require dogs to be fast and agile and shows for dogs that don't require as much physical effort for those less athletically inclined. Many types of competitions are only for certain breeds, focusing on the attributes that they were bred for, such as herding trials for Border Collies, Corgis, and Australian Shepherds. Other examples of sports for certain breeds are lure coursing for sighthound breeds—such as Greyhounds, Afghans, and Borzois—earthdog competitions for terriers, and trials for dog breeds developed for hunting. I find it is useful to know some general considerations and guidelines for active dogs, which areas of the body tend to accumulate tension, what type of problems or possible injuries are common with different sports, and which Masterson Method Techniques to use to help with any problems.

As with the large number of different dog breeds, there are so many recognized types of competitions for dogs that I cannot discuss all of them. In the material that follows, I will reference the most common.

Pre-Competition Bodywork

In general, when doing bodywork on a dog before a competition or event, remember that you just want to "loosen him up," so take it easy when you find a problem area. We tend to want to "fix" an issue, but just before going into a competition ring is *not* the time to do this. When a muscle has been very tight or restricted for some time, it may be sensitive or sore once the tension is released—something to be avoided right before competing. If you find an area of excessive tension, pain, or restriction just prior to an event, pass over it lightly and go back to it later, after the competition is over.

The *Releases* you can get may be deeper than you think, so it may take your dog a little while to adjust to the changes in his body and his movement. Allow enough time before an event for this possibility. If the dog has never had any bodywork done before, I recommend working on him at least 48 to 72 hours before a competition or show. If he is used to bodywork, then for a full Masterson Method session, I would recommend 12 to 24 hours prior to the event, and some light follow-up shortly before the competition should be fine.

Individual dogs respond differently to bodywork. Most will be more flexible and looser, and have more energy, but some may be sleepy or sore, have decreased energy levels, and need a day off afterward. When doing Masterson Method with a dog before or during an event, I recommend he be yours or a dog you are familiar with and that is used to the work to avoid any potential issues. Be light with your touch, and the less you do the better, in most cases.

Below are general guidelines for techniques I recommend to loosen up your dog and help with warming up the muscles, whatever kind of activity or competition you do with him. Remember to watch for the dog's *Responses,* as they will guide your work.

1 *Bladder Meridian* (p. 36): This may be a good place to start to help balance the body and may help with focus and reducing tension prior to an event.

2 Go lightly over the occiput, atlas, and neck using light touch and *Lateral Cervical Microflexion* (p. 63).

3 *Scapula and Forelimb Movements* (p. 80) may be done, if the dog accepts these techniques and relaxes.

4 Address the *Lumbosacral-Pelvic Junction and Hind Limb Points* (p. 110) for a short time—no more than a minute or two on either side.

5 *Hind Limb Movements* (p. 112) should allow the dog to relax into the positions.

6 Try *Lateral Body Rocking* (p. 142), taking a little time for the dog to relax into the motion.

Tips

Perform all techniques gently, for a short time, and keep in mind you are only looking for an improvement—you are not fixing anything.

- If you find an area of excessive tightness or restriction, pass over it lightly. Do not try to fix it just before an event.
- Don't spend more than 30 minutes working on a dog before an event; 10 to 15 minutes is probably all you need.
- While using the techniques, spend less time asking for movement and more time allowing the dog to relax into the positions.
- Spend more time on light work, like the *Bladder Meridian,* and focus on the various *Release Points*, rather than on the movement techniques, especially if a dog tends to get excited before a competition.
- Don't rush through the techniques. Dogs can tell when you are hurrying and won't relax, and they may only get more tense.

Masterson Method for Different Competitions and Sporting Events

Conformation

This is what most people think of as "dog shows." Dogs are judged by their looks and movement based on how they exemplify or conform to the standards for their breed. They are first judged against others of their same breed, but then are judged against other breeds to pick the "best in show."

Show dogs are highly pampered, but they spend a lot of time in kennels at shows and traveling between shows, so can develop stiffness, restrictions, and muscle tension. Dog shows can also be very stressful with a lot of dogs kenneled close together and no room for the dogs to be able to run or move freely for several days at a time.

With being stressed and kept in a kennel so much, show dogs will accumulate a lot of tension in the occiput, atlas, and neck, just like people do when they are tense. The dog's shoulders and hind end should be kept loose so he can move freely in the show ring. Also work on the mid-back to allow proper movement and get rid of any tension that can result from confinement.

Agility

Agility is one of the most popular sports competitions for dogs. It is a timed obstacle course for dogs. Courses usually have 14 to 20 obstacles that may include jumps, tunnels, weave poles, tires, and seesaws. Dogs are trained to go around the course by watching their owners' or trainers' hand signals, cues, and body language. It is an exciting and fun sport to participate in or just to watch.

With the speed involved and different types of obstacles on an agility course, dogs will develop muscle tightness and tension, and injuries may occur. When an agility dog is having problems with the weave poles, I pay particular attention to the neck, shoulders, and C7-T1 Junction. The hind end and mid-back can also be a problem in these instances, but I check the front end first.

When a dog is refusing to jump, adding steps in before a jump, or pulling poles when jumping, I think more about the hind end, hind legs, or possibly the back being the location of tension or restrictions. When a dog has problems with climbing up the A-frame, look for hind end problems; if hesitant going down, then look closely at the neck and front end. Regular Masterson Method over the whole body will keep your agility dog in good condition and may also help prevent injuries.

Flyball

Flyball is a relay race between two teams of four dogs. The dogs race side by side along a 51 foot long course, have to jump four jumps, release a tennis ball from a flyball box, retrieve the ball, and carry it back over the four jumps and across the finish line. The next dog on the team can go once the previous dog crosses the finish line with the ball. The first team to have all four dogs complete the course cleanly and bring back the ball is the winner.

As with any speed event, there is a possibility for injuries, including cranial cruciate ligament (CCL) tears, other ligament injuries, and muscle or tendon strains and sprains that may require veterinary attention. Muscle tension and restrictions are common with flyball dogs because of the repetitive motions involved with the sport. Neck, shoulder, and lower front limb tension and restrictions are common from the way dogs "hit" the flyball box to release the ball. They may have issues with the hind end or hind legs from jumping as well. Consider all of these particular areas when doing Masterson Method work with your dog, and as always, keep the dog's back relaxed, releasing any tension due to compensations from front-end or hind-end issues. Regular Masterson Method bodywork will help keep your flyball dog in top racing form.

Speed Events: Lure Coursing, CAT, Fast CAT

Lure coursing is a sport that is only for sighthounds—such as Greyhounds, Afghan Hounds, and Borzois—testing their natural ability to chase down prey by sight. Dogs follow a lure made of a plastic bag dragged over the ground in an erratic pattern, simulating a real chase. Dogs run in groups of three over a 600-foot-long course.

Coursing Ability Test (CAT) is a non-competitive race over a 300- or 600-foot-long course open for any breed of dog and designed for beginners to test a dog's ability to run and chase a lure. Only one dog runs at a time and must complete the course in a certain time. CAT is a great event to see if your dog may be up for and interested in speed competitions.

Fast CAT is a timed 100-yard dash for individual dogs running on a closed course chasing a lure. This is a relatively new and rapidly growing sport because any dog may compete, as long as he is over a year old.

Routine bodywork will help keep your speed event dog running his best. By keeping the neck and shoulders free from tension, as well as the hind legs, dogs will be able to maintain top form. Injuries can occur in these speed events that may require more attention. When lure coursing with inexperienced dogs, there is a possibility of dogs running into each other. I have seen and treated dogs with shoulder and carpal sprains and rib bruising. As with any dog sport, there is always a possibility of cranial cruciate ligament (CCL) injury.

Scent Work Events

Dogs have a sense of smell 10,000 to 100,000 times more sensitive than people. Dogs love sniffing to find crumbs you may have dropped, to see where you have been all day, and if you have been "cheating on them" by petting another dog! There are multiple types of competitive events related to scent. Any breed or mixed breed of dog may compete in most of these sports, except earthdog events, which are limited to Terriers and Dachshunds.

Nose work is a fun sport where the dog is in control, rather than the handler. The dog must detect where the target scent is hidden and alert the handler once it's found. Although this sport does not require as much athleticism as some of the other sports I've talked about, Masterson Method Techniques to keep the occiput, atlas, and neck relaxed will help keep these canine detectives at their best.

Barn hunt and earthdog competitions both utilize dogs' ability to sniff out mice or rats. Both of these events are timed and have different levels of competition. When doing bodywork for these dogs, make sure to keep the occiput, atlas, and neck relaxed, as well as pay attention to tension in the C7-T1 Junction area. These dogs must crawl through burrows or tunnels in competition and use their hind legs to push themselves along, so make sure that you spend time releasing the hind end and addressing any compensations for either a tight neck or tension in the hind end.

Service and Working Dogs

Dogs have long been used for protection and in police work for aiding in apprehension of criminals on the run, tracking, bomb detection, drug detection, search-and-rescue, and cadaver detection. Guard dogs are commonly used to protect businesses and personal property. Common breeds for these jobs are German Shepherds, Belgian Malinois, Labrador Retrievers, and Dobermans. Service dogs include therapy dogs and those trained to be companions and assist people with disabilities, sight impairments, or other health problems.

It is best to only do bodywork on a service dog that is your own or whose handler is present. You must have the handler's and dog's permission prior to touching the dog. Never pet or touch any of these dogs while they are working.

That said, once these dogs get used to bodywork, they enjoy "spa days." Often these dogs are walking and on their feet for long periods of the day, so special attention to keeping their front legs, hind legs, and paws relaxed and free from muscle tension will keep them working at their best. Also relax the neck and back. Regular whole-body sessions utilizing all the Masterson Method Techniques will be beneficial and can be of particular use in decreasing stress accumulated from the work these dogs do on a regular basis.

Good for All

In general, any dog, whether a "couch potato" family pet, a top-level competitive sporting dog, or a hard-working police dog, will benefit from the Masterson Method. Plus, petting dogs has been shown to decrease blood pressure and stress levels in people, so you will receive health benefits from using these techniques, too!

APPENDIX II

Your Dog's Personality and Constitution with Dr. Robin Robinett

I would like to explain a little about Traditional Chinese Veterinary Medicine (TCVM) and your dog's personality. The more insight you as an owner can have into your dog's personality and constitution, the better you may be able to interpret how your dog may respond to any situation or interaction, including the Masterson Method.

One of the principal theories of TCVM is the *Five Element Theory*. The Five Element Theory defines personalities or constitutions of individuals into different elements or categories. The fve elements are *Wood, Earth, Metal, Water,* and *Fire*.

The Wood Element

Wood-type animals are the "alpha" or leaders. They are dominant over other dogs and can be very bossy. They generally like massage on their terms and like to be asked for permission prior to touching. They like to be *worked with* rather than *worked on*. Wood-type dogs may take longer before showing any release of tension with bodywork, since they don't like to show weakness, because of their role as "leader." They do not like their paws being touched in general. When these dogs are having physical problems or are unbalanced in some way, they can become irritable or angry and may lash out.

Any breed of dog may be a Wood type, but Dobermans, Rottweilers, German Shepherds, Malinois, and other "protection-type" breeds are most common.

The Fire Element

Fire-type animals are everyone's friend; they love to be the center of attention and to be petted, so they love massage and bodywork like the Masterson Method. These dogs tend to have anxiety issues and can become scared and panicky if unbalanced. They may lash out when stressed, but it is not directed at you, it is just to help them "prepare to run away."

Any breed may be a Fire type, but I especially see it in toy and small breeds.

The Metal Element

Metal-type animals are friendly but aloof. They take some time to totally warm up to strangers, but once they do, they are *very* friendly. They like order, schedules, and things to be done in a specific way. They like bodywork, but at first may only like a small amount and should be allowed to leave when they are ready to do so. Metal types may be prone to lung and breathing problems or allergies.

Any breed may be a Metal type, but I find that

a lot of the herding breeds, such as Border Collies, Australian Shepherds, Shetland Sheepdogs, and Blue Heelers, are common. Sighthounds, such as Greyhounds, Afghan Hounds, Borzoi, and Whippets, tend to be Metal types as well.

The Earth Element

Earth-type animals are easy-going, friendly dogs. They love attention, petting, and any type of bodywork and massage. They are wonderful companions. Earth types may have gastrointestinal problems from internalizing stress because they don't want to show it.

Any breed dog may be an Earth type, but in general, think of the laid-back, sweet Labrador Retriever as an example.

The Water Element

Water types are the "fear-biter" dogs. They love their immediate family but fear everyone else, and they may try to bite or can just be very submissive and try to run away. In a veterinary office, these are the dogs hiding under the owner's chair or behind the owner in the exam room. They usually do okay with bodywork over time, but you have to go very slow with them in order to gain their trust. Water types tend to have kidney and bladder problems.

Any breed may fit into this category.

Applying the Five Element Theory

When you start to recognize your dog's personality type, then you can better predict how he may react in different situations, as well as how he may react to Masterson Method bodywork. This can be useful in ensuring your dog remains happy and comfortable in all that you do together.

APPENDIX III

Contraindications to Bodywork with Dr. Robin Robinett

The Masterson Method Techniques for dogs are intended to enhance performance and mobility in the healthy dog. This bodywork is not meant to treat any type of disease and is not a substitute for proper veterinary care and treatment. If you have any doubts or questions about the physical health of your dog, please consult your veterinarian, especially in cases of the following.

Arthritis

Light bodywork can make the arthritic dog more

comfortable and improve his mobility and quality of life. Less may be more for these older guys, so don't do too much bodywork at a time; do short sessions with a very light touch. Consult with your veterinarian regarding bodywork for an older arthritic pet before working on him.

Pregnancy

The Masterson Method may be done on pregnant dogs to make them more comfortable, but check with your veterinarian prior to beginning any bodywork for their recommendations related to your dog.

Acute Injury

Bodywork like the Masterson Method is not recommended for dogs with acute injuries. Heat, inflammation, pain, and swelling are indications of an acute injury and need to be examined and treated by a veterinarian as soon as possible. Your veterinarian can formulate a treatment plan and recommend the appropriate time to start with bodywork after the acute phase has passed.

Chronic Injury

Most dogs with a chronic injury benefit from bodywork to help with the compensations due to the old injury. Consult with your veterinarian for any recommendations prior to beginning to apply Masterson Method Techniques.

Infectious Disease

During the early stages of an infectious disease, most bodywork on dogs may not be appropriate, but in the recovery stages of a disease, bodywork may make him more comfortable. Consult with your veterinarian for recommendations.

Allergic Reaction

Dogs suffering from an allergic reaction, such as hives, need to be seen by a veterinarian and treated as soon as possible. After treatment, they may be too sensitive to touch for Masterson Method Techniques to be effective, or they may appreciate a very light touch. Experiment with the levels of touch to see what your dog may like.

Cage Rest

If your dog is on "cage rest" due to an injury or while recovering from surgery, consult your veterinarian before performing Masterson Method. Depending on the injury, gentle bodywork, in most cases, can help keep him flexible, improve mobility, increase circulation, reduce muscle tension, and make him feel better overall. Be careful around surgical sites as they may be painful and the dog could be reactive; either avoid the area or experiment with a very light touch.

When a dog has an injured leg, he may not be able to support himself well, so work on him while he is lying down, if possible.

Note: The above list is by no means complete. If you have any doubts regarding the health or condition of your dog and whether bodywork is safe to apply, please consult your veterinarian.

APPENDIX IV

Recommended Reading from Dr. Robin Robinett

Dog Anatomy

Color Atlas of Veterinary Anatomy, Volume 3, The Dog and Cat, 2nd edition, by Stanley H. Done, Peter C. Goody, Susan A. Evans, and Neil C. Strickland (Mosby, 2009).

Dog Anatomy Coloring Book by Anatomy Academy (Muze Publishing, 2020).

Canine Wellness

Accelerate Canine Performance Through Conditioning: A Step-by-Step Guide by Lin McGonagle and Lin Gelbman (Morning Star Farms, 2014).

The Well Connected Dog: A Guide to Canine Acupressure by Amy Snow and Nancy Zidonis (Tallgrass Publishers, LLC, 1999).

The Healthy Way to Stretch Your Dog by Sasha Foster (Dogwise Publishing, 2009).

The Forever Dog by Rodney Habib and Dr. Karen Shaw Becker (Harper Wave, 2021).

Where Does My Dog Hurt: Find the Source of Behavioral Issues or Pain: A Hands on Guide by Renee Tucker, DVM (Trafalgar Square Books, 2022).

Canine Training and Conditioning

Kyra's Canine Conditioning by Kyra Sundance (Quarry Books, 2019).

Canine Cross Training: Building Balance Strength and Endurance for Your Dog by Sasha Foster (Dogwise Publishing, 2013).

Care of the Canine Athlete by Lowri Davies (First Stone Publishing).

Canine Good Citizen: The Official AKC Guide, 2nd edition, by Mary R. Burch (Companion House Books, 2020).

Acknowledgments from Jim Masterson

The same applies to this book *Beyond Dog Massage* as to its precursor *Beyond Horse Massage:*

"For anyone thinking of taking on the challenge of accumulating whatever body of knowledge he or she might have and writing a book, let this be fair warning that it's nowhere near a one-man job—neither in the accumulation of the knowledge, nor the writing of the book."

I have to start by acknowledging everyone involved in both the accumulation of knowledge and the writing of *Beyond Horse Massage.* Without those people, this book, *Beyond Dog Massage,* wouldn't have happened.

For helping me overcome the unexpected (again!) challenge of putting *this* book together, I thank:

Robin Robinett, DVM, for taking on the challenge, and Masterson Method Instructor Becky Tenges for bringing us together and getting this thing rolling. With Dr. Robinett's many years' experience, knowledge of healing, Traditional Chinese Veterinary Medicine background, the fact that she has been successfully using Masterson Method techniques with her clients for years, and especially her openness and willingness to share her knowledge, I knew that this was going to be a good fit.

Martha Cook, Managing Director at Trafalgar Square Books, and Managing Editor Rebecca Didier (aka "Thelma" and "Louise") for prodding me to write this book and for doing such an amazing job with the last one.

Stephanie Goddard, Masterson Method Certified Practitioner, photographer (www.White-horse-photography.com), and dog wizard. Thanks for taking on this project and making the photographing process so much fun.

Friend and photographer Geoff Northridge for (as is becoming his habit) pinch-hitting at a moment's notice to provide critical photography.

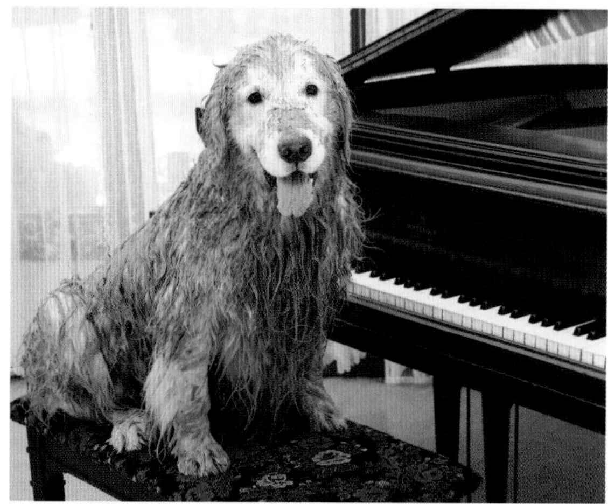

Warning! Working with a large, muddy dog on the soft furniture can result in an accumulation of unwanted tension in the spouse!

I'd also like to acknowledge Masterson Method Certified Practitioner Stef Watts. Stef has been working with dogs in the United Kingdom and helped to get this idea going before the pandemic put us all in the dog house. We're out now, Stef!

A special thanks to our doggy models and their owners.

At home in Iowa:

- Anna Sika and her Red Doberman, Izzy
- Weda Boolos and her Poodle-Bichon mix, Jojo
- Jane Fleshman and her Corgi, Barry
- Kaitlin Willard and her black Pomeranian-Poodle-Shih Tzu cross, Yoshi (a long description for such a tiny dog)

In Missouri:

- Amanda Brooks and her Jack Russell-Rat Terrier cross, Tito
- Kelly Midkiff and her Dachshund, Reese
- Deb Litzelfelner and her sometimes soggy Golden Retriever, Leo.

Also, to my previous Red Aussie, Ruby, and current Red Aussie (used in this book), Popper—my companions at home and on the road for many seasons, working on horses at the Winter Equestrian Festival in Wellington, Florida.

And a special thanks to my wife Conley, mom to our Shepherd-cross doggy model Nellie, and writing, organizing, life and inspirational partner, without whom I couldn't and wouldn't have done this. You made it happen.

Acknowledgments from Robin Robinett, DVM

First, I would like to dedicate this to the memory of my father, John Henry Robinett, who put me through veterinary school and always told me I could do anything I wanted to do if I was willing to do the work. I also want to thank my mom, Joyce Frichette, who has been my number one supporter.

I would like to acknowledge some of the people and dogs that helped me in the undertaking of writing and in gaining the knowledge outlined in this book:

Without my friend Becky Tenges, imparting her knowledge to me and introducing me to the Masterson Method and to Jim Masterson, this book would not have been possible.

The experience of working and collaborating with Jim Masterson has been wonderful. His ability to translate his Masterson Method techniques into words and accurately describe how to perform each one was amazing. Most of our work together took place during the COVID-19 pandemic, and we would talk on ZOOM. He would ask me how I performed a certain technique, so I would use one of my dogs to show him, and then he would translate it into words. Jim is an amazing person with a wonderful sense of humor, and he made the writing experience seem easier. I am honored to have been able to work with him, and I love to see how dogs respond to him and his methods.

I need to recognize my partner in life and partner at work, Jerri O'Donohoe-Robinett. She keeps our clinic, Veterinary Chiropractic and Rehabilitation Clinic (VCRC), running, takes care of my schedule, and keeps up with me and our dogs. Without all her hard work keeping me organized, I would not have been able to do this project.

I also would like to mention my wonderful employees at VCRC, who all helped, allowing me to use their dogs for photography sessions, taking videos, or just listening and critiquing my thoughts and ideas: Chelsey Michelsen, DVM; Kasey Guillory; Leslie Hood; Lizet Corona; Dana Bogatin; and Dayna Marie Dority. Also, thank you to Angie McCubbins and Donnette Rodriguez, who no longer work with us but helped with the process and hopefully may return in the future.

Special thanks to my talented friend, hairdresser, and photographer, Amanda Barnett-Guidry for her amazing photos. Also, thank you for all your encouragement and support for all of my projects.

Thank you to all of the dogs I have known, owned, and worked on who have taught me so much! The dog models in this book include:

My dogs: Drew, the Golden Retriever/Yellow Lab mix; Cora, the Corgi; and Stella, the French Bulldog.

Leslie Hood's dogs: Kizzy, the Malamute/Cattle Dog mix, and Huckleberry, the Cattle Dog mix.

Index

Page numbers in *italics* indicate illustrations.

Interested in Learning More About the

Masterson Method?

Additional instructional books and videos available at
www.mastersonmethod.com

Masterson Method also provides online and hands-on training in The Masterson Method. Find out more about educational courses at **www.mastersonmethod.com**

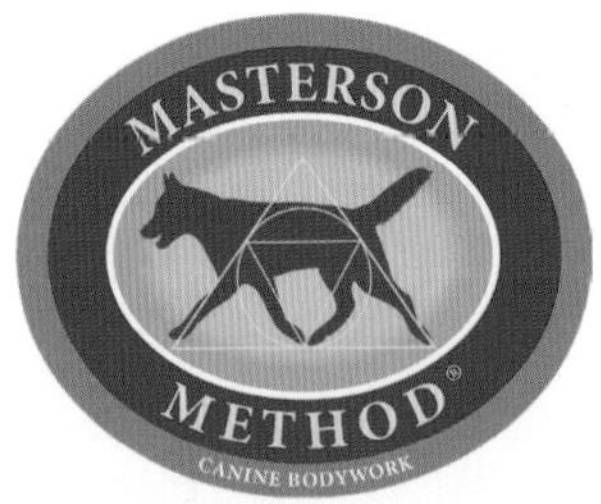